American
Heart
Association®

GO FRESH

ALSO BY THE AMERICAN HEART ASSOCIATION

American Heart Association The Go Red For Women Cookbook

American Heart Association Eat Less Salt

American Heart Association Healthy Slow Cooker Cookbook

American Heart Association Quick & Easy Cookbook, 2nd Edition

American Heart Association Low-Salt Cookbook, 4th Edition

American Heart Association No-Fad Diet, 2nd Edition

The New American Heart Association Cookbook, 8th Edition

American Heart Association Quick & Easy Meals

American Heart Association Complete Guide to Women's Heart Health

American Heart Association Healthy Family Meals

American Heart Association Low-Fat, Low-Cholesterol Cookbook, 4th Edition

American Heart Association Low-Calorie Cookbook

American Heart Association One-Dish Meals

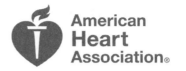

GO FRESH

A HEART-HEALTHY COOKBOOK WITH SHOPPING AND STORAGE TIPS

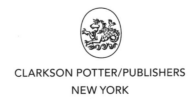

CLARKSON POTTER/PUBLISHERS

NEW YORK

ACKNOWLEDGMENTS

AMERICAN HEART ASSOCIATION CONSUMER PUBLICATIONS

Director: Linda S. Ball

Managing Editor: Deborah A. Renza

Senior Editor: Robin P. Loveman

Assistant Managing Editor: Roberta W. Sullivan

RECIPE DEVELOPERS

Ellen Boeke

Janice Cole

Nancy S. Hughes

Amelia Levin

Diane A. Welland, M.S., R.D.

NUTRITION ANALYST

Tammi Hancock, R.D.

Published in the United States by Clarkson Potter/Publishers, an imprint of the Crown Publishing Group, a division of Random House LLC, a Penguin Random House Company, New York.
www.crownpublishing.com
www.clarksonpotter.com

CLARKSON POTTER is a trademark and POTTER with colophon is a registered trademark of Random House LLC.

Your contributions to the American Heart Association support research that helps make publications like this possible. For more information, call 1-800-AHA-USA1 (1-800-242-8721) or contact us online at www.heart.org.

Library of Congress Cataloging-in-Publication Data is available upon request.

ISBN 978-0-307-88806-8
eBook ISBN 978-0-307-88808-2

Printed in the United States of America
Design by La Tricia Watford
Front cover photograph © Klenova/Veer
Interior photographs and back cover by Ben Fink

DEDICATED TO

Kelly Chapman Meyer

Passionate activist for children's health and family wellness
Cofounder of the American Heart Association's Teaching Gardens*
National champion of the American Heart Association's Fruit and Vegetable Initiative

*The American Heart Association has planted hundreds of AHA Teaching Gardens across America.

PREFACE

If you want to enjoy good health, then it makes sense to focus on the wholesome, nutritious foods that support your goal and to limit the overly processed ones. In fact, the more you include minimally processed, fresh-from-the-farm food in your diet, the easier it is to meet the American Heart Association's recommendations for good nutrition. Having grown up on a farm in Michigan myself, I'm pleased that our American Heart Association guidelines, based on a review of the best available science, support the importance of eating a wide variety of vegetables, fruits, whole grains, and other nutrient-dense foods that help keep your heart healthy.

Although many factors influence your well-being, scientific research has clearly established that what you eat affects your overall health. At the American Heart Association, we understand how eating an unbalanced diet—one that is high in sodium, added sugar, or harmful fats, or is higher in calories than you need—can increase your risk of developing cardiovascular disease, while eating a heart-healthy varied diet can actually reduce your risk and increase your chances for a longer, disease-free life. Having that diet be delicious is a great bonus!

As a nation, recent concerns about where our food comes from and how it is produced, along with a growing interest in better nutrition and healthier food, are changing the way we think about what we eat. People are asking more questions and shopping smarter. From the vegetable garden at the White House to the American Heart Association's Teaching Gardens at schools across the country, we can see that the spotlight is shining more brightly than ever on the benefits and importance of fresh-off-the-vine or plucked-from-the-earth foods.

Not everyone can grow fresh vegetables in their backyard, of course, but the renewed focus on fresh and healthy food has led to many options you can explore. We encourage you to shop frequently at your local farmers' market and the fresh produce section in your favorite grocery store. Try a new heirloom vegetable or fruit, experiment with a sustainable but unfamiliar fish, and ask the butcher for unadulterated, lean meat and skinless poultry. Visit a pick-your-own farm to experience a harvest of fruits and vegetables from the field, or take part in a local community gardening project. We hope you take advantage of the great variety of nutritious and delicious foods available to you. Using the recipes in our *Go Fresh* cookbook is the perfect *fresh* start to eating well and keeping your heart healthy.

Rose Marie Robertson, M.D., FAHA
Chief Science and Medical Officer
American Heart Association/American Stroke Association

CONTENTS

FRESH, FAST, AND HEALTHY

If you're looking to move away from heavily processed foods that rely on preservatives, salt, and sugar and to take advantage of nature's bounty of flavor and nutrition, this is the book for you. We'll show you how to easily combine fresh ingredients with fast cooking techniques to create delicious and healthy meals.

Why focus on fresh? First, because fresh is healthy. The less time spent to move food from the farm to the table, the less time for important nutrients to be lost. When you buy local produce in season, chances are better that those vegetables and fruits have been left to ripen on the plant longer and are at their flavor peak. Fresh also can be economical. Building menus around in-season foods allows you to take advantage of the best buys on produce at your local markets. Foods that are easily available and plentiful cost less than produce that must be shipped halfway around the globe.

Fresh food can be fast food, too. **Fresh vegetables, fruits, and herbs inherently taste good,** so you don't need to spend a lot of time or add much to get them ready for the table. In a few easy steps, you can prepare a nutritious, delicious meal every night of the week in less time than it takes to pick up takeout. In fact, most of the recipes in this book take less than 20 minutes to put together and less than 30 minutes to cook. **If minimal prep for maximum flavor is your goal,** you'll find just what you're looking for in our *Go Fresh* cookbook.

Fresh also means flavorful. Compare the flavor of fresh green beans with that of canned cut beans, for example, and it may seem as if you're eating two different vegetables. Canning involves processing and sterilization by heat, so although most essential nutrients remain, the taste and texture of vegetables and fruits are altered along the way. If fresh choices aren't always available, be sure to choose frozen or canned versions without added sauce, salt, or sugar.

Our recipes particularly **showcase fresh at its finest.** Dishes such as Butternut Squash Pasta (page 184) let the full flavors of winter squash and sugar snap peas come through, enhanced by a sprinkling of fresh sage. Soups made from simple ingredients—tomatoes, bell peppers, cucumber, and red onion in Garden-Fresh Gazpacho (page 77)—impart both comfort and the clean flavor of vegetables grown in the sun. Family favorites such as Country Thyme Chicken Strips (page 149) come alive when made with the freshest of herbs instead of dried, and interesting new pairings, such as Mustard-Crusted Pork Medallions with Celery Root Purée (page 179), will show you **how to use less-familiar ingredients with confidence.**

Food should be more than just sustenance. Fresh-tasting, home-cooked meals can please your palate, allow you to experience new flavor profiles, and bring your family together at the table. The foods you choose to eat become part of the habits and traditions that you establish at home. You can take advantage of all the goodness nature has to offer by **making fresh, fast, and healthy meals** part of *your* family culture.

SHOPPING FOR AND STORING FRESH FOODS

When selecting from the array of produce and other fresh foods available, it pays to know how to pick the best of the bunch. It's also important to be able to protect your purchases when you get home by properly storing them to maintain freshness and follow food safety guidelines. In general, heat and moisture encourage the growth of bacteria that destroy the quality of fresh food. Exposure to air and light also can deteriorate flavor, texture, and nutritional value. Whenever it's practical, use a cooler or insulated reusable totes to transport foods that should be kept cold, such as fresh fish, meat, and delicate vegetables like lettuce. If that's not possible, sack your groceries so you keep cold items together to help them stay colder.

VEGETABLES AND HERBS

Vegetables are nutritional powerhouses that are low in calories yet provide essential nutrients, minerals, and fiber. Fresh, tasty vegetables can be found in abundance in most supermarkets nowadays, and farmers' markets can be found in just about any town or city. With greater access to whole foods, it's simple to throw together a tasty veggie dish in just a few minutes. (For information on timing for specific vegetables, see Appendix B: At-a-Glance Vegetable Cooking Times, page 304.) With so many options available, however, shopping can be confusing unless you know how to make the best choices.

Shopping: To make the most of the fresh vegetables and herbs you buy, follow a few simple guidelines to maximize nutritional value, flavor, texture, and color.

- Shop for different types of vegetables in a variety of colors. The deeper the color and the more variety you eat, the greater the range of nutritional benefits.

- Look for locally grown vegetables for the best flavor and quality; they are more likely to be harvested recently.

- Choose vegetables that look firm and appealing, not dried out or damaged.

- Pass over vegetables that have browned, have started to sprout, or are dented, bruised, or moldy. Don't buy leafy vegetables, such as spinach, that seem either dried out or slimy.

- Select herbs that are vibrant-looking and robust. When buying delicate, leafy herbs such as basil, look for bright green leaves that are deeply indented, and watch out for limp, yellowing, or spotted leaves. Parsley and cilantro should be crisp with no yellow or wilted sprigs. Hardy herbs, such as rosemary and thyme, should have firm stems. All herbs should be free of mold.

Storing: Once harvested, vegetables and herbs begin to lose quality as they deplete their water and food reserves. You can slow this aging process by preventing moisture loss. (An exception is the tomato, which is actually a fruit. Tomatoes need to be ripened and stored as described on page 302.) Different varieties need different conditions for best results; refer to Appendix A: At-a-Glance Food Storage Guide (page 300), for information on specific vegetables.

- Prep vegetables by removing any damaged areas or leaves and packaging, such as rubber bands or plastic ties.

- Because excess moisture causes spoiling, in most cases it's best to wait and rinse vegetables just before you use them. If you do rinse before storing, be sure to dry the produce enough to leave it slightly moist but not wet.

- To keep produce with a high water content (such as lettuce, celery, cucumber, and zucchini) from shriveling, store it in the refrigerator in the original packaging or plastic bags in your refrigerator's crisper. Try to leave enough air in the bags to keep the plastic from directly touching the food in many areas; lack of air circulation can cause waterlogging and rotting at the surface. Reduce the humidity in your crisper by adjusting the vents to let in more cold air.

- Some types of fresh produce, such as onions, garlic, shallots, and potatoes, are sensitive to cold. To prevent sprouting, keep these vegetables dry and at room temperature, preferably in the dark.

- To extend the life of fragile fresh herbs, such as parsley, dill, and cilantro, cut the stems and place the herbs in a juice glass half filled with water, cover loosely with a plastic bag, and refrigerate. Just as you would for flowers in a vase, change the water every few days and remove spoiled leaves. This trick works for basil as well, but it is cold-sensitive and is best kept in water at room temperature.

- For more sturdy herbs, such as oregano, rosemary, and thyme, trim away damaged leaves and remove rubber bands or ties. Rinse and spread the herbs on a paper towel or plate and let dry at room temperature.

- If you refrigerate herbs in the plastic containers they came in, watch carefully for signs of mold or rot.

FRUIT

Chock-full of important nutrients and fiber, fruit is an important component of a well-rounded diet. Almost all fruit tastes best when it's been left on the plant long enough to develop the most flavor. Some fruits, such as peaches and bananas, continue to ripen after being harvested, but others, such as grapes and citrus fruit, don't. Most fruit destined to be shipped for sale is picked before it can ripen so it will be less prone to damage and will keep longer without spoiling. The result is that finding ripe and truly delicious fruit can be challenging—unless you know what to look for when you shop and how to store fruit so it can reach its peak flavor potential.

Shopping: When it's not practical to buy fruit that has been allowed to ripen on the plant, such as local fruits in season and heirloom varieties, or if it is unavailable where you shop, use these general guidelines to find the best your market offers.

- Choose fruit that is firm, bright, and "alive" looking. If a fruit appears artificially shiny, it may have been coated with wax to make it last longer on the shelf, and it may look fresher than it is. Most fruits do have some natural wax, which is less noticeable but will become shiny when gently rubbed.

- Skip over fruit that is dented, bruised, or wrinkled or has become leathery or moldy. Especially check the berries in the bottoms of clear plastic baskets; without adequate air circulation, they can become moldy very quickly.

- Compare several fruit by weight and choose those that are heavier for their size. Select small- to medium-size fruit over the very large ones, which often taste bland and watery in comparison.

- Take advantage if your store offers tasting samples of fresh fruit; it's the best way to know exactly what you are buying.

Storing and ripening: Even more than vegetables, different types of fruit do better in very different conditions. Depending on the fruit, proper storage both allows fruit to ripen and keeps the fruit from spoiling. Use the following guidelines for best results; Appendix A: At-a-Glance Food Storage Guide (page 300), also provides specific information for most common fruits.

- Be careful not to crush or damage fruit when you bring it home from the store.

- Take just-purchased fruit that is fully ripe out of bags and baskets to provide air and minimize moisture on the surface. Arrange the fruit in a single layer if possible.

- Fruits ripen when exposed to the gas ethylene, which they emit naturally. To speed up the process, seal unripe fruit in a paper bag, with a ripe piece of fruit if possible, and store in a warm place for several days. (Unless perforated, plastic bags will suffocate the fruit and cause it to spoil rather than ripen.) This method is recommended for fruit such as apricots, avocados, bananas, kiwifruit, mangoes, pears, peaches, and nectarines.

- Don't refrigerate fruits until they are fully ripe. After that point, to slow further ripening, put them in the produce compartment or plastic bags and refrigerate for another few days.

- Allow chilled fruit to warm up for several hours before eating it, for best flavor and aroma.

- You can freeze most raw fruit for long-term storage. Just wash and prepare as needed, place on a baking sheet, freeze until hard, and transfer to airtight freezer containers.

FISH AND SHELLFISH

Fish, particularly those varieties rich in heart-healthy omega-3 fatty acids, such as salmon, trout, and herring, is a delicious source of protein and other important nutrients. An added bonus is that most fish cooks very quickly, so it's a natural go-to for busy nights.

Shopping: Unless you buy seafood straight from the fisherman, the term "fresh fish" can be confusing. Often the fish on display at the supermarket seafood counter was frozen right after it was caught, then transported and thawed for sale. Conventional wisdom has always been that you should choose fresh fish over frozen, but newer methods of immediately freezing fresh-caught fish have made it possible to retain the quality and texture of fresh fish. The best approach is to ask a lot of questions so you know exactly what you are buying.

- Check with the fishmonger to find the freshest catch of the day.

- Look for firm, clear flesh with no fishy smell. Fillets should have good color, and whole fish should also have clear eyes and gills that are bright red.

- Look for fresh varieties, preferably those that are local, abundant, and caught or farmed in environmentally friendly ways. To view a current list of sustainable seafood, visit www.seafoodwatch.org.

- Avoid fish that has been dipped in saltwater or a sodium solution to extend shelf life; check packaging labels or ask at the seafood counter.

- Buy fish at the end of your shopping trip and keep it on ice if available.

Storing: Ideally, fish should be eaten just after it is caught, without being stored at all. For most people, however, that's not practical, so it is important to know how to best preserve the quality and freshness. Check Appendix A: At-a-Glance Food Storage Guide (page 300), for details.

- When possible, purchase fish on the same day that you plan to eat it. Keep it in the refrigerator until you are ready to prepare it. If you want to keep it for more than a day or two, freeze it.

- Wrap fish in plastic wrap, then in paper or aluminum foil to keep out oxygen and light, which can turn flavor.

- Keep cleaned shrimp refrigerated, wrapped well and buried in ice, for up to two days.

- Refrigerate live lobsters and crabs for up to 24 hours. Live lobsters and crabs should have some leg movement; only live lobsters and crabs should be selected and prepared. Live crawfish should be prepared as soon as possible. Inspect crawfish before they are prepared and discard dead crawfish, bait, and other debris. Refrigerate live clams, mussels, and oysters for up to one or two days. Live clams, mussels, and oysters will close up when the shell is lightly tapped; if they do not close when tapped, discard them. Store mollusks on top of (not under) ice or wrapped in a damp cloth; be sure they are not immersed in water or wrapped in plastic, which will kill them.

MEAT AND POULTRY

Meat and poultry are often expensive, so it's especially important to know what you're buying and how to keep it fresh and delicious. If you, like many people, plan most of your meals around your meat and poultry purchases, protect your investment by buying and storing these foods carefully.

Shopping: In general, the best way to choose meat and poultry is to judge by appearance: Beef should be bright red; the darker the color, the more flavor. Pork should appear pink, and chicken and turkey should have pale skin with whitish flesh.

- Choose heart-healthy lean cuts of meat (for example, sirloin, 95% lean ground beef, and pork tenderloin) and skinless poultry.

- Ask your butcher to grind or cut your meat and poultry to order for best results. Pre-ground meat that is exposed to air and light, such as the loose hamburger on display, or shrink-wrapped and piled up in the meat section, can lose flavor.

- Don't buy meats that are gray, brown, or off-color in any way.

- Avoid "enhanced" poultry or pre-seasoned meat. Although you may think of these foods as fresh, they contain added brines or salt-based flavorings that contain as much sodium as you would find in a processed product. Read the ingredient labels carefully to be sure what you buy is free of salt and other additives.

- Pick up meat and poultry at the end of your shopping trip to lessen the time they spend in transit from your cart to your refrigerator.

Storing: As is true for fish, oxygen, light, and heat can deteriorate the quality of meat and poultry. The general information below and in Appendix A: At-a-Glance Food Storage Guide (page 300), will give you specifics on how to keep these foods delicious and safe to eat.

- Store meat and poultry in the meat compartment or the coldest part of your refrigerator, which is usually at the back. Check to be sure the temperature registers 40°F or lower.

- Use most meat and poultry within a day or two of purchase. If you know that won't be possible, freeze the food right away. (You can make an exception to this guideline for cuts of beef that improve with aging, such as steaks, chops, and roasts. Refrigerate them sealed in their original packaging for up to five days at home.)

DAIRY PRODUCTS

As a delicious and important part of a nutritious diet, fat-free, 1% fat, and low-fat dairy products should be chosen and stored with the same care as other types of fresh food.

Shopping: Most dairy foods are highly perishable and require correct handling from farm to market. Fresh dairy products especially need careful refrigeration to minimize the growth of bacteria, so it's wise to follow some basic guidelines when you go shopping.

- Know the various types of milk available: Pasteurized means the milk has been heated to kill bacteria; homogenized means the fat content has been broken down into smaller particles so it stays suspended rather than rising to the top as cream; raw means the milk has been neither pasteurized nor homogenized.

- Always check the labels for sell-by dates and choose the product with the longest time to expiration.

- Choose items from the coldest area of the display case or refrigerated section.

- Buy dairy foods packaged in opaque containers when possible because exposure to light can destroy flavor and nutrients.

- Shop for dairy products toward the end of your shopping trip to minimize the time they are unrefrigerated.

Storing: Most dairy products are best kept in the coldest part of your refrigerator, at 40°F or lower. Don't be tempted to store milk in the door compartments for convenience; this area of the refrigerator is the warmest spot. For more tips on storing dairy, see Appendix A: At-a-Glance Food Storage Guide (page 300).

- Keep milk in the fridge as much as possible. Even a few minutes on the counter in warm room air can speed up the spoiling process.

- Smell dairy products before you use them and, if needed, taste them to be sure they have not soured.

- Freeze hard cheese to keep it fresh for months. Wrap tightly in several layers of plastic wrap to keep out air.

TAKING A FRESH APPROACH TO YOUR TIME IN THE KITCHEN

Making meals with fresh ingredients rather than opening up cans or boxes does not mean taking extra time in the kitchen. With the 250 recipes in this book, we show you how to easily cook fresh food fast. With each recipe, you'll find both prep and cooking times (rounded to the nearest five minutes), so you'll know how to work a particular recipe into your schedule. Of course, each cook works at an individual rate, so use these times as estimates. Our prep time means you can be ready to cook in 20 minutes or less from the minute you grab the first ingredient to when you turn on the heat or the blender. Once your prep work is complete, your food will be finished cooking and ready to eat in 30 minutes or less. From start to finish, the two add up to no more than an hour—and in many cases much less—leaving you more time to enjoy your delicious, fresh-tasting meal.

QUICK PREP STEPS
for speed and efficiency

- Put a damp paper towel or dish towel under your cutting board to keep it from sliding.

- Use a food processor or mandoline to slice or chop large amounts of vegetables easily and quickly.

- Try a garlic peeler (a rubber cylinder that rubs off the peel) or rubber jar opener to speed up this sometimes tedious step, or simply press garlic cloves with the flat side of a knife to break the skin.

- Grate cheese or lemon peel over wax paper or a bendable cutting mat so you can just pour what you need into a measuring cup or spoon.

- Put parsley, cilantro, and other herbs in a cup and snip them with kitchen scissors rather than using a knife to chop them.

- Cover pots to bring liquids to a faster boil.

- Measure dry ingredients before wet ones if the recipe allows so you can reuse measuring spoons and cups without having to wash them between steps.

- Lightly spray cups, measuring spoons, and other utensils with cooking spray before filling them with sticky ingredients such as honey or molasses. The ingredient will slide out and the utensil will be easier to clean.

- Put raw meat or poultry in the freezer for 10 to 15 minutes to harden it slightly—it will be much easier to slice.

QUICK COOKING METHODS
to keep things moving

- **Broiling and grilling** both require direct exposure of food to the heat source, browning the outside and leaving the inside moist and tender. Both allow fat to drip away and air to circulate, helping food to cook faster. For a quick and complete meal, cook vegetables and fruits right along with your meat, poultry, or seafood.

- **Microwaving** can cut cooking time to a third or even a quarter of the time allotted for a conventional recipe. Because this method requires no added oils and very little, if any, liquid to keep food from drying out, it is a healthy way to prepare food.

- **Sautéing and stir-frying** both involve quickly cooking food over direct heat, using a small amount of hot oil. Vegetables quickly become tender-crisp in the high heat, and as the surface of meat, poultry, and seafood is seared, natural juices are sealed in. Stir-frying moves fast, so prepare ingredients and sauces before you begin cooking.

- **Steaming** food in a basket over simmering liquid helps retain flavor, color, and nutrients. In addition to vegetables, you can also prepare fish, chicken breasts, and any other foods that can be quickly cooked this way.

- **Poaching**, or gently immersing foods in almost-simmering liquid, is especially good for delicate foods, such as fish and fruit. You can use any poaching liquid, such as wine, fat-free, low-sodium broth, or water; the liquid is often reduced to make a sauce after the food is removed.

QUICK KITCHEN TIPS
to save time

- Organize your pantry, freezer, and fridge so you can find what you need quickly. Group similar canned items together, such as vegetables, soups, and beans, for example. Reconsider your storage options to make the most of the space you have.

- Get rid of clutter but keep the items you use every day within easy reach. You should be able to find knives, measuring spoons, whisks, and other basic utensils without rooting through a crowded drawer.

- Group cooking equipment according to how it is used, and designate specific areas for certain tasks.

- Keep tools and appliances clean and in good working order.

- Read a recipe all the way through before you decide to make it! Nothing is more frustrating than discovering in the middle of prep time that you are out of an essential ingredient. For really efficient prep, use the classic technique of professional chefs called *mise en place*: Measure and put out every ingredient and tool needed for your recipe before you start cooking. (This method was used in calculating the prep and cooking times for the recipes in this book.)

CULTIVATING FRESH AND HEALTHY EATING HABITS

For good nutrition, it's important to make it a habit to eat a wide variety of healthy foods. These choices will give your body the key nutrients it needs. At the same time, the more you focus on foods that promote better health, the less likely you are to eat the foods that can contribute to heart disease and stroke.

WHY IS VARIETY SO IMPORTANT?

Wholesome foods don't come with a scorecard. Each has its own unique profile of important nutrients; some are rich in one or two specific vitamins, while others contain valuable combinations of minerals and vitamins that act together for the most benefit. To be sure you get the widest possible range of those benefits from all potential sources, it's best to eat a variety of foods rather than to focus on just a few "superfoods." You want to be sure you are getting enough of all the essentials, such as potassium, calcium, magnesium, vitamin C, folate, carotenoids, iron, and fiber. As you plan your meals, be sure to include foods from each of the following categories:

Vegetables and fruits: Eating many different types of vegetables and fruits is a cornerstone of good health. The broad range of vitamins and minerals they provide, especially the deeply colored ones, is difficult to find in any other food.

GOOD NUTRITION IN A NUTSHELL

So, what *should* you eat? To judge how much of each type of food from each category you need, start by gauging how many daily calories you can eat to maintain a healthy weight. This differs for each individual, of course, depending on his or her level of physical activity and metabolic rate. If your daily calorie needs are higher or lower than 2,000 calories, the number of daily servings from each food group will vary.

- **VEGETABLES:** 4 to 5 servings each day

- **FRUITS:** 4 to 5 servings each day

- **FAT-FREE, 1%, AND LOW-FAT DAIRY PRODUCTS:** 2 to 3 servings each day

- **FIBER-RICH WHOLE GRAINS:** 6 to 8 servings each day

- **FISH RICH IN OMEGA-3 FATTY ACIDS:** 2 servings each week

- **LEAN MEATS AND SKINLESS POULTRY:** less than 6 (cooked) ounces each day

- **LEGUMES, NUTS, AND SEEDS:** 4 to 5 servings each week

- **HEALTHY OILS AND FATS:** 2 to 3 servings each day

Fat-free, 1% fat, and low-fat dairy products: Dairy-based foods, such as milk and cheese, contain many important nutrients, especially calcium and protein. Select fat-free or low-fat options as often as you can; the full-fat and 2% fat varieties are high in saturated fat and cholesterol.

Fiber-rich whole grains: Grains provide an essential complex of nutrients as well as both soluble and insoluble fiber. The edible kernels of grains can be ground into flour for bread (wheat and corn, for example) or eaten whole (rice, barley, quinoa, and others) or in cereal. For the best nutrition, at least half of your grains should be whole; whole grains retain the germ and outer bran, where the greatest concentration of nutrients and fiber is found. Eating fiber from whole grains can help reduce blood cholesterol levels, and because grains help you feel more satisfied, they can help you control your weight as well.

Fish rich in omega-3 fatty acids: Eating fish that contain high levels of healthy oils, called omega-3 fatty acids, can help reduce the risk of heart disease. Aim to eat at least two servings of these fish, such as salmon, tuna, or trout, every week.

Lean meats and skinless poultry: An excellent source of protein, meats and poultry have an important place at the table, but most adults don't need more than 3 to 6 ounces cooked weight (about the size of a deck of cards), which is 4 to 8 ounces when raw, each day. Choose lean cuts of meat and remove the skin from poultry before eating to reduce your intake of harmful saturated fat and cholesterol.

Legumes, nuts, and seeds: Legumes and lentils provide plant protein and a variety of nutrients, and they are rich in dietary fiber. Nuts and seeds have helpful unsaturated fats but are also high in calories. Common legumes include beans (kidney, pinto, black, lima, and others), peas (green, split, black-eyed, and chickpeas), edamame (green soybeans), and peanuts.

Healthy fats and oils: Unsaturated fats are essential to a balanced diet. Like any fat, they are high in calories, so it's a good idea to use them in moderation. To avoid saturated and trans fats, use liquid vegetable oils or soft light tub margarine instead of butter or stick margarines.

CUT BACK TO HELP YOUR HEART

In addition to choosing the right foods, it's a good idea to eat fewer of the foods that add calories without adding nutrients, are high in sodium, or contain unhealthy fats. Focusing on fresh, minimally processed foods will help you avoid these dietary dangers, each of which can increase your risk of heart disease and stroke.

Added sugars: To keep your weight at a healthy level, cut back on the empty calories that come from foods with no real nutritional value. Examples include soft drinks, candy, and desserts, which all contain large amounts of sugar added during processing. Women should aim to limit added sugar to no more than 100 calories per day (about six teaspoons) and men should aim for no more than 150 calories per day (about nine teaspoons). For some perspective, just one 12-ounce can of regular soda contains eight teaspoons of sugar, or 130 calories, with no nutritional value at all. Both men and women should limit sugar-sweetened beverages to no more than 450 calories (36 ounces) a week. To determine how many grams of added sugar are in one serving of a particular product (if that product contains little or no milk or fruit, which both provide natural sugars), use the "Sugars" number on a product's nutrition facts panel. Divide the number of sugar grams by 4 to get the number of teaspoons of sugar per serving; multiply the grams by 4 to calculate the number of calories from sugar.

Sodium: Too much sodium in your diet can lead to high blood pressure, a serious condition that can damage the circulatory system and, if left uncontrolled, puts you at higher risk for heart disease and stroke. The American Heart Association's current recommendation for daily sodium intake is no more than 1,500 milligrams, but the average American consumes more than twice that amount. Three-quarters of that sodium comes from the salt added to processed food products. To cut back on sodium, choose products with the least amount of sodium you can find in your store. Watch how much sodium you add to your meals in the form of condiments, dressings, and sauces. Finally, educate yourself about how much sodium your favorite foods—especially restaurant meals—contain and decide what you can do without and what you can replace with alternatives that contain less sodium.

Harmful fats: Eating a diet high in saturated fat and trans fat increases your risk for high blood cholesterol, which in turn increases risk of heart disease. To avoid eating saturated fat, cut back on animal-based foods, such as full-fat dairy products (butter, whole milk, full-fat cheese), meat and poultry, and certain tropical oils (coconut, cocoa butter, palm, and palm kernel). Trans fat, perhaps the most damaging of harmful fats, is found primarily in commercial products such as baked goods, fried foods, and stick margarine. Try to eliminate trans fat from your diet by choosing foods made with vegetable-based oils that are not partially hydrogenated. Like saturated and trans fats, dietary cholesterol can increase blood cholesterol; therefore, it's wise to limit your intake of dietary cholesterol to no more than 300 milligrams each day.

Restaurant meals: Eating out frequently can test your best intentions to eat healthy, especially if you're trying to cut back on sodium, but you can enjoy a restaurant meal and also follow the basic guidelines for good nutrition. One good strategy is to ask that your food be grilled, broiled, steamed, or baked instead of fried, and prepared with less salt or sauce. Order dishes that offer lots of vegetables and whole grains, and split your entrée with your dining partner or take half home. These approaches will help you keep the sodium, sugar, unhealthy fats, and calories in check.

LEADING A HEALTHY LIFESTYLE

When it comes to preventing heart disease and stroke, eating fresh, healthy foods is only part of the equation. Although some risk factors, such as age, family history, and ethnicity, can't be changed, many of the most damaging risk factors are things you can control.

Move more: Getting regular physical activity can help prevent or control high blood pressure, high blood cholesterol, and diabetes. It's also an important part of reaching and maintaining a healthy weight. By exercising for as little as 30 minutes a day, you can reduce your risk of heart disease. Adults should aim each week for at least 150 minutes (2 hours and 30 minutes) of moderate-intensity activity or 75 minutes (1 hour and 15 minutes) of vigorous-intensity activity, or a combination of both. Thirty minutes a day, five days a week, is an easy goal to remember, but you will also benefit if you divide your time into two or three 10- to 15-minute segments per day. Physical activity is anything that makes you move your body and burn calories, such as climbing stairs or playing sports. Aerobic exercise, such as walking, jogging, swimming, or biking, benefits your heart. Strength and stretching exercises are best for overall stamina and flexibility. The simplest positive change you can make to effectively improve your heart health is to start walking. It's free, fun, easy, and can be done alone or with your family and friends. To locate American Heart Association-designated walking paths in your area or to find—or create—a walking club, visit www.startwalkingnow.org.

Maintain a healthy weight: To best manage your weight, you need to eat the right amount of calories for you and engage in regular physical activity. People who are overweight or obese have a much higher risk of heart disease and stroke, even if they have no other risk factors. Losing just 10 percent of your body weight will help lower your risk.

Avoid tobacco smoke: Smoking is the number one preventable cause of premature death in the United States. Smoking makes blood vessels stiff, greatly increasing your risk of cardiovascular disease and stroke. A smoker's risk of dying from coronary heart disease is two to three times that of a nonsmoker's. The good news is that when you do stop smoking—no matter how long or how much you've smoked—your risk of heart disease and stroke drops rapidly. If you don't smoke, don't start. If you do smoke, stop now!

Limit alcohol: Drinking too much alcohol can raise blood pressure, increase the risk of heart failure and stroke, produce irregular heartbeats, and contribute to many other diseases. If you do drink, do so in moderation, which means no more than one drink per day for women and two drinks per day for men. One drink is the equivalent of 12 ounces of beer, 4 ounces of wine, or 1½ ounces of 80-proof spirits. If you don't drink, don't start.

RECIPES

This book was created to help give you the opportunity to use fresh ingredients as often as possible, but we know there are times when you may not have a certain food on hand. If you need to substitute a frozen or canned product for a fresh ingredient in one of our recipes, be sure to choose one that contains no sauce or added salt or sugar. To make shopping for our recipes easier, we have compiled a list of approximate equivalents in weight and volume for the most common vegetables and fruits, which you can find in Appendix C: Ingredient Equivalents on page 306.

EACH RECIPE in the book includes a nutritional analysis so you can decide how that dish fits with your dietary needs. These guidelines will give you some details on how the analyses were calculated.

- Each analysis is for a *single* serving; garnishes or optional ingredients are *not* included unless noted.

- Because of the many variables involved, the nutrient values provided should be considered approximate. When figuring portions, remember that the serving sizes are approximate also.

- When ingredient options are listed, the first one is analyzed. When a range of amount is given, the average is analyzed.

- Values other than fats are rounded to the nearest whole number. Fat values are rounded to the nearest half gram. Because of the rounding, values for saturated, trans, monounsaturated, and polyunsaturated fats may not add up to the amount shown for total fat value.

- All the recipes are analyzed using unsalted or low-sodium ingredients whenever possible. In some cases, we call for unprocessed foods or no-salt-added and low-sodium products, then add table salt sparingly for flavor.

- We specify canola, corn, and olive oils in these recipes, but you can also use other heart-healthy unsaturated oils, such as safflower, soybean, and sunflower.

- Meats are analyzed as lean, with all visible fat discarded. Values for ground beef are based on lean meat that is 95 percent fat free.

- When meat, poultry, or seafood is marinated and the marinade is discarded, the analysis includes all of the sodium from the marinade but none of the other nutrients from it.

- If alcohol is used in a cooked dish, we estimate that most of the alcohol calories evaporate as the food cooks.

- Because product labeling in the marketplace can vary and change quickly, we use the generic terms "fat-free" and "low-fat" throughout to avoid confusion.

- We use the abbreviations *g* for gram and *mg* for milligram.

APPETIZERS, SNACKS, AND BEVERAGES

Creamy Avocado-Chive Dip

SERVES 8
¼ cup per serving

PREP TIME
15 minutes

Oversized slices of red, orange, and yellow bell peppers make colorful "scoops" for this easily prepared dip. You can also serve this with blanched broccoli florets, baby carrots, and unsalted baked tortilla or pita chips. Try the dip as a spread on a turkey sandwich or burger rather than the usual condiments to add an unexpected layer of flavor.

1 medium garlic clove

2 medium avocados, diced

½ cup fat-free plain Greek yogurt

1 tablespoon fresh lime juice

¼ teaspoon salt

⅛ to ¼ teaspoon cayenne

2 tablespoons chopped fresh chives

1. With the motor running, drop the garlic through the feed tube of a food processor. Process until finely chopped.

2. Add the remaining ingredients except the chives. Process until smooth.

3. Add the chives. Pulse just until the chives are blended in.

TIPS, TRICKS & TIMESAVERS: This dip may be made up to 2 hours in advance. To prevent browning, place a piece of plastic wrap directly on the surface of the dip and refrigerate.

SHOP & STORE: Ripe avocados yield to firm but gentle pressure. If the avocado is firm and does not yield, let it ripen for a few days at room temperature. Very soft or mushy avocados are overripe.

PER SERVING: Calories 89 • Total Fat 7.5 g • Saturated Fat 1.0 g • Trans Fat 0.0 g
Polyunsaturated Fat 1.0 g • Monounsaturated Fat 5.0 g • Cholesterol 0 mg
Sodium 82 mg • Carbohydrates 5 g • Fiber 3 g • Sugars 1 g • Protein 2 g
DIETARY EXCHANGES: 1 vegetable, 1½ fat

Dill Dip

SERVES 4
¼ cup per serving

PREP TIME
5 minutes

1 cup fat-free plain Greek yogurt

4 medium green onions, finely chopped

¼ cup chopped fresh dillweed

⅛ teaspoon salt

You will love that you can easily throw together this four-ingredient dip in five minutes. Serve it with an array of fresh vegetables, such as grape tomatoes, celery or jícama sticks, or cucumber spears.

In a small bowl, whisk together all the ingredients. Serve immediately or cover and refrigerate for up to two days.

PER SERVING: Calories **40** • Total Fat **0.0 g** • Saturated Fat **0.0 g** • Trans Fat **0.0 g** • Polyunsaturated Fat **0.0 g** • Monounsaturated Fat **0.0 g** • Cholesterol **0 mg** • Sodium **99 mg** • Carbohydrates **4 g** • Fiber **1 g** • Sugars **3 g** • Protein **5 g**
DIETARY EXCHANGES: ½ fat-free milk

Lemon-Ginger Dip

SERVES 4
2 tablespoons
per serving

PREP TIME
5 minutes

1 teaspoon grated lemon zest

⅓ cup fresh lemon juice

3 tablespoons sugar

1½ to 2 tablespoons water

1 teaspoon grated peeled gingerroot

This citrusy, gingery dip is the perfect complement to fresh summer fruits, such as sliced, hulled strawberries and cubed watermelon and cantaloupe. Put this on the table as a no-cook, no-fuss appetizer while dinner is grilling on a hot summer night or as a cool, refreshing, light dessert to end the meal.

In a small bowl, whisk together all the ingredients until the sugar is dissolved. Serve immediately or cover and refrigerate for up to two days.

PER SERVING: Calories **42** • Total Fat **0.0 g** • Saturated Fat **0.0 g** • Trans Fat **0.0 g** • Polyunsaturated Fat **0.0 g** • Monounsaturated Fat **0.0 g** • Cholesterol **0 mg** • Sodium **1 mg** • Carbohydrates **11 g** • Fiber **0 g** • Sugars **10 g** • Protein **0 g**
DIETARY EXCHANGES: ½ other carbohydrate

Creole "Caviar"

The hot sauce and "holy trinity" of onion, bell pepper, and celery give these black-eyed peas a classic Creole taste. Serve the "caviar" as a dip with whole-grain pita chips, atop crisp toasted baguette slices, alongside sandwiches, or as a topper for grilled fish, chicken, or pork chops.

In a medium bowl, stir together all the ingredients. Serve immediately or cover and refrigerate for up to four days.

COOK'S TIP ON BLACK-EYED PEAS: Also called field peas or cowpeas, these legumes are a traditional food to eat on New Year's Day to bring good luck for the year ahead. The pea has a prominent black dot, resembling a tiny eye, on its interior curve. Black-eyed peas are a great source of fiber.

PER SERVING: Calories **43** • Total Fat **0.0 g** • Saturated Fat **0.0 g** • Trans Fat **0.0 g**
Polyunsaturated Fat **0.0 g** • Monounsaturated Fat **0.0 g** • Cholesterol **0 mg**
Sodium **107 mg** • Carbohydrates **8 g** • Fiber **2 g** • Sugars **3 g** • Protein **2 g**
DIETARY EXCHANGES: ½ starch

½ **15.5-ounce can no-salt-added black-eyed peas, rinsed and drained**

¼ **cup finely chopped celery**

¼ **cup diced red onion**

¼ **cup finely chopped green bell pepper**

¼ **cup finely chopped red bell pepper**

2 **tablespoons chopped fresh parsley**

1½ **teaspoons sugar**

1 **teaspoon Louisiana-style hot sauce**

1 **teaspoon cider vinegar**

½ **medium garlic clove, minced**

¼ **teaspoon salt**

SERVES 4
3 wraps per serving

PREP TIME
20 minutes

Asian Veggie Wraps

These wraps hold big flavor in a small package. Spicy peanut sauce tops cool, crunchy cucumber, fresh herbs, and ginger—all wrapped up in tender Boston lettuce leaves. *(See photo insert.)*

SAUCE

2 tablespoons
  low-sodium smooth
  peanut butter

2 tablespoons fresh lime
  juice

2 tablespoons water

1 tablespoon sugar

1 teaspoon soy sauce
  (lowest sodium
  available)

1/8 teaspoon crushed red
  pepper flakes

FILLING

1 medium cucumber,
  peeled, seeded, and
  diced

1/4 cup finely chopped
  red onion

2 tablespoons chopped
  fresh mint

2 tablespoons chopped
  fresh cilantro

2 teaspoons grated
  peeled gingerroot

* * *

12 small Boston or Bibb
  lettuce leaves

1. In a small microwaveable bowl, microwave the peanut butter on high (100 percent power) for 20 to 25 seconds, or until slightly melted. Whisk in the remaining sauce ingredients until smooth.

2. In a separate small bowl, stir together the filling ingredients. Spoon 2 tablespoons of filling onto the center of each lettuce leaf. Spoon 1½ teaspoons of sauce over the filling in each bundle.

3. Fold the lettuce around the filling.

COOK'S TIP ON LEFTOVER MINT: Use leftover mint to flavor unsweetened iced tea, or chop the leaves and add them to fruit salad or cooked green peas.

PER SERVING: Calories **76** • Total Fat **4.0 g** • Saturated Fat **0.5 g** • Trans Fat **0.0 g**
Polyunsaturated Fat **1.0 g** • Monounsaturated Fat **2.0 g** • Cholesterol **0 mg**
Sodium **53 mg** • Carbohydrates **9 g** • Fiber **1 g** • Sugars **6 g** • Protein **3 g**
DIETARY EXCHANGES: ½ other carbohydrate, 1 fat

Baked Nachos

Here's a fresh take on a family favorite. These crispy, cheesy nachos are high in flavor but low in fat and salt. Once you see how quick and easy it is to make your own baked chips, you may never buy the bagged kind again.

1. Preheat the oven to 350°F.

2. Put the tortillas on a cutting board. Brush one side of each tortilla with the oil. Stack the tortillas. Cut into 6 equal triangles for a total of 12. Arrange in a single layer on a baking sheet. Sprinkle with the cumin.

3. Bake the chips for 10 minutes, or until lightly browned on the edges and beginning to crisp. Turn off the oven.

4. Meanwhile, in a medium bowl, gently stir together the remaining ingredients except the salt.

5. Spread the bell pepper mixture on the chips. Sprinkle with the salt. Return to the oven. Let stand in the oven for 3 to 4 minutes, or until the Cheddar is slightly melted.

PER SERVING: Calories **42** • Total Fat **2.0 g** • Saturated Fat **0.5 g** • Trans Fat **0.0 g** Polyunsaturated Fat **0.5 g** • Monounsaturated Fat **1.0 g** • Cholesterol **1 mg** Sodium **119 mg** • Carbohydrates **5 g** • Fiber **1 g** • Sugars **1 g** • Protein **2 g** DIETARY EXCHANGES: ½ starch

SERVES 4
3 wedges
per serving

PREP TIME
5 minutes

COOKING TIME
10 minutes

STANDING TIME
3 to 4 minutes

2 6-inch corn tortillas

1 teaspoon canola or corn oil

½ teaspoon ground cumin

¼ cup diced red bell pepper

1 medium green onion, finely chopped

3 tablespoons shredded low-fat sharp Cheddar cheese

2 tablespoons chopped fresh cilantro

⅛ teaspoon salt

1 large jalapeño
(see Cook's Tip,
page 261)

1 teaspoon olive oil and
1 tablespoon olive oil,
divided use

2 cups chopped
portobello or baby
bella mushrooms

4 medium garlic cloves,
minced

6 ounces spinach

1 teaspoon finely
chopped fresh
rosemary

12 2-inch mini whole-grain
pitas, each separated
into top and bottom
rounds

Spicy Mini Pitas with Spinach and Mushrooms

A roasted jalapeño and a hint of fresh rosemary kick up the flavor of these mini pita snacks. Toasting the pita rounds gives them a pleasant crunchiness.

1. Preheat the broiler.

2. Put the jalapeño on a small baking sheet or round baking stone. Broil about 4 to 6 inches from the heat for 6 to 7 minutes, or until the skin is brown and blistered, turning every 2 minutes. Turn off the broiler. Transfer the jalapeño to a small paper bag. Close the bag. Set aside.

3. Preheat the oven to 400°F.

4. In a medium saucepan, heat 1 teaspoon oil over medium-high heat for 5 minutes, swirling to coat the bottom. Cook the mushrooms and garlic for 5 minutes, or until the mushrooms begin to soften and release their juices, stirring frequently.

5. Add the spinach (you may need to do this in two batches). Reduce the heat to medium. Cook, covered, for 5 minutes, or until the spinach is wilted, stirring frequently. Set aside.

6. Meanwhile, in a small microwaveable bowl, stir together the rosemary and the remaining 1 tablespoon oil. Microwave on 100 percent power (high) for 40 seconds, or until the oil is fragrant.

7. Place the pita rounds with the rough interior side up on a large baking sheet or rectangular baking stone. Brush the tops with the rosemary mixture. Bake the pitas for 2 to 3 minutes, or until they begin to crisp.

8. Meanwhile, remove the jalapeño from the bag. Discard the stem, skin, seeds, and ribs. Finely chop the flesh.

9. Remove the baking sheet with the pitas from the oven. Top each pita with 1 heaping tablespoon of the spinach mixture. Sprinkle with the jalapeño.

10. Bake the pitas at 400°F for 3 minutes to heat through. Serve immediately.

PER SERVING: Calories 80 • Total Fat 0.5 g • Saturated Fat 0.0 g • Trans Fat 0.5 g
Polyunsaturated Fat 0.5 g • Monounsaturated Fat 2.5 g • Cholesterol 0 mg
Sodium 100 mg • Carbohydrates 10 g • Fiber 2 g • Sugars 1 g • Protein 3 g
DIETARY EXCHANGES: ½ starch, ½ fat

SERVES 6
4 pieces per serving

PREP TIME
15 minutes

COOKING TIME
5 minutes

3 whole-grain round sandwich thins (lowest sodium available), halved and toasted

1 medium pear, thinly sliced

¾ teaspoon chopped fresh thyme

2 tablespoons chopped walnuts, dry-roasted

¼ cup plus 2 tablespoons shredded smoked mozzarella cheese, shredded Gruyère, or crumbled low-fat blue cheese

Smoky Pear Melts

This appetizer gets its sweetness from fresh pear, savoriness from aromatic thyme, crunchiness from toasted walnuts, and creaminess from melted cheese. These warm delights are fast to prepare and even faster to cook.

1. Preheat the broiler.

2. Place the sandwich-thin halves with the cut sides up on a baking sheet. Top with the pear slices. Sprinkle, in order, with the thyme, walnuts, and mozzarella. Broil about 4 inches from the heat for 1 minute, or until the mozzarella is melted. Cut into quarters. Serve warm.

COOK'S TIP ON CORING PEARS: Pears are an excellent source of fiber and vitamin C. To core the fruit, halve it lengthwise and use a melon baller to scoop out the core. Use the melon baller or a paring knife to remove the stem.

PER SERVING: Calories **105** • Total Fat **4.0 g** • Saturated Fat **1.0 g** • Trans Fat **0.0 g** • Polyunsaturated Fat **1.5 g** • Monounsaturated Fat **0.5 g** • Cholesterol **6 mg** • Sodium **115 mg** • Carbohydrates **15 g** • Fiber **3 g** • Sugars **4 g** • Protein **4 g** • DIETARY EXCHANGES: 1 starch, ½ fat

Blueberry Crostini

SERVES 4
4 crostini
per serving

PREP TIME
10 minutes

If you like blueberry crisp, then you're sure to be a fan of this appetizer. A blueberry-ricotta mixture that has a smidge of sweetness and a touch of tartness tops warm whole-grain toast. Crunchy granola adds a hint of nuttiness.

1. In a small bowl, stir together the ricotta, honey, lemon zest, and cinnamon. Stir in the blueberries.

2. Spread the toast with the ricotta mixture. Sprinkle with the granola. Cut each piece of toast diagonally into quarters.

COOK'S TIP: These crostini also make for a delicious side dish for breakfast or brunch with scrambled eggs and fresh orange juice.

¼ cup fat-free ricotta cheese or fat-free vanilla yogurt

1 tablespoon honey

½ teaspoon grated lemon zest

⅛ teaspoon ground cinnamon

1 cup blueberries

4 slices whole-grain bread (lowest sodium available), toasted

¼ cup low-fat granola

PER SERVING: Calories **141** • Total Fat **1.5 g** • Saturated Fat **0.5 g** • Trans Fat **0.0 g**
Polyunsaturated Fat **0.5 g** • Monounsaturated Fat **0.5 g** • Cholesterol **1 mg**
Sodium **153 mg** • Carbohydrates **27 g** • Fiber **3 g** • Sugars **12 g** • Protein **6 g**
DIETARY EXCHANGES: 1½ starch, ½ fruit

Triple Citrus Refresher

SERVES 4
½ cup per serving

PREP TIME
5 minutes

2 cups fresh orange juice

2 to 3 tablespoons fresh lime juice

2 tablespoons sugar

1 tablespoon plus 1 teaspoon fresh lemon juice

Wake up your morning orange juice with splashes of lemon and lime that are sure to add a bit of zest to your breakfast.

In a medium pitcher, stir together all the ingredients.

PER SERVING: Calories 83 • Total Fat **0.5 g** • Saturated Fat **0.0 g** • Trans Fat **0.0 g** Polyunsaturated Fat **0.0 g** • Monounsaturated Fat **0.0 g** • Cholesterol **0 mg** Sodium **2 mg** • Carbohydrates **20 g** • Fiber **0 g** • Sugars **17 g** • Protein **1 g** DIETARY EXCHANGES: 1 fruit, ½ other carbohydrate

Spicy Mexican-Style Tomato Juice

SERVES 4
½ cup per serving

PREP TIME
10 minutes

2 cups grape tomatoes

¼ cup chopped fresh cilantro

3 tablespoons fresh lime juice

1 to 2 medium jalapeños, seeds and ribs discarded (see Cook's Tip, page 261)

1 teaspoon Worcestershire sauce (lowest sodium available)

1 teaspoon cider vinegar

⅛ teaspoon salt

The south-of-the-border combination of lime, cilantro, and jalapeño adds a new level of flavor to plain tomato juice. With the addition of Worcestershire sauce and vinegar, this drink is similar to a Mexican Bloody Mary (but without the alcohol). To get the desired level of heat, experiment with the amount of jalapeño.

In a food processor or blender, process all the ingredients until smooth.

PER SERVING: Calories 30 • Total Fat **0.5 g** • Saturated Fat **0.0 g** • Trans Fat **0.0 g** Polyunsaturated Fat **0.0 g** • Monounsaturated Fat **0.0 g** • Cholesterol **0 mg** Sodium **90 mg** • Carbohydrates **7 g** • Fiber **1 g** • Sugars **4 g** • Protein **1 g** DIETARY EXCHANGES: 1 vegetable

Sweet Green Smoothie

SERVES 2
1 cup per serving

PREP TIME
5 minutes

Avocado and Greek yogurt make this beverage thick and creamy. Along with the spinach and flax seed, they also provide protein, making this perfect for breakfast or an afternoon pick-me-up. *(See photo insert.)*

In a food processor or blender, process all the ingredients until smooth.

> **SHOP & STORE:** Flax seed meal—ground flax seed that is usually found in the health food section of the market—is a rich source of fiber, omega-3 fatty acids, calcium, iron, niacin, and vitamin E. When mixed with liquid, it becomes gelatinous and adds body to drinks like smoothies. Store flax seed meal in the refrigerator or freezer.

2 cups tightly packed baby spinach

1 cup 100% white grape juice, chilled

½ cup fat-free plain Greek yogurt

½ medium avocado

1 tablespoon flax seed meal

1 tablespoon honey

PER SERVING: Calories **245** • Total Fat **9.0 g** • Saturated Fat **1.0 g** • Trans Fat **0.0 g**
Polyunsaturated Fat **2.0 g** • Monounsaturated Fat **5.0 g** • Cholesterol **0 mg**
Sodium **55 mg** • Carbohydrates **36 g** • Fiber **5 g** • Sugars **29 g** • Protein **8 g**
DIETARY EXCHANGES: 1½ fruit, 1 vegetable, ½ fat-free milk, 1½ fat

Honeydew Smoothie

SERVES 5
1 cup per serving

PREP TIME
5 minutes

4 cups 1-inch cubes of honeydew melon

1 cup fat-free plain yogurt

1 cup ice cubes

1 cup unsweetened low-fat vanilla almond milk

1 tablespoon honey

Do try this smoothie, which gets its sweetness from potassium-rich honeydew melon and a touch of honey. Its creaminess comes from tangy yogurt and rich vanilla almond milk.

In a food processor or blender, process all the ingredients until smooth.

PER SERVING: Calories 97 • Total Fat 1.0 g • Saturated Fat 0.0 g • Trans Fat 0.0 g Polyunsaturated Fat 0.0 g • Monounsaturated Fat 0.0 g • Cholesterol 1 mg Sodium 98 mg • Carbohydrates 20 g • Fiber 1 g • Sugars 18 g • Protein 4 g DIETARY EXCHANGES: 1 fruit, ½ other carbohydrate

Strawberry-Kiwi Cooler

SERVES 4
1 cup per serving

PREP TIME
5 minutes

3 cups hulled strawberries

2 cups fat-free vanilla yogurt

2 medium kiwifruit, peeled

1 to 2 tablespoons sugar

1 tablespoon lime juice (optional)

1 teaspoon vanilla extract

Here's a fruity, refreshing drink for any time of day. The sweet-tart kiwifruit adds some tropical flair and a hefty dose of vitamin C.

In a food processor or blender, process all the ingredients until smooth.

COOK'S TIP: The sweetness of strawberries varies, so start with just 1 tablespoon of sugar and taste the cooler before you add more.

PER SERVING: Calories 182 • Total Fat 0.5 g • Saturated Fat 0.0 g • Trans Fat 0.0 g Polyunsaturated Fat 0.5 g • Monounsaturated Fat 0.0 g • Cholesterol 2 mg Sodium 86 mg • Carbohydrates 38 g • Fiber 3 g • Sugars 33 g • Protein 7 g DIETARY EXCHANGES: 1 fat-free milk, 1 fruit, ½ other carbohydrate

Rise-and-Shine Shake

SERVES 4
1 cup per serving

PREP TIME
5 minutes

Punch up your morning glass of orange juice by adding smooth yogurt and luscious strawberries, peaches, and bananas for a fruit explosion that will surely get your day off to a healthy start.

In a food processor or blender, process all the ingredients until smooth.

PER SERVING: Calories **163** • Total Fat **0.5 g** • Saturated Fat **0.0 g** • Trans Fat **0.0 g** Polyunsaturated Fat **0.0 g** • Monounsaturated Fat **0.0 g** • Cholesterol **0 mg** Sodium **33 mg** • Carbohydrates **32 g** • Fiber **3 g** • Sugars **25 g** • Protein **9 g** DIETARY EXCHANGES: 2 fruit, 1 lean meat

2 cups hulled strawberries

1½ cups fat-free plain Greek yogurt

2 medium unpeeled peaches, halved

1 medium banana, cut into large chunks

⅓ cup fresh orange juice

2 tablespoons sugar

1½ teaspoons vanilla extract

Coconut-Peach Breeze

SERVES 4
¾ cup per serving

PREP TIME
10 minutes

An abundance of coconut flavor gives this creamy beverage true tropical flair.

In a food processor or blender, process all the ingredients until smooth. Serve over ice if desired.

SHOP & STORE: Unsweetened coconut milk beverage is not the same as coconut milk. The beverage has about 50 calories per cup versus more than 400 per cup for regular coconut milk, and even about 150 per cup for lite coconut milk.

2 cups chopped unpeeled peaches

¾ cup unsweetened coconut milk beverage

½ cup fat-free vanilla yogurt or fat-free coconut yogurt

¼ cup coconut water

PER SERVING: Calories **70** • Total Fat **1.0 g** • Saturated Fat **1.0 g** • Trans Fat **0.0 g** Polyunsaturated Fat **0.0 g** • Monounsaturated Fat **0.0 g** • Cholesterol **1 mg** Sodium **40 mg** • Carbohydrates **13 g** • Fiber **1 g** • Sugars **12 g** • Protein **3 g** DIETARY EXCHANGES: ½ fruit, ½ other carbohydrate

1 cup sliced unpeeled
  nectarine

1 cup pineapple cubes

1 cup fat-free milk

¾ cup sliced banana

2 tablespoons flax seed
  meal

⅛ teaspoon almond
  extract

1 cup ice cubes

Nectarine-Pineapple Chill

A shot of protein, mostly from dairy and flax, makes this chill an a.m. energy booster or a p.m. pick-me-up on a warm summer day. You'll also add fiber to your diet, with just over a serving of fruit in every cup. Use the ripest fruit you can find for the sweetest flavor. *(See photo insert.)*

In a food processor or blender, process all the ingredients except the ice until smooth. Add the ice. Process until smooth.

COOK'S TIP ON PEELING AND CORING A PINEAPPLE: Lay a pineapple on its side on a cutting board. Cut off the top and bottom. Stand the pineapple up on one of its ends. Cutting vertically, carefully remove the skin, leaving as much of the flesh as possible. Remove any "eye spots." Use a pineapple corer to remove the core, or cut the pineapple into slices and use a knife to remove the core from each slice.

PER SERVING: Calories **103** • Total Fat **2.0 g** • Saturated Fat **0.0 g** • Trans Fat **0.0 g**
Polyunsaturated Fat **1.5 g** • Monounsaturated Fat **0.5 g** • Cholesterol **1 mg**
Sodium **26 mg** • Carbohydrates **20 g** • Fiber **3 g** • Sugars **13 g** • Protein **4 g**
DIETARY EXCHANGES: 1 fruit, ½ fat-free milk

Fruit Frappé

Trade in your usual breakfast cereal for this breakfast in a glass. Thanks to the fruit and wheat germ, the beverage is full of fiber. Plus, you get about three servings of fruit as a great start to your day.

In a food processor or blender, process all the ingredients except the wheat germ until smooth. Pour into glasses. Sprinkle with the wheat germ.

2 cups chopped cantaloupe

2 cups hulled strawberries

1 cup fresh orange juice

2 medium peaches or apricots or 1 large nectarine, halved

1 medium banana

2 tablespoons sugar

3 tablespoons toasted wheat germ

SHOP & STORE: Stop bananas from ripening too quickly by storing them for a few days in the refrigerator crisper. The outer skin will darken, but the banana will stay firm longer.

PER SERVING: Calories 178 • Total Fat 1.5 g • Saturated Fat 0.0 g • Trans Fat 0.0 g Polyunsaturated Fat 0.5 g • Monounsaturated Fat 0.0 g • Cholesterol 0 mg Sodium 15 mg • Carbohydrates 41 g • Fiber 5 g • Sugars 31 g • Protein 4 g DIETARY EXCHANGES: 3 fruit

SERVES 4
¾ cup per serving

PREP TIME
5 minutes

2 cups whole hulled strawberries

1 medium peeled pear, halved

1 cup ice cubes

½ cup fresh grapefruit juice

¼ cup chopped fresh mint

2 tablespoons sugar

Strawberry-Pear Slush

The hottest days of summer will seem cooler when you drink this icy slush. The grapefruit juice adds a subtle tartness to balance out the pervasive sweetness of the berries and pear.

In a food processor or blender, process all the ingredients until smooth.

HEALTHY SWAP: Substitute ½ cup water for the ice cubes to make a juice drink instead of a slush.

COOK'S TIP ON GRAPEFRUIT: Grapefruit can interact with a number of medications, including many heart medicines. Be sure to check with your doctor or pharmacist if you take any medication, and use orange juice as an alternative ingredient if necessary.

PER SERVING: Calories **88** • Total Fat **0.5 g** • Saturated Fat **0.0 g** • Trans Fat **0.0 g**
Polyunsaturated Fat **0.0 g** • Monounsaturated Fat **0.0 g** • Cholesterol **0 mg**
Sodium **4 mg** • Carbohydrates **22 g** • Fiber **3 g** • Sugars **16 g** • Protein **1 g**
DIETARY EXCHANGES: 1½ fruit

Peanutty Chocolate-Banana Freezer

SERVES 4
¾ cup per serving

PREP TIME
5 minutes

Chocolate and banana are a classic combination, made even better with the addition of peanut butter.

In a food processor or blender, process all the ingredients until smooth.

HEALTHY SWAP: Stir in 1 to 2 teaspoons instant coffee granules to deepen the chocolaty flavor of your shake.

1½ cups fat-free chocolate milk

1 cup fat-free frozen vanilla yogurt or fat-free vanilla ice cream

2 medium bananas

2 tablespoons low-sodium smooth peanut butter

2 tablespoons unsweetened dark cocoa powder

PER SERVING: Calories 217 • Total Fat **5.0 g** • Saturated Fat **1.0 g** • Trans Fat **0.0 g** Polyunsaturated Fat **1.0 g** • Monounsaturated Fat **2.0 g** • Cholesterol **2 mg** Sodium **87 mg** • Carbohydrates **38 g** • Fiber **3 g** • Sugars **28 g** • Protein **8 g** DIETARY EXCHANGES: 1 fat-free milk, 1 fruit, ½ other carbohydrate, ½ fat

SOUPS

Cauliflower-Carrot
Soup 44

Roasted Onion Soup 45

Indian-Spiced
Pumpkin-Apple Soup 46

Parmesan-Spinach
Soup 48

Summer Zucchini
Soup 49

Butternut Squash Soup
with Sage Cream 50

Lemony Brown Rice
Soup 51

Chilled Cucumber-Melon
Soup 52

Creamy Peach-Berry
Soup 53

Caribbean Fish Stew 54

Shiitake Mushroom and
Spinach Soup with
Shrimp 55

Mexican Tortilla Soup with
Tilapia 56

Asparagus-Sausage Soup
with Quinoa 58

Chicken-Escarole
Soup 59

Chicken and Red Lentil
Soup 60

Chicken and Rotini Soup
with Vegetables 61

Verde Chicken Soup 62

Turkey and Wild Rice
Soup 63

White Bean Soup with Spicy
Turkey Meatballs, Leeks, and
Kale 64

SERVES 4
¾ cup per serving

PREP TIME
10 minutes

COOKING TIME
15 minutes

Cauliflower-Carrot Soup

This creamy soup, with a hint of nutmeg, goes well with your favorite chicken or turkey sandwich. The cayenne adds a dash of heat.

1 teaspoon canola or
  corn oil

1 cup diced onion

1½ cups small cauliflower
  florets

1 cup water

½ cup diced carrots

½ teaspoon sugar

¼ teaspoon ground
  nutmeg

Dash of cayenne

¾ cup fat-free
  half-and-half

1 tablespoon light tub
  margarine

⅛ teaspoon salt

1. In a medium saucepan, heat the oil over medium-high heat, swirling to coat the bottom. Cook the onion for 3 minutes, or until soft, stirring frequently.

2. Stir in the cauliflower, water, carrots, sugar, nutmeg, and cayenne. Increase the heat to high and bring to a boil. Reduce the heat and simmer, covered, for 8 to 9 minutes, or until the carrots are tender. Remove from the heat.

3. Add the half-and-half, margarine, and salt, stirring until the margarine has melted. Just before serving, sprinkle with additional nutmeg if desired.

COOK'S TIP: Be sure to cut your vegetables to the same size for even cooking.

PER SERVING: Calories 86 • Total Fat 2.5 g • Saturated Fat 0.0 g • Trans Fat 0.0 g
Polyunsaturated Fat 0.5 g • Monounsaturated Fat 1.5 g • Cholesterol 0 mg
Sodium 167 mg • Carbohydrates 14 g • Fiber 2 g • Sugars 7 g • Protein 4 g
DIETARY EXCHANGES: 1 vegetable, ½ fat-free milk, ½ fat

Roasted Onion Soup

SERVES 4
¾ cup per serving

PREP TIME
10 minutes

COOKING TIME
30 minutes

Roasting the onions brings out their natural sweetness in a fraction of the time it would take to caramelize them on the stovetop. You'll save half the time but still enjoy all the oniony goodness. Partner this soup with Grilled Portobello Burgers with Spicy Avocado Sauce (page 202).

1. Preheat the oven to 425°F. Line a large baking sheet with aluminum foil. Lightly spray the foil with cooking spray.

2. Put the yellow and red onions, shallots, and garlic on the foil. Pour the oil over the vegetables. Stir to coat. Arrange the vegetables in a single layer.

3. Roast for 20 minutes, or until richly browned, stirring once halfway through.

4. Transfer the onion mixture to a medium saucepan. Stir in the remaining ingredients. Bring to a boil over high heat. Reduce the heat and simmer for 1 minute.

PER SERVING: Calories **96** • Total Fat **3.5 g** • Saturated Fat **0.5 g** • Trans Fat **0.0 g**
Polyunsaturated Fat **0.5 g** • Monounsaturated Fat **2.5 g** • Cholesterol **0 mg**
Sodium **121 mg** • Carbohydrates **15 g** • Fiber **2 g** • Sugars **7 g** • Protein **2 g**
DIETARY EXCHANGES: 3 vegetable, ½ fat

Cooking spray

1 cup chopped yellow onion

1 cup chopped red onion

½ cup thinly sliced shallots

4 medium garlic cloves, peeled

1 tablespoon extra-virgin olive oil

2½ cups water

4 packets (1 tablespoon plus 1 teaspoon) salt-free instant beef bouillon

1 teaspoon sugar

1 teaspoon chopped fresh rosemary

1 teaspoon Worcestershire sauce (lowest sodium available)

⅛ teaspoon salt

SERVES 4
1 cup per serving

PREP TIME
15 minutes

COOKING TIME
30 minutes

Indian-Spiced Pumpkin-Apple Soup

Garam masala gives this creamy pumpkin soup its spicy Indian-flavored edge, while cinnamon rounds out the apple and onion flavors, providing a subtle sweetness. Cook this soup on a cold day when you want something warm and comforting. If you like a more exotic taste, try substituting curry powder for the cinnamon.

1 teaspoon canola or corn oil

2 peeled apples, such as Fuji or Gala, chopped into 1-inch pieces

1 medium onion, chopped into 1-inch pieces

1/4 cup water, up to 1/4 cup water, and 1/2 cup water, divided use

2 cups canned solid-pack pumpkin (not pie filling)

1 1/2 cups fat-free, low-sodium vegetable broth

1 tablespoon garam masala

1/4 teaspoon ground cinnamon

1/2 cup fat-free milk

1/4 cup fat-free sour cream (optional)

1 tablespoon plus 1 teaspoon unsalted shelled pumpkin seeds, dry-roasted

1. In a medium saucepan, heat the oil over medium-high heat, swirling to coat the bottom. Cook the apples and onion for 5 minutes, or until soft, stirring frequently.

2. Pour in 1/4 cup water. Cook, covered, for 7 minutes, or until the apples and onion are very soft, uncovering only once or twice to add 2 tablespoons of water as needed to prevent sticking (adding no more than 1/4 cup water total).

3. Gently stir in the pumpkin, broth, garam masala, cinnamon, and the remaining 1/2 cup water. Increase the heat to high and bring to a boil. Reduce the heat and simmer, covered, for 10 minutes.

4. In a food processor or blender (vent the blender lid), process the soup in batches for 10 to 15 seconds, or until slightly chunky. Carefully return to the pan.

5. Slowly pour in the milk, stirring until blended. Cook over medium heat for 30 seconds, or until heated through.

6. Garnish each serving with the sour cream and pumpkin seeds.

TIPS, TRICKS & TIMESAVERS: This soup tastes even better the next day because the flavors blend. To make the soup the day before, prepare the recipe through the blender step and then cover and refrigerate for 8 to 12 hours. Just before reheating, stir in the milk. Cook over medium heat for 5 minutes, or until heated through, stirring gently. Don't let the soup boil.

SHOP & STORE: A blend of dry-roasted ground spices, garam masala is often used in Indian cooking. There are many variations, each containing as many as 12 spices, such as pepper, cinnamon, cloves, coriander, cumin, cardamom, fennel, mace, and nutmeg. Look for it in the ethnic section of your grocery store or in Indian supermarkets.

PER SERVING: Calories **130** • Total Fat **3.0 g** • Saturated Fat **0.5 g** • Trans Fat **0.0 g**
Polyunsaturated Fat **1.0 g** • Monounsaturated Fat **1.0 g** • Cholesterol **1 mg**
Sodium **44 mg** • Carbohydrates **24 g** • Fiber **7 g** • Sugars **16 g** • Protein **5 g**
DIETARY EXCHANGES: 1 starch, ½ fruit, ½ fat

Parmesan-Spinach Soup

SERVES 4
¾ cup per serving

PREP TIME
10 minutes

COOKING TIME
5 minutes

Chopped spinach and a squeeze of lemon add freshness to our version of *stracciatella*, which is an Italian egg-drop soup. It's also known as rag soup because *stracciatto* means "torn apart" and the whisked egg white in the broth looks like small torn or shredded rags.

3 cups water

4 packets (1 tablespoon plus 1 teaspoon) salt-free instant chicken bouillon

⅛ teaspoon ground nutmeg (optional)

1 large egg white

1 cup spinach, coarsely chopped

⅓ cup chopped fresh basil

¼ cup chopped fresh parsley

1 tablespoon plus 1 teaspoon olive oil

1 teaspoon chopped fresh rosemary

⅛ teaspoon salt

1 tablespoon plus 1 teaspoon shredded or grated Parmesan cheese

1 medium lemon, cut into 4 wedges

1. In a medium saucepan, bring the water, bouillon, and nutmeg to a rolling boil over high heat. Whisk in the egg white. Boil for 30 seconds. Remove from the heat.

2. Stir in the spinach, basil, parsley, oil, rosemary, and salt. Sprinkle each serving with the Parmesan. Serve with the lemon wedges.

PER SERVING: Calories 65 • Total Fat **5.0 g** • Saturated Fat **1.0 g** • Trans Fat **0.0 g** • Polyunsaturated Fat **0.5 g** • Monounsaturated Fat **3.5 g** • Cholesterol **1 mg** • Sodium **128 mg** • Carbohydrates **3 g** • Fiber **0 g** • Sugars **0 g** • Protein **2 g**
DIETARY EXCHANGES: 1 fat

Summer Zucchini Soup

Flecks of carrot add color and texture to this easy zucchini-basil soup. At the end of cooking, stir in lemon zest and fresh basil to bring out the flavors, and add a bit of milk for some creaminess. Enjoy the soup with a dark green leafy salad for a light, summery meal.

SERVES 6
1 cup per serving

PREP TIME
10 minutes

COOKING TIME
20 minutes

1. In a large saucepan, heat the oil over medium-high heat, swirling to coat the bottom. Cook the onion and garlic for 2 minutes, or until the onion begins to soften, stirring constantly.

2. Stir in the zucchini, broth, water, and carrots. Bring to a simmer, covered. Simmer for 15 minutes, or until the vegetables are tender.

3. In a food processor or blender (vent the blender lid), process the soup for 10 to 15 seconds, or until almost smooth but with some flecks of vegetable. Add the basil. Pulse 6 or 7 times, or until the basil is chopped. Carefully return the soup to the pan.

4. Gently stir in the remaining ingredients. Reduce the heat to medium and cook for 30 seconds to reheat. Don't let the soup boil. Serve immediately.

1 tablespoon canola or corn oil

½ medium onion, chopped into ½-inch pieces

2 medium garlic cloves, minced

3 medium zucchini (1 pound total), cut into ½-inch pieces

2 cups fat-free, low-sodium chicken broth or fat-free, low-sodium vegetable broth

1½ cups water

2 small carrots, peeled and cut into ½-inch pieces

½ cup tightly packed basil, coarsely chopped

½ cup plus 2 tablespoons unsweetened soy milk or fat-free milk

1 teaspoon grated lemon zest

¼ teaspoon salt

⅛ teaspoon freshly ground pepper

TIPS, TRICKS & TIMESAVERS: This soup can be served hot, at room temperature, or chilled. To chill, cover and refrigerate for 3 to 8 hours. The soup will keep in the refrigerator for up to six days.

PER SERVING: Calories 59 • Total Fat 3.0 g • Saturated Fat 0.5 g • Trans Fat 0.0 g
Polyunsaturated Fat 1.0 g • Monounsaturated Fat 1.5 g • Cholesterol 0 mg
Sodium 146 mg • Carbohydrates 6 g • Fiber 2 g • Sugars 4 g • Protein 3 g
DIETARY EXCHANGES: 1 vegetable, ½ fat

SERVES 4
¾ cup per serving

PREP TIME
15 minutes

COOKING TIME
25 to 30 minutes

Cooking spray

⅓ cup chopped shallots

⅓ cup chopped carrots

1 small garlic clove, minced

1¾ cups fat-free, low-sodium vegetable broth

12 ounces butternut squash, cut into ¾-inch pieces

1 tablespoon chopped fresh sage and 2 tablespoons chopped fresh sage, divided use

⅛ teaspoon pepper

Dash of ground allspice

2 tablespoons fat-free half-and-half and ½ cup fat-free half-and-half, divided use

2 tablespoons fat-free plain yogurt

Butternut Squash Soup with Sage Cream

This soup is a complementary first course to poultry or pork entrées, such as Turkey Cutlets with Cranberry-Pineapple Relish (page 154) or Pork Tenderloin with Roasted Apple (page 176). Fresh sage and a pinch of allspice highlight the nutty flavor of the squash. A drizzle of pale green sage cream makes for a color-contrasting and silky finishing touch.

1. Lightly spray a large saucepan with cooking spray. Cook the shallots and carrots over medium heat for 3 minutes, or until beginning to soften, stirring occasionally. Stir in the garlic. Cook for 30 seconds, or until fragrant.

2. Stir in the broth, squash, 1 tablespoon sage, the pepper, and allspice. Increase the heat to high and bring to a boil. Reduce the heat and simmer, partially covered, for 20 minutes, or until the vegetables are tender. Remove from the heat.

3. Meanwhile, in a small food processor or blender, process 2 tablespoons half-and-half, the yogurt, and the remaining 2 tablespoons sage until the mixture is pale green and almost smooth. Set aside.

4. Using an immersion blender, purée the soup until smooth. Stir in the remaining ½ cup half-and-half. Or let the soup stand until slightly cooled. Using a food processor or blender (vent the blender lid), process the soup in batches, filling the blender no more than halfway full. Carefully return the soup to the pan and stir in the remaining ½ cup half-and-half.

5. If the soup has cooled too much, cook over medium heat for 3 minutes, or until heated through, stirring occasionally. Garnish each serving with the sage cream.

PER SERVING: Calories **88** • Total Fat **0.0 g** • Saturated Fat **0.0 g** • Trans Fat **0.0 g**
Polyunsaturated Fat **0.0 g** • Monounsaturated Fat **0.0 g** • Cholesterol **0 mg**
Sodium **64 mg** • Carbohydrates **20 g** • Fiber **3 g** • Sugars **7 g** • Protein **5 g**
DIETARY EXCHANGES: 1 starch, 1 vegetable

Lemony Brown Rice Soup

SERVES 4
1 generous cup
per serving

PREP TIME
5 minutes

COOKING TIME
20 minutes

This creamy, sunshine-yellow soup is a healthy take on Greek egg-lemon soup, *avgolemono* (ahv-goh-LEH-moh-noh). The traditional soup is made with chicken broth, whole eggs or egg yolks, lemon juice, and rice. Our recipe uses Greek yogurt instead of eggs to thicken the soup. Perfect for lunch, this soup is a tasty match for Grilled Summer Veggie Salad with Hummus Dressing (page 108) or a basic Greek salad.

1. In a medium saucepan, bring the broth to a boil over high heat. Stir in the rice. Reduce the heat and simmer, covered, for 10 to 12 minutes, or until the rice is tender. Remove from the heat.

2. In a food processor or blender (vent the blender lid), process 2 cups of the broth mixture, the watercress, yogurt, lemon zest, and lemon juice until smooth. Carefully return the mixture to the pan.

3. Stir in the dillweed and turmeric. Cook the soup over medium heat for 3 to 5 minutes, or until heated through, stirring frequently.

4 cups fat-free, low-sodium chicken broth

½ cup uncooked instant brown rice

1½ cups tightly packed watercress

1 cup fat-free plain Greek yogurt

1 teaspoon grated lemon zest

1 to 2 tablespoons fresh lemon juice

2 tablespoons chopped fresh dillweed

¼ teaspoon ground turmeric

COOK'S TIP ON BLENDING HOT LIQUIDS: Be careful when blending hot liquids. Venting the blender lid prevents heat and steam from popping off the lid. Most blender lids have a center section that can be removed. You can even place a kitchen towel over the opening to avoid splatters. Begin blending at the lowest speed and increase to the desired speed, holding the lid down firmly.

PER SERVING: Calories **86** • Total Fat **0.5 g** • Saturated Fat **0.0 g** • Trans Fat **0.0 g**
Polyunsaturated Fat **0.0 g** • Monounsaturated Fat **0.0 g** • Cholesterol **0 mg**
Sodium **89 mg** • Carbohydrates **12 g** • Fiber **1 g** • Sugars **3 g** • Protein **8 g**
DIETARY EXCHANGES: 1 starch, 1 lean meat

Chilled Cucumber-Melon Soup

SERVES 4
¾ cup per serving

PREP TIME
10 minutes

CHILLING TIME
20 to 30 minutes

¼ cup fat-free plain Greek yogurt

4 cups cubed very ripe cantaloupe

1 cup peeled, sliced English, or hothouse, cucumber

1 tablespoon fresh lime juice

¼ cup chopped fresh mint

1 medium serrano pepper, seeds and ribs discarded, minced (see Cook's Tip, page 261)

Lime juice, mint, and serrano pepper perk up the cooling cantaloupe and cucumber, while Greek yogurt brings a touch of richness to this soup.

1. In a food processor or blender, process the yogurt until smooth. Add the cantaloupe, cucumber, and lime juice. Process for 1 to 2 minutes, or until smooth. Transfer the soup to a glass bowl. Cover and freeze for 20 to 30 minutes, or until chilled but not frozen.

2. Just before serving, sprinkle the soup with the mint and serrano.

SHOP & STORE: A ripe cantaloupe gives off a sweet smell and will be golden or orange, with little or no green. Cantaloupe continues to ripen off the vine, so if your melon isn't ready yet, just leave it on the kitchen counter for a few days.

PER SERVING: Calories **70** • Total Fat **0.5 g** • Saturated Fat **0.0 g** • Trans Fat **0.0 g** • Polyunsaturated Fat **0.0 g** • Monounsaturated Fat **0.0 g** • Cholesterol **0 mg** • Sodium **35 mg** • Carbohydrates **15 g** • Fiber **2 g** • Sugars **13 g** • Protein **3 g**
DIETARY EXCHANGES: 1 fruit

Creamy Peach-Berry Soup

SERVES 4
¾ cup per serving

PREP TIME
5 minutes

Here's a fast and easy way to make a light meal using two popular summer fruits. This soup is so creamy, it's like a smoothie in a bowl!

1. In a food processor or blender, process all the ingredients except the yogurt until smooth.

2. Pour into a medium bowl. Whisk in 1 cup yogurt.

3. Top each serving with 2 tablespoons of the remaining ½ cup yogurt.

1½ cups 100% cherry-pomegranate juice

2 medium peaches, peeled if desired

1 cup raspberries

2 tablespoons sugar

1 cup fat-free vanilla yogurt and ½ cup fat-free vanilla yogurt, divided use

SHOP & STORE: When buying raspberries, look for unblemished berries in unstained containers. The berries should be medium to bright red, depending on the variety, and free of surface moisture. They have a very short shelf life, so don't buy them more than a day or two before you plan to use them. To store them in the refrigerator, remove them from the container as soon as you get them home, discarding any moldy berries. Blot the berries with paper towels to remove any moisture. Spread them in a shallow pan or on a plate and cover them with paper towels. Wrap the pan or plate in plastic wrap. Rinse just before serving.

PER SERVING: Calories 206 • Total Fat 0.5 g • Saturated Fat 0.0 g • Trans Fat 0.0 g
Polyunsaturated Fat 0.0 g • Monounsaturated Fat 0.0 g • Cholesterol 1.5 mg
Sodium 76 mg • Carbohydrates 46 g • Fiber 3 g • Sugars 40 g • Protein 6 g
DIETARY EXCHANGES: 1 fruit, 1 fat-free milk, 1 other carbohydrate

Caribbean Fish Stew

SERVES 6
1½ cups per serving

PREP TIME
15 minutes

COOKING TIME
30 minutes

2 teaspoons olive oil

1 cup chopped onion

1 cup chopped carrot

2 medium garlic cloves, minced

1 medium sweet potato, peeled and cut into ½-inch cubes

1 to 2 serrano peppers, seeds and ribs discarded, finely chopped (see Cook's Tip, page 261)

4 cups fat-free, low-sodium vegetable broth

1 pound thin mild white fish fillets, such as cod, sole, tilapia, or halibut, rinsed, patted dry, and cut into 1-inch cubes

1 13.5- to 13.75-ounce can lite coconut milk

½ cup chopped fresh cilantro

¼ cup fresh lime juice

Robust chiles, cooling coconut milk, and earthy sweet potatoes harmonize with mild fish in this island stew.

1. In a large saucepan, heat the oil over medium heat, swirling to coat the bottom. Cook the onion, carrot, and garlic for 6 minutes, or until the onion is very soft, stirring occasionally.

2. Stir in the sweet potato and serrano. Cook for 5 minutes, stirring occasionally.

3. Pour in the broth. Bring to a boil over medium-high heat. Reduce the heat, and simmer, partially covered, for 10 minutes, or until the sweet potato is tender. Stir in the fish and coconut milk. Cook for 5 to 6 minutes, or until the fish flakes easily when tested with a fork, stirring occasionally. Stir in the cilantro and lime juice.

COOK'S TIP ON TESTING THE HEAT LEVEL OF HOT CHILES: Chiles are a great healthy flavor booster, but they vary in how much kick they have. For this recipe, use one or two serranos depending on how spicy yours are and how much heat you like. To test the hotness of a chile, cut a small piece and touch it with your tongue.

PER SERVING: Calories 191 • Total Fat 5.5 g • Saturated Fat 2.5 g • Trans Fat 0.0 g
Polyunsaturated Fat 0.5 g • Monounsaturated Fat 1.0 g • Cholesterol 33 mg
Sodium 128 mg • Carbohydrates 20 g • Fiber 3 g • Sugars 6 g • Protein 16 g
DIETARY EXCHANGES: 1 starch, 1 vegetable, 2 lean meat

Shiitake Mushroom and Spinach Soup with Shrimp

SERVES 4
1 cup per serving

PREP TIME
10 minutes

COOKING TIME
10 minutes

The citrus notes of cilantro, snap of ginger, and tang of lime make this quick-to-fix soup come alive with Asian flavors. Just cook the mushrooms for a couple of minutes, toss in the shrimp for a few more minutes, then remove from the heat and stir in the rest—done!

1. In a medium saucepan, heat 1 teaspoon oil over medium-high heat, swirling to coat the bottom. Cook the mushrooms for 2 minutes, stirring frequently.

2. Stir in the shrimp, water, and bouillon. Increase the heat to high and bring to a boil. Reduce the heat and simmer, covered, for 4 minutes, or until the shrimp are pink on the outside. Remove from the heat.

3. Stir in the spinach, cilantro, onion, gingerroot, soy sauce, salt, and the remaining 2 teaspoons oil. Serve with the lime wedges.

PER SERVING: Calories **114** • Total Fat **4.5 g** • Saturated Fat **0.5 g** • Trans Fat **0.0 g**
Polyunsaturated Fat **1.5 g** • Monounsaturated Fat **1.5 g** • Cholesterol **107 mg**
Sodium **375 mg** • Carbohydrates **6 g** • Fiber **1 g** • Sugars **2 g** • Protein **13 g**
DIETARY EXCHANGES: 1 vegetable, 2 lean meat

1 teaspoon toasted sesame oil and 2 teaspoons toasted sesame oil, divided use

3½ ounces shiitake mushrooms (stems discarded), thinly sliced

12 ounces raw medium shrimp, peeled, rinsed, and patted dry

1 cup water

2 packets (2 teaspoons) salt-free instant chicken bouillon (optional)

1½ cups loosely packed spinach, coarsely chopped

¾ cup chopped cilantro

½ to ¾ cup finely chopped red onion

1½ tablespoons grated peeled gingerroot

1 tablespoon soy sauce (lowest sodium available)

⅛ teaspoon salt

1 medium lime, cut into 4 wedges

SERVES 4
1½ cups per serving

PREP TIME
15 minutes

COOKING TIME
30 minutes

1 teaspoon canola or corn oil

1 medium onion, chopped into 1-inch pieces

1 large rib of celery, chopped into 1-inch pieces

1 medium garlic clove, minced

2 cups fat-free, low-sodium chicken broth

1½ cups corn kernels, cut from 2 or 3 medium ears of corn, husks and silk discarded

4 medium plum (Roma) tomatoes, chopped into 1-inch pieces

1 cup water

1 teaspoon ground cumin

¼ teaspoon chipotle powder

2 6-inch corn tortillas, cut into thin strips

Cooking spray

8 ounces tilapia fillets, rinsed, patted dry, and cut into 1-inch pieces

1 tablespoon fresh lime juice

(continued)

Mexican Tortilla Soup with Tilapia

Our Mexican tortilla soup uses meaty tilapia instead of chicken or shrimp to bolster the chile-and-lime scented broth. We also substitute baked corn tortilla strips for fried tortilla chips. Fresh toppings of avocado, yogurt, and cilantro make for a lush presentation.

1. Preheat the oven to 425°F. Line a small baking sheet with aluminum foil. Set aside.

2. In a large saucepan, heat the oil over medium-high heat, swirling to coat the bottom. Cook the onion, celery, and garlic, covered, for 5 minutes, or until the vegetables are soft, stirring frequently.

3. Stir in the broth, corn, tomatoes, water, cumin, and chipotle powder. Increase the heat to high and bring to a boil, covered. Reduce the heat and simmer, covered, for 15 minutes.

4. Meanwhile, arrange the tortilla strips on the baking sheet. Lightly spray with cooking spray. Bake for 15 minutes, or until lightly browned and crisp, stirring once halfway through. Transfer the baking sheet to a cooling rack and cool completely.

5. When the soup is cooked, gently stir in the fish and lime juice. Simmer for 3 minutes, or until the fish flakes easily when tested with a fork.

6. Sprinkle each serving with the tortilla strips. Top with the avocado and yogurt. Sprinkle with the cilantro.

¼ medium avocado, cubed

¼ cup fat-free plain Greek yogurt

¼ cup chopped fresh cilantro

COOK'S TIP: This soup is even more delicious the next day. The flavors have more time to "ripen" and blend.

COOK'S TIP ON CHIPOTLE POWDER: Chipotle powder is made from ground chipotle peppers, which are dried, smoked jalapeños. Regular chili powder is made from dried chile peppers (any variety) and doesn't have that smoky flavor.

PER SERVING: Calories **189** • Total Fat **5.0 g** • Saturated Fat **1.0 g** • Trans Fat **0.0 g**
Polyunsaturated Fat **1.0 g** • Monounsaturated Fat **2.5 g** • Cholesterol **28 mg**
Sodium **108 mg** • Carbohydrates **22 g** • Fiber **4 g** • Sugars **8 g** • Protein **17 g**
DIETARY EXCHANGES: 1 starch, 1 vegetable, 2 lean meat

SERVES 4
1½ cups per serving

PREP TIME
10 minutes

COOKING TIME
25 to 30 minutes

2 teaspoons olive oil

1 cup chopped onion

1 medium garlic clove, minced

8 ounces asparagus, trimmed and cut diagonally into 1-inch pieces

2 2.5-ounce cooked chicken andouille sausage links, finely chopped

4 cups fat-free, low-sodium chicken broth

1 cup water

⅓ cup uncooked quinoa, rinsed and drained

¼ teaspoon cracked pepper

Asparagus-Sausage Soup with Quinoa

A small amount of spicy smoked chicken andouille sausage, common in Cajun cooking, is used to give big flavor to this soup. Enjoy this taste of the bayou with a hint of sweet from Peach-Perfect Muffins (page 272) as a side or Broiled Vanilla Peaches Topped with Meringue (page 298) for dessert.

1. In a large saucepan, heat the oil over medium heat, swirling to coat the bottom. Cook the onion and garlic for 4 to 6 minutes, or until the onion is soft, stirring occasionally.

2. Increase the heat to medium high. Stir in the asparagus and sausages. Cook for 5 to 6 minutes, or until the onion, asparagus, and sausages are lightly browned on the edges, stirring frequently.

3. Pour in the broth and water. Bring to a boil. Stir in the quinoa. Reduce the heat and simmer for 16 to 18 minutes, or until the quinoa is tender. Stir in the pepper.

PER SERVING: Calories **149** • Total Fat **5.0 g** • Saturated Fat **1.5 g** • Trans Fat **0.0 g**
Polyunsaturated Fat **1.5 g** • Monounsaturated Fat **2.5 g** • Cholesterol **9 mg**
Sodium **243 mg** • Carbohydrates **16 g** • Fiber **3 g** • Sugars **4 g** • Protein **12 g**
DIETARY EXCHANGES: ½ starch, 1 vegetable, 1½ lean meat

Chicken-Escarole Soup

SERVES 4
1 cup per serving

PREP TIME
10 minutes

COOKING TIME
20 minutes

STANDING TIME
5 minutes

Escarole is a variety of endive, but with a milder, less bitter flavor. As with spinach and other leafy greens, escarole wilts quickly when exposed to heat, so add it at the very end and let it rest for only a few minutes so it can soak up the flavors of this full-bodied soup.

1. In a medium saucepan, heat 1 teaspoon canola oil over medium heat, swirling to coat the bottom. Cook the chicken for 2 minutes, or until white on the outside but still pink in the center (the chicken won't be done at this point), stirring frequently. Transfer to a plate.

2. In the same pan, heat the remaining 1 teaspoon canola oil, swirling to coat the bottom. Cook the bell peppers for 4 minutes, or until tender-crisp, stirring frequently. Stir in the water, tomatoes, sugar, bouillon, and chicken and any accumulated juices. Increase the heat to high and bring to a boil. Reduce the heat and simmer, covered, for 10 minutes, or until the bell peppers are soft. Remove from the heat.

3. Stir in the remaining ingredients. Let stand for 5 minutes so the flavors blend.

PER SERVING: Calories **198** • Total Fat **8.5 g** • Saturated Fat **1.0 g** • Trans Fat **0.0 g** Polyunsaturated Fat **1.5 g** • Monounsaturated Fat **4.5 g** • Cholesterol **54 mg** Sodium **421 mg** • Carbohydrates **11 g** • Fiber **2 g** • Sugars **7 g** • Protein **19 g** DIETARY EXCHANGES: 1 vegetable, ½ other carbohydrate, 2½ lean meat

1 teaspoon canola or corn oil and 1 teaspoon canola or corn oil, divided use

12 ounces boneless, skinless chicken breasts, all visible fat discarded, diced

1½ cups diced green bell peppers

1½ cups water

1 cup grape tomatoes, halved

1 tablespoon sugar

2 packets (2 teaspoons) salt-free instant chicken bouillon

3 ounces escarole, tough stems discarded, chopped

1 tablespoon chopped fresh oregano

1 tablespoon olive oil

1 tablespoon Worcestershire sauce (lowest sodium available)

1 teaspoon balsamic vinegar

¼ teaspoon salt

SERVES 6
1½ cups per serving

PREP TIME
10 minutes

COOKING TIME
30 to 35 minutes

4 cups fat-free, low-sodium chicken broth

2 cups water

1 cup uncooked red or yellow lentils, sorted for stones and shriveled lentils, rinsed, and drained

1 tablespoon olive oil

1 cup chopped onion

1 cup chopped carrot

½ cup sliced celery

2 teaspoons cumin seeds

1 medium garlic clove, minced

1 pound boneless, skinless chicken breasts, all visible fat discarded, cut into ½-inch cubes

1 cup chopped red bell pepper

¼ teaspoon pepper

Chicken and Red Lentil Soup

Red lentils cook to a beautiful golden color, making this soup as pleasing to the eyes as it is to the palate. They also cook faster than most other lentil varieties, so this legume-rich meal is sure to be done in no time.

1. In a large saucepan, bring the broth and water to a boil over high heat. Stir in the lentils. Reduce the heat and simmer, covered, for 12 to 15 minutes, or until tender.

2. Meanwhile, in a large nonstick skillet, heat the oil over medium heat, swirling to coat the bottom. Cook the onion, carrot, celery, cumin seeds, and garlic for 8 to 10 minutes, or until the vegetables are tender, stirring occasionally. Stir the onion mixture into the lentils.

3. In the same skillet, cook the chicken for 5 to 7 minutes, or until no longer pink in the center, stirring occasionally.

4. Stir the chicken, bell pepper, and pepper into the lentil mixture. Bring to a simmer and simmer for 10 minutes so the flavors blend, stirring occasionally.

PER SERVING: Calories 262 • Total Fat **4.5 g** • Saturated Fat **1.0 g** • Trans Fat **0.0 g**
Polyunsaturated Fat **0.5 g** • Monounsaturated Fat **2.5 g** • Cholesterol **48 mg**
Sodium **155 mg** • Carbohydrates **28 g** • Fiber **6 g** • Sugars **5 g** • Protein **28 g**
DIETARY EXCHANGES: 1½ starch, 1 vegetable, 3 lean meat

Chicken and Rotini Soup with Vegetables

SERVES 4
1 cup per serving

PREP TIME
10 minutes

COOKING TIME
15 to 20 minutes

Why choose between chicken soup and vegetable soup when you can have both? Our recipe departs from ordinary chicken soup by using rotini instead of noodles and incorporating bell pepper, cauliflower, and broccoli for color and texture. *(See photo insert.)*

1. In a medium saucepan, heat the canola oil over medium-high heat, swirling to coat the bottom. Cook the onion for 2 minutes, stirring frequently. Stir in the chicken, bell pepper, and garlic. Cook for 1 minute, stirring frequently.

2. Increase the heat to high. Stir in the water, pasta, and bouillon. Bring to a boil. Reduce the heat and simmer, covered, for 4 minutes.

3. Stir in the broccoli and cauliflower. Cook, covered, over medium heat for 4 to 5 minutes, or until the vegetables are just tender. Remove from the heat.

4. Stir in the remaining ingredients.

COOK'S TIP: Don't underestimate the power of a small amount of margarine. It's just enough to round out the flavors of the other ingredients.

PER SERVING: Calories **205** • Total Fat **8.0 g** • Saturated Fat **1.0 g** • Trans Fat **0.0 g**
Polyunsaturated Fat **1.5 g** • Monounsaturated Fat **5.0 g** • Cholesterol **36 mg**
Sodium **381 mg** • Carbohydrates **18 g** • Fiber **3 g** • Sugars **3 g** • Protein **16 g**
DIETARY EXCHANGES: ½ starch, 1 vegetable, 2 lean meat, ½ fat

1 teaspoon canola or corn oil

½ cup diced onion

8 ounces boneless, skinless chicken breasts, all visible fat discarded, cut into bite-size pieces

½ cup diced red bell pepper

2 medium garlic cloves, minced

2 cups water

2 ounces dried whole-grain rotini

2 packets (2 teaspoons) salt-free instant chicken bouillon

1 cup small broccoli florets

1 cup small cauliflower florets

1 tablespoon plus 1 teaspoon olive oil

1 teaspoon fresh thyme

1 teaspoon light tub margarine

½ teaspoon salt

SERVES 4
1¾ cups per serving

———

PREP TIME
15 minutes

———

COOKING TIME
20 to 25 minutes

1 tablespoon olive oil

½ cup chopped onion

½ cup sliced celery

1 medium jalapeño, seeds and ribs discarded, finely chopped (see Cook's Tip, page 261)

2 medium garlic cloves, minced

1 pound boneless, skinless chicken breasts, all visible fat discarded, cut into bite-size pieces

8 ounces tomatillos, papery husks discarded, chopped

4 cups fat-free, low-sodium chicken broth

1 tablespoon chopped fresh oregano

1 teaspoon ground cumin

½ teaspoon chili powder

½ medium avocado, diced

¼ cup shredded radishes

¼ cup chopped fresh cilantro

1 medium lime, cut into 4 wedges (optional)

Verde Chicken Soup

This soup gets its *verde* color from fresh tomatillos (tohm-ah-TEE-ohs), also known as Mexican green tomatoes. The tartness from the tomatillos, the heat from the jalapeño and chili powder, the bite from the radishes, and the tang from the lime make for a full-flavored dish.

1. In a large saucepan, heat the oil over medium heat, swirling to coat the bottom. Cook the onion, celery, jalapeño, and garlic for 4 to 6 minutes, or until the onion is soft and the celery, jalapeño, and garlic are tender, stirring occasionally.

2. Stir in the chicken and tomatillos. Cook for 5 to 6 minutes, or until the chicken is no longer pink in the center, stirring occasionally. Stir in the broth, oregano, cumin, and chili powder. Increase the heat to medium high and bring to a boil. Reduce the heat and simmer for 10 minutes, stirring occasionally.

3. Top each serving with the avocado, radishes, and cilantro. Serve with the lime wedges.

PER SERVING: Calories **246** • Total Fat **11.0 g** • Saturated Fat **2.0 g** • Trans Fat **0.0 g**
Polyunsaturated Fat **1.5 g** • Monounsaturated Fat **6.0 g** • Cholesterol **73 mg**
Sodium **215 mg** • Carbohydrates **9 g** • Fiber **4 g** • Sugars **4 g** • Protein **28 g**
DIETARY EXCHANGES: 2 vegetable, 3 lean meat, ½ fat

Turkey and Wild Rice Soup

SERVES 6
1½ cups per serving

PREP TIME
10 minutes

COOKING TIME
30 to 35 minutes

This soup is redolent with the aromas of a Thanksgiving meal. Why wait until November when you can enjoy this holiday turkey dinner in a bowl any time of the year?

1. In a large nonstick skillet, heat the oil over medium-high heat, swirling to coat the bottom. Cook the leeks, carrots, bell pepper, and garlic for 4 to 6 minutes, or until tender, stirring frequently. Transfer the leek mixture to a large saucepan.

2. Pour in the broth and water. Increase the heat to high and bring to a boil.

3. Meanwhile, in the large skillet, still over medium-high heat, cook the turkey for 5 to 6 minutes, or until no longer pink in the center, stirring occasionally. Stir the turkey into the soup.

4. Return the soup to a boil. Stir in the rice, sage, and pepper. Reduce the heat and simmer, covered, for 20 to 25 minutes, or until the rice is tender.

1 tablespoon olive oil

2 small leeks, sliced

1 cup chopped carrot

¾ cup chopped red bell pepper

1 medium garlic clove, minced

4 cups fat-free, low-sodium chicken broth

2 cups water

1 pound boneless, skinless turkey breast fillets, all visible fat discarded, cut into ½-inch cubes

6 ounces uncooked long grain and wild rice blend, seasoning packet discarded, or ¾ cup uncooked instant brown rice

2 tablespoons chopped fresh sage

¼ teaspoon pepper

SHOP & STORE: Leeks, which look like large green onions, are milder in flavor than yellow onions so they blend in rather than overpower. To prepare them, discard the root ends. Cut a 3- to 4-inch section from the cut end of each leek, including a little of the green part. Halve the sections lengthwise, then cut them crosswise into thin slices. Transfer the leeks to a small colander. Rinse well under cold water. Drain well.

PER SERVING: Calories 227 • Total Fat 3.0 g • Saturated Fat 0.5 g • Trans Fat 0.0 g
Polyunsaturated Fat 0.5 g • Monounsaturated Fat 1.5 g • Cholesterol 47 mg
Sodium 101 mg • Carbohydrates 26 g • Fiber 2 g • Sugars 3 g • Protein 23 g
DIETARY EXCHANGES: 1½ starch, 1 vegetable, 2½ lean meat

SERVES 4
1½ cups per serving

PREP TIME
15 minutes

COOKING TIME
20 to 25 minutes

White Bean Soup with Spicy Turkey Meatballs, Leeks, and Kale

A leafy green vegetable belonging to the family that includes cabbage, collards, and brussels sprouts, kale adds an earthy flavor and a nutritional boost to this meal in a bowl.

12 ounces ground skinless turkey breast

1 tablespoon chopped fresh thyme and 2 tablespoons chopped fresh thyme, divided use

¾ teaspoon paprika (smoked preferred)

1 teaspoon crushed red pepper flakes

¼ teaspoon salt

1½ teaspoons olive oil and 1½ teaspoons olive oil, divided use

1 cup chopped leeks

2 medium garlic cloves, minced

4 cups fat-free, low-sodium chicken broth

1 15.5-ounce can no-salt-added cannellini or Great Northern beans, rinsed and drained

3 cups coarsely chopped kale, any large stems discarded

1. In a medium bowl, using your hands or a spoon, combine the turkey, 1 tablespoon thyme, the paprika, red pepper flakes, and salt until well blended. Using 1 level tablespoon of the turkey mixture for each, shape into 24 meatballs, each about ¾ inch in diameter. Transfer to a plate.

2. In a large nonstick skillet, heat 1½ teaspoons oil over medium heat, swirling to coat the bottom. Cook the meatballs for 3 minutes (you may need to cook them in two batches). Turn over. Cook for 2 minutes, or until browned on both sides (the meatballs won't be done at this point). Transfer the meatballs to a separate large plate.

3. Meanwhile, in a large saucepan, heat the remaining 1½ teaspoons oil, swirling to coat the bottom. Cook the leeks and garlic for 4 minutes, or until softened, stirring frequently.

4. Stir in the broth and meatballs and any accumulated juices. Increase the heat to high and bring to a boil. Reduce the heat and simmer for 5 minutes, stirring frequently and scraping to dislodge any browned bits.

5. Stir in the beans, kale, and the remaining 2 tablespoons thyme. Return to a simmer and simmer for 5 minutes, or until the meatballs are no longer pink in the center and the kale is tender-crisp.

PER SERVING: Calories **265** • Total Fat **5.5 g** • Saturated Fat **0.5 g** • Trans Fat **0.0 g**
Polyunsaturated Fat **0.5 g** • Monounsaturated Fat **2.5 g** • Cholesterol **53 mg**
Sodium **309 mg** • Carbohydrates **24 g** • Fiber **6 g** • Sugars **2 g** • Protein **30 g**
DIETARY EXCHANGES: 1 starch, 2 vegetable, 3 lean meat

Beef and Noodle Broth

Asian flavors abound in this broth, which is similar to the Vietnamese noodle soup known as *pho*. Serve it in a large shallow bowl in order to appreciate all its colors and textures.

1. Put the beef in a large bowl. Add the soy sauce, stirring to coat.

2. In a large nonstick skillet, heat the oil over medium-high heat, swirling to coat the bottom. Cook the beef for 4 to 6 minutes, or until no longer pink in the center, stirring frequently.

3. Meanwhile, in a large saucepan, bring the broth and water to a boil over high heat. Stir in the beef, bok choy, and bell pepper. Return to a boil.

4. Stir in the pasta. Return to a boil and boil for 5 to 6 minutes, or until the pasta is tender, stirring occasionally. Remove from the heat.

5. Stir in the green onions and basil. Serve the soup with the chili sauce on the side.

COOK'S TIP: The optional chili garlic sauce adds 70 milligrams of sodium to the soup.

SHOP & STORE: Bok choy, a leafy Chinese cabbage with a crisp texture and neutral flavor, is a good source of calcium and vitamin C. It is commonly used in stir-fries and as a complementary ingredient in soups. To store it, wrap it in paper towels and refrigerate it in the vegetable bin for up to one week.

SERVES 6
1²/₃ cups per serving

PREP TIME
15 minutes

COOKING TIME
15 minutes

1 pound flank steak, all visible fat discarded, thinly sliced and cut into bite-size pieces

1 tablespoon soy sauce (lowest sodium available)

2 teaspoons toasted sesame oil

4 cups fat-free, low-sodium beef broth

2 cups water

3 cups shredded bok choy

1 medium red bell pepper, cut into bite-size strips (about 1¼ cups)

4 ounces dried whole-grain angel hair pasta, broken into small pieces

½ cup diagonally sliced green onions

¼ cup chopped fresh basil

1½ teaspoons chili garlic sauce or paste, or to taste (optional)

PER SERVING: Calories 211 • Total Fat 6.5 g • Saturated Fat 2.0 g • Trans Fat 0.0 g
Polyunsaturated Fat 1.0 g • Monounsaturated Fat 3.0 g • Cholesterol 32 mg
Sodium 202 mg • Carbohydrates 17 g • Fiber 3 g • Sugars 3 g • Protein 20 g
DIETARY EXCHANGES: 1 starch, 2½ lean meat

1 teaspoon canola or
   corn oil

12 ounces extra-lean
   ground beef

1 large green bell pepper,
   diced

1 cup diced onion

1 medium carrot, thinly
   sliced crosswise

4 medium tomatoes,
   chopped

1½ cups water

¼ cup uncooked quick-
   cooking barley

3 ounces green beans,
   trimmed and cut into
   1-inch pieces

2 tablespoons no-salt-
   added tomato paste

1 tablespoon balsamic
   vinegar

3 packets (1 tablespoon)
   salt-free instant beef
   bouillon

1 cup spinach or arugula

½ teaspoon salt

Beef Barley Vegetable Soup

Thanks to a handful of different vegetables—including powerhouse spinach—and a whole grain, this bowl full of goodness is not only nutritious but also delicious. This satisfying "super soup" freezes well, so keep it on hand for those evenings when you get home from a long day and need to put a hot entrée on the table—pronto. Orange-Soaked Apple Wedges (page 249) are a pleasing go-with.

1. In a large saucepan, heat the oil over medium-high heat. Cook the beef for 3 minutes, or until browned on the outside, stirring frequently to turn and break up the beef. Stir in the bell pepper, onion, and carrot. Cook for 3 to 4 minutes, or until the onion is soft, stirring frequently.

2. Stir in the tomatoes, water, barley, green beans, tomato paste, vinegar, and bouillon. Increase the heat to high and bring to a boil. Reduce the heat and simmer, covered, for 15 minutes, or until the vegetables are very tender. Remove from the heat.

3. Stir in the spinach and salt.

PER SERVING: Calories 230 • Total Fat 6.0 g • Saturated Fat 2.0 g • Trans Fat 0.5 g
Polyunsaturated Fat 1.0 g • Monounsaturated Fat 2.5 g • Cholesterol 47 mg
Sodium 395 mg • Carbohydrates 24 g • Fiber 5 g • Sugars 10 g • Protein 22 g
DIETARY EXCHANGES: ½ starch, 3 vegetable, 2½ lean meat

Minute Steak Soup with Pasta and Vegetables

SERVES 4
1½ cups per serving

PREP TIME
10 minutes

COOKING TIME
20 minutes

STANDING TIME
5 minutes

Using less than a pound of an economical cut of beef, this soup goes easy on the budget but not on the flavor. Adding instant coffee pulls out the beefy flavors and gives the soup more depth and richness. Whole-grain rotini and a variety of vegetables round out this robust meal.

1. In a large saucepan, heat 1 teaspoon oil over medium-high heat, swirling to coat the bottom. Cook the beef for 1½ minutes, or until browned, stirring occasionally. Transfer to a plate.

2. In the same pan, heat the remaining 1 teaspoon oil, swirling to coat the bottom. Cook the bell pepper and onion for 3 to 4 minutes, or until soft, stirring frequently. Stir in the water. Increase the heat to high and bring to a simmer. Stir in the carrot and pasta. Return to a simmer. Reduce the heat and simmer, covered, for 6 minutes.

3. Stir in the broccoli and cauliflower. Cook, covered, for 4 minutes, or until tender-crisp. Remove from the heat.

4. Stir in the beef and any accumulated juices and the remaining ingredients. Let stand, covered, for 5 minutes so the flavors blend.

PER SERVING: Calories 221 • Total Fat **4.5 g** • Saturated Fat **1.0 g** • Trans Fat **0.0 g** Polyunsaturated Fat **1.0 g** • Monounsaturated Fat **2.0 g** • Cholesterol **27 mg** Sodium **390 mg** • Carbohydrates **28 g** • Fiber **5 g** • Sugars **10 g** • Protein **18 g** DIETARY EXCHANGES: 1 starch, 3 vegetable, 2 lean meat

1 teaspoon canola or corn oil and 1 teaspoon canola or corn oil, divided use

8 ounces very thin round steak, all visible fat discarded, cut into ½-inch cubes

1 medium green bell pepper, diced

1 cup diced onion

3 cups water

1 medium carrot, sliced crosswise

2 ounces dried whole-grain rotini

2 cups small broccoli florets

2 cups small cauliflower florets

¼ cup no-salt-added ketchup

3 packets (1 tablespoon) salt-free instant beef bouillon

1½ teaspoons Worcestershire sauce (lowest sodium available)

1 teaspoon instant coffee granules

½ teaspoon salt

1 teaspoon canola or
corn oil, 1 teaspoon
canola or corn oil, and
1 teaspoon canola or
corn oil, divided use

1 pound boneless sirloin
steak, all visible fat
discarded, cut into
½-inch cubes

½ teaspoon ground
cinnamon

⅛ teaspoon cayenne

½ cup thinly sliced
shallots (about
4 medium)

4 medium garlic cloves,
minced

2 cups water

3 medium tomatoes,
chopped

2 medium carrots, thinly
sliced crosswise

1 tablespoon sugar

3 packets (1 tablespoon)
salt-free instant beef
bouillon

(continued)

Sweet and Spicy Beef Soup with Vegetables

The secret to success for this soup is to brown the meat briefly, bringing out its natural flavors while keeping it extra tender. A light dusting of cinnamon and cayenne atop the meat imparts a harmonious balance of sweetness and spiciness, making the beef command center stage in your soup bowl.

1. In a large saucepan, heat 1 teaspoon oil over medium-high heat, swirling to coat the bottom. Add half the beef. Sprinkle half the cinnamon and cayenne over the beef. Cook for 1½ minutes, or until browned on the outside but still pink in the center. Don't stir the beef during the first minute of cooking time. Transfer to a plate. Repeat with 1 teaspoon oil and the remaining beef, cinnamon, and cayenne. Set aside.

2. Heat the remaining 1 teaspoon oil, swirling to coat the bottom. Cook the shallots for 1 to 2 minutes, or until golden, stirring frequently. Stir in the garlic. Cook for 15 seconds, stirring constantly.

3. Stir in the water, tomatoes, carrots, sugar, bouillon, and vinegar. Increase the heat to high and bring to a simmer. Reduce the heat and simmer, covered, for 10 minutes, or until the carrots are tender. Remove from the heat.

4. Stir in the beef and any accumulated juices and the remaining ingredients. Let stand, covered, for 3 minutes to heat through.

2 teaspoons balsamic
   vinegar

½ cup frozen green peas

¼ cup chopped fresh mint

2 teaspoons grated
   peeled gingerroot

½ teaspoon salt

PER SERVING: Calories **267** • Total Fat **8.5 g** • Saturated Fat **2.0 g** • Trans Fat **0.0 g**
Polyunsaturated Fat **1.5 g** • Monounsaturated Fat **4.5 g** • Cholesterol **60 mg**
Sodium **416 mg** • Carbohydrates **19 g** • Fiber **4 g** • Sugars **11 g** • Protein **28 g**
DIETARY EXCHANGES: ½ starch, 2 vegetable, 3 lean meat

SERVES 6
1½ cups per serving

PREP TIME
10 minutes

COOKING TIME
20 minutes

Pork and Pinto Bean Soup

You'll be pleasantly surprised by the addition of orange juice and a hint of ground cloves to this pork and bean soup. A garnish of orange zest and parsley makes for a pop of bright flavor right on top.

1 tablespoon olive oil

1 pound pork tenderloin, all visible fat discarded, cut into ½-inch cubes

¾ cup chopped red or green bell pepper

½ cup chopped onion

2 medium garlic cloves, minced

4 cups fat-free, low-sodium chicken broth

1 15.5-ounce can no-salt-added pinto beans, rinsed and drained

2 teaspoons grated orange zest

½ cup fresh orange juice

¼ teaspoon pepper

⅛ teaspoon ground cloves

¼ cup chopped fresh parsley

1. In a large saucepan, heat the oil over medium-high heat, swirling to coat the bottom. Cook the pork, bell pepper, onion, and garlic for 6 to 8 minutes, or until the pork is no longer pink in the center, stirring occasionally.

2. Stir in the broth, beans, orange juice, pepper, and cloves. Bring to a boil. Reduce the heat and simmer for 10 minutes so the flavors blend.

3. In a small bowl, stir together the parsley and orange zest. Sprinkle the mixture over each serving.

PER SERVING: Calories **189** • Total Fat **4.0 g** • Saturated Fat **1.0 g** • Trans Fat **0.0 g** • Polyunsaturated Fat **0.5 g** • Monounsaturated Fat **2.5 g** • Cholesterol **49 mg** • Sodium **92 mg** • Carbohydrates **15 g** • Fiber **4 g** • Sugars **3 g** • Protein **21 g**
DIETARY EXCHANGES: 1 starch, 2½ lean meat

Hearty Pork and Cabbage Soup

A variation of the robust French vegetable soup, *garbure*, this one-dish meal has a hefty helping of vegetables surrounding pieces of lean pork. Whole sprigs of fresh thyme season it while the soup simmers.

SERVES 4
1½ cups per serving

PREP TIME
15 minutes

COOKING TIME
20 to 25 minutes

STANDING TIME
3 minutes

1. Lightly spray a large saucepan with cooking spray. Heat over medium-high heat. Cook half the pork for 3 to 4 minutes, or until browned on the outside and slightly pink in the center, stirring frequently. Transfer to a plate. Repeat with the remaining pork.

2. Reduce the heat to medium. Cook the onion and garlic for 3 minutes, or until the onion just begins to soften, stirring frequently.

3. Stir in the cabbage, potatoes, carrot, and thyme. Cook for 1 minute, stirring frequently. Stir in the broth and pepper. Increase the heat to high and bring to a boil, stirring and scraping to dislodge any browned bits.

4. Reduce the heat and simmer, partially covered, for 10 minutes, or until the vegetables are tender, stirring occasionally. Stir in the pork. Cook for 1 to 2 minutes, or until the pork is heated through. Discard the thyme sprigs before serving.

Cooking spray

4 boneless pork loin chops (about 4 ounces each), all visible fat discarded, cut into slices about 3/8 inch thick, slices halved crosswise

1 large onion, coarsely chopped

3 large garlic cloves, minced

8 ounces green cabbage, thinly sliced

8 ounces red potatoes, cut into 1/2-inch cubes

1 large carrot, halved lengthwise, then sliced crosswise

2 sprigs of fresh thyme, about 3 inches long

4 cups fat-free, low-sodium chicken broth

1/4 teaspoon pepper

TIPS, TRICKS & TIMESAVERS: To save time, you can substitute 3 cups of packaged shredded cabbage.

PER SERVING: Calories 261 • Total Fat 8.0 g • Saturated Fat 3.0 g • Trans Fat 0.0 g Polyunsaturated Fat 0.5 g • Monounsaturated Fat 3.5 g • Cholesterol 64 mg Sodium 141 mg • Carbohydrates 20 g • Fiber 4 g • Sugars 7 g • Protein 27 g DIETARY EXCHANGES: 1/2 starch, 2 vegetable, 3 lean meat

SERVES 6
1½ cups per serving

PREP TIME
15 minutes

COOKING TIME
20 minutes

1 tablespoon olive oil

1 pound assorted mushrooms, such as button, brown (cremini), shiitake (stems discarded), or portobello, trimmed and sliced

½ cup finely chopped onion

3 tablespoons all-purpose flour

1 tablespoon paprika

4 cups fat-free, low-sodium beef or vegetable broth

12 ounces fat-free evaporated milk

1 medium russet potato, peeled and chopped into ¼-inch pieces

1 tablespoon chopped fresh dillweed

¼ teaspoon salt

¼ teaspoon pepper

¼ cup plus 2 tablespoons fat-free sour cream (optional)

Dash of cayenne (optional)

Mixed-Mushroom Soup

Using a variety of mushrooms gives this soup a deep, rich flavor. If you have just a few extra minutes, bake some pumpernickel croutons (see Cook's Tip) for a crunchy soup topper that adds texture.

1. In a large saucepan, heat the oil over medium-high heat, swirling to coat the bottom. Cook the mushrooms and onion for 6 to 8 minutes, or until the mushrooms are tender and the onion is very soft. Reduce the heat to medium. Stir in the flour and paprika. Cook for 30 seconds, stirring constantly.

2. Stir in the broth, evaporated milk, and potato. Increase the heat to medium high and bring to a boil. Reduce the heat and simmer for 8 to 10 minutes, or until the potato is tender, stirring occasionally.

3. Stir in the dillweed, salt, and pepper. Top each serving with the sour cream and cayenne.

COOK'S TIP: If you use shiitake mushrooms, be sure to discard the tough, woody stems. If you wish, you can save them for later use. They add lots of flavor to homemade vegetable stock.

COOK'S TIP ON PUMPERNICKEL CROUTONS: To make pumpernickel croutons, preheat the oven to 350°F. Cut 2 slices of pumpernickel bread (lowest sodium available) into ¾-inch cubes. Arrange in a single layer on a baking sheet. Lightly spray the cubes with olive oil cooking spray. Bake for 5 minutes, or until toasted. Transfer the baking sheet to a cooling rack.

PER SERVING: Calories 144 • Total Fat 3.0 g • Saturated Fat 0.5 g • Trans Fat 0.0 g Polyunsaturated Fat 0.5 g • Monounsaturated Fat 1.5 g • Cholesterol 3 mg Sodium 260 mg • Carbohydrates 21 g • Fiber 2 g • Sugars 10 g • Protein 10 g DIETARY EXCHANGES: ½ starch, ½ fat-free milk, 1 vegetable, ½ fat

Coconut Curry Chickpea Soup

SERVES 4
1½ cups per serving

PREP TIME
15 minutes

COOKING TIME
20 minutes

Mixing the coconut milk with fat-free half-and-half helps keep this soup rich and creamy, and the jalapeños make it come alive. If you don't relish the heat, discard some or all of the jalapeño seeds.

1. In a large saucepan, heat the oil over medium-high heat, swirling to coat the bottom. Cook the onion, bell peppers, jalapeño, and garlic for 3 to 4 minutes, or until soft, stirring frequently.

2. Stir in the chickpeas, water, tomato, sugar, and curry powder. Increase the heat to high and bring to a boil. Reduce the heat and simmer, covered, for 10 minutes, or until the vegetables are very tender. Remove from the heat.

3. Gradually whisk in the half-and-half and coconut milk, ¼ cup at a time, to prevent curdling. Whisk in the cilantro and salt.

PER SERVING: Calories **291** • Total Fat **5.5 g** • Saturated Fat **2.0 g** • Trans Fat **0.0 g**
Polyunsaturated Fat **0.5 g** • Monounsaturated Fat **1.0 g** • Cholesterol **0 mg**
Sodium **393 mg** • Carbohydrates **50 g** • Fiber **6 g** • Sugars **16 g** • Protein **16 g**
DIETARY EXCHANGES: 2 starch, 2 vegetable, 1 fat-free milk, ½ lean meat

1 teaspoon canola or corn oil

1 cup diced onion

1 cup diced yellow bell pepper

1 cup diced orange bell pepper

1 to 2 medium jalapeños, ribs discarded, finely chopped (see Cook's Tip, page 261)

2 medium garlic cloves, minced

1 15.5-ounce can no-salt-added chickpeas, rinsed and drained

¾ cup water

1 medium tomato, diced

1½ to 2 teaspoons sugar

1 teaspoon curry powder

2 cups fat-free half-and-half

1 cup lite coconut milk

¾ cup chopped fresh cilantro

⅜ teaspoon salt

SERVES 6
1½ cups per serving

PREP TIME
20 minutes

COOKING TIME
25 to 30 minutes

Italian-Style Vegetable Soup

An excellent use for extra vegetables from a bulk purchase or your garden, this versatile soup includes a variety of vegetables, beans, and pasta. If you're missing a veggie in the ingredients list, just substitute with something you have on hand.

1 tablespoon olive oil

1½ cups sliced zucchini (halved lengthwise before slicing crosswise)

1½ cups sliced mushrooms, such as button, brown (cremini), portobello, or shiitake (stems discarded)

½ cup chopped yellow or red bell pepper

½ cup chopped onion

2 medium garlic cloves, minced

4 cups fat-free, low-sodium vegetable broth

2 cups shredded green cabbage

1 15.5-ounce can no-salt-added cannellini beans, rinsed and drained

1 large tomato, seeded and chopped

1 tablespoon chopped fresh oregano

½ teaspoon salt

¼ to ½ teaspoon pepper

½ cup dried tiny pasta, such as ditalini, rings (anellini), stars, or ancini di pepe

¼ cup chopped fresh Italian (flat-leaf) parsley

1. In a large saucepan, heat the oil over medium heat, swirling to coat the bottom. Cook the zucchini, mushrooms, bell pepper, onion, and garlic for 10 to 12 minutes, or until the zucchini, mushrooms, and bell pepper are tender and the onion is very soft, stirring occasionally.

2. Stir in the broth, cabbage, beans, tomato, oregano, salt, and pepper. Increase the heat to medium high and bring to a boil. Stir in the pasta. Reduce the heat and simmer for 8 to 10 minutes, or until the pasta is tender, stirring occasionally. Stir in the parsley.

COOK'S TIP: If the pasta has absorbed too much liquid while cooking and you prefer your soup more brothy, add water until the soup is the desired consistency.

PER SERVING: Calories 157 • Total Fat 3.5 g • Saturated Fat 0.5 g • Trans Fat 0.0 g Polyunsaturated Fat 0.5 g • Monounsaturated Fat 1.5 g • Cholesterol 0 mg Sodium 244 mg • Carbohydrates 26 g • Fiber 5 g • Sugars 5 g • Protein 8 g DIETARY EXCHANGES: 1½ starch, 1 vegetable, ½ fat

Soba Noodle Soup with Vegetables and Tofu

SERVES 4
1½ cups per serving

PREP TIME
15 minutes

COOKING TIME
15 minutes

This quick and easy take on a traditional Japanese noodle soup combines a savory broth with fresh vegetables and toothsome noodles. In Japanese culture, it's a compliment to the chef to slurp your soup.

1. In a large deep skillet over high heat, bring the water, broth, and gingerroot to a boil. Stir in the noodles. Reduce the heat and simmer for 1 to 2 minutes, or just until the noodles begin to soften, stirring frequently.

2. Stir in the snow peas, carrots, mushrooms, and bok choy. Return to a simmer and simmer for 5 minutes, stirring once halfway through.

3. Stir in the tofu, green onions, and soy sauce. Simmer for 2 minutes, or until heated through. Remove from the heat.

4. Stir in the sesame oil.

5. Sprinkle each serving with the cilantro. Serve with the chile sauce.

SHOP & STORE: Dried soba noodles can be found in the ethnic section of most supermarkets. Made with buckwheat flour, soba noodles have fewer calories and more fiber than regular noodles.

3 cups water

2 cups fat-free, low-sodium vegetable broth

1 tablespoon finely grated peeled gingerroot

2 ounces dried soba noodles

1 cup matchstick-size strips of snow peas

½ cup very thinly sliced carrots

4 ounces shiitake mushrooms, stems discarded, thinly sliced

2 heads baby bok choy, cut crosswise into 1½-inch strips

10 ounces light firm tofu, drained, patted dry, and cut into ¾-inch pieces

2 medium green onions, diagonally sliced into ¼-inch pieces

2 tablespoons soy sauce (lowest sodium available)

1 tablespoon toasted sesame oil

¼ cup chopped fresh cilantro

½ teaspoon hot chile sauce (sriracha preferred) (optional)

PER SERVING: Calories 160 • Total Fat 5.0 g • Saturated Fat 0.5 g • Trans Fat 0.0 g
Polyunsaturated Fat 2.5 g • Monounsaturated Fat 1.5 g • Cholesterol 0 mg
Sodium 293 mg • Carbohydrates 20 g • Fiber 3 g • Sugars 5 g • Protein 11 g
DIETARY EXCHANGES: 1 starch, 1 vegetable, 1 lean meat

SERVES 4
2 cups per serving

PREP TIME
15 minutes

COOKING TIME
20 minutes

2 teaspoons olive oil

1 large onion, chopped

2½ pounds large
  tomatoes, chopped

2 cups fat-free, low-
  sodium vegetable
  broth

¼ teaspoon salt

14 ounces light soft tofu,
  drained and patted
  dry

¼ cup chopped fresh
  dillweed

Tomato Soup with Tofu and Fresh Dill

Chopped tomatoes and bright green dillweed add fresh-from-the-garden flavor to this soup. It's dairy-free, with its decadent creaminess coming from puréed tofu.

1. In a large saucepan, heat the oil over medium heat, swirling to coat the bottom. Cook the onion for 5 minutes, or until lightly browned, stirring frequently and reducing the heat if the onion begins to brown too quickly.

2. Stir in the tomatoes, broth, and salt. Increase the heat to medium high and bring to a boil. Reduce the heat and simmer for 10 minutes, or until the tomatoes are soft, stirring occasionally.

3. Meanwhile, in a food processor or blender, process the tofu until smooth. Stir the tofu and dillweed into the soup. Cook for 1 to 2 minutes, or until heated through, stirring occasionally.

COOK'S TIP ON TOFU: Soft tofu has a creamy consistency, making it just right for use in dips, spreads, smoothies, and creamy soups. Firm or extra-firm tofu holds its shape while cooking and is the best choice for use in sautés and stir-fries. Both types are a good source of calcium.

PER SERVING: Calories **150** • Total Fat **4.5 g** • Saturated Fat **0.5 g** • Trans Fat **0.0 g**
Polyunsaturated Fat **1.5 g** • Monounsaturated Fat **2.0 g** • Cholesterol **0 mg**
Sodium **225 mg** • Carbohydrates **17 g** • Fiber **5 g** • Sugars **11 g** • Protein **12 g**
DIETARY EXCHANGES: 3 vegetable, 1 lean meat, ½ fat

Garden-Fresh Gazpacho

No heat is required for this soup! Gazpacho is the ultimate summertime vegetarian dish because it maximizes the garden's bounty and it's served at room temperature or chilled. *(See photo insert.)*

1. In a food processor or blender, process the chopped tomatoes, 1½ cups vegetable juice, the red bell pepper, onion, basil, lemon juice, garlic, and cayenne until smooth. Transfer to a large bowl.

2. Stir in the remaining 1 cup vegetable juice and the remaining ingredients. Serve immediately or cover and refrigerate until serving time.

COOK'S TIP: To make a complete meal, increase the serving size to 1½ cups and serve the soup with grilled chicken or shrimp and crusty whole-grain bread.

PER SERVING: Calories **56** • Total Fat **0.5 g** • Saturated Fat **0.0 g** • Trans Fat **0.0 g** Polyunsaturated Fat **0.0 g** • Monounsaturated Fat **0.0 g** • Cholesterol **0 mg** Sodium **69 mg** • Carbohydrates **12 g** • Fiber **3 g** • Sugars **8 g** • Protein **2 g** DIETARY EXCHANGES: 2 vegetable

2½ cups chopped, seeded tomatoes

1½ cups chilled low-sodium spicy mixed-vegetable juice and 1 cup chilled low-sodium spicy mixed-vegetable juice, divided use

½ cup chopped red bell pepper

¼ cup finely chopped red onion

¼ cup loosely packed fresh basil

1 tablespoon fresh lemon juice

1 medium garlic clove, minced

¼ teaspoon cayenne (optional)

1 cup chopped seeded cucumber

1 cup quartered yellow pear tomatoes or red cherry tomatoes

¼ cup finely chopped green bell pepper

¼ cup chopped fresh parsley

SALADS AND SALAD DRESSINGS

SERVES 6
1½ cups salad and
1 tablespoon
dressing per serving

PREP TIME
15 minutes

Mango and Butter Lettuce Salad with Curry-Dijon Vinaigrette

A hint of curry gives this salad a deep, exotic flavor. Serve it as a refreshing complement to grilled chicken or pork.

2 heads butter lettuce, leaves torn into pieces (about 8 cups)

2 medium mangoes, peeled and cut into cubes (about 2½ cups)

½ cup slivered red onion

DRESSING

2 tablespoons walnut oil or canola oil

2 tablespoons white wine vinegar

2 tablespoons 100% mango-orange juice

½ teaspoon curry powder

½ teaspoon Dijon mustard (lowest sodium available)

¼ teaspoon salt

¼ teaspoon pepper

* * *

¼ cup chopped walnuts, dry-roasted

1. In a large bowl, toss together the lettuce, mangoes, and onion.

2. In a small bowl, whisk together the dressing ingredients. Pour over the salad, tossing gently to coat. Just before serving, sprinkle with the walnuts.

TIPS, TRICKS & TIMESAVERS: To dry-roast nuts in the oven, place them in a shallow baking pan. Roast them at 350°F for 10 to 15 minutes, stirring occasionally. You can roast extra and freeze them in an airtight freezer container so they can be ready at a moment's notice. You don't even need to thaw the nuts before using them.

PER SERVING: Calories **129** • Total Fat **8.0 g** • Saturated Fat **1.0 g** • Trans Fat **0.0 g** • Polyunsaturated Fat **5.5 g** • Monounsaturated Fat **1.5 g** • Cholesterol **0 mg** • Sodium **110 mg** • Carbohydrates **14 g** • Fiber **2 g** • Sugars **11 g** • Protein **2 g**
DIETARY EXCHANGES: 1 fruit, 1½ fat

Salad Greens with Blue Cheese and Italian Herb Vinaigrette

SERVES 4
2 cups salad
and scant
1½ tablespoons
dressing per serving

PREP TIME
10 minutes

In every bite, this sprightly salad offers a forkful of greens dressed with the sweet notes of white balsamic vinegar, the zing of lemon zest, a profusion of fresh herbs, and a hint of sharp blue cheese.

1. In a large bowl, combine the salad greens and onion.

2. In a small bowl, whisk together the dressing ingredients. Pour over the salad, tossing gently to coat. Sprinkle with the blue cheese.

PER SERVING: Calories 83 • Total Fat **6.0 g** • Saturated Fat **1.5 g** • Trans Fat **0.0 g**
Polyunsaturated Fat **1.5 g** • Monounsaturated Fat **3.5 g** • Cholesterol **4 mg**
Sodium **113 mg** • Carbohydrates **5 g** • Fiber **2 g** • Sugars **2 g** • Protein **3 g**
DIETARY EXCHANGES: 1 vegetable, 1 fat

8 ounces mixed baby salad greens or spring greens
½ cup thinly sliced red onion

DRESSING

2 tablespoons chopped fresh basil

1 tablespoon plus 1 teaspoon canola or corn oil

1 tablespoon plus 1 teaspoon white balsamic vinegar

2 teaspoons chopped fresh oregano

½ teaspoon chopped fresh rosemary

½ teaspoon grated lemon zest

* * *

1 ounce low-fat blue cheese, crumbled

SERVES 4
2 cups salad and
2 tablespoons
dressing per serving

PREP TIME
10 minutes

Spinach-Apple Salad with Cherry-Ginger Vinaigrette

The cherry-pomegranate juice in this vinaigrette takes ordinary oil-and-vinegar dressing to a new flavor profile. The sweetness of the juice marries well with the bitterness of the spinach, while the creaminess of the goat cheese highlights the crunch of the spinach and apple.

DRESSING

⅓ cup 100% cherry-pomegranate juice

2 tablespoons white balsamic vinegar

1 tablespoon canola or corn oil

2 teaspoons sugar

2 teaspoons grated peeled gingerroot

* * *

6 ounces baby spinach

1 large unpeeled red apple (about 6 ounces), such as Jazz or Ambrosia, thinly sliced

½ cup thinly sliced red onion

1 ounce crumbled soft goat cheese

1. In a small bowl, whisk together the dressing ingredients.

2. Put the spinach on plates. Arrange the apple and onion on top.

3. Pour the dressing over the salad. Sprinkle with the goat cheese.

HEALTHY SWAP: You can also try this dressing on arugula and crisp pears, stirred into fruit salad, or simply spooned over slices of melon or another favorite fruit.

PER SERVING: Calories **115** • Total Fat **5.5 g** • Saturated Fat **1.5 g** • Trans Fat **0.0 g** Polyunsaturated Fat **1.0 g** • Monounsaturated Fat **2.5 g** • Cholesterol **3 mg** Sodium **66 mg** • Carbohydrates **16 g** • Fiber **2 g** • Sugars **12 g** • Protein **3 g** DIETARY EXCHANGES: 1 fruit, 1 fat

Baby Spinach and Tomato Salad with Warm Olive Vinaigrette

SERVES 4
1½ cups per serving

PREP TIME
5 minutes

COOKING TIME
5 minutes

When heirloom tomatoes are in season, use any two red and yellow varieties in this simple salad for a beautiful presentation. Year-round, cherry tomatoes provide a bit more sweetness.

1. In a large bowl, toss together the spinach and romaine. Transfer the greens to salad plates. Arrange the tomato on the greens.

2. In a small saucepan, heat the oil over medium-low heat, swirling to coat the bottom. Cook the garlic for 1 minute, or until fragrant, stirring constantly.

3. Stir in the olives. Cook for 1 to 2 minutes, or just until warmed, stirring frequently. Remove from the heat.

4. Stir in the vinegar. Spoon the dressing over the salads. Sprinkle with the basil and pepper.

PER SERVING: Calories 91 • Total Fat **6.5 g** • Saturated Fat **1.0 g** • Trans Fat **0.0 g**
Polyunsaturated Fat **1.0 g** • Monounsaturated Fat **4.5 g** • Cholesterol **0 mg**
Sodium **120 mg** • Carbohydrates **8 g** • Fiber **2 g** • Sugars **4 g** • Protein **2 g**
DIETARY EXCHANGES: 1 vegetable, 1½ fat

2 cups baby spinach

2 cups torn romaine

1 large yellow tomato, cut into 8 wedges, or 6 mini yellow tomatoes, halved

1 large red tomato, cut into 8 wedges, or 6 cherry tomatoes, halved

1½ tablespoons extra-virgin olive oil

2 medium garlic cloves, minced

⅓ cup thickly sliced, canned natural green ripe olives, rinsed and drained

1½ tablespoons balsamic vinegar

½ cup thinly sliced basil

Freshly ground pepper

½ small head red or
green cabbage,
shredded (about
3 cups)

1 medium carrot, halved
lengthwise, thinly
sliced crosswise

½ medium red bell
pepper, diced

½ cup shelled green peas
or frozen green peas,
thawed

2 tablespoons sugar

2 tablespoons cider
vinegar

1 tablespoon canola or
corn oil

Crunchy Coleslaw with Peas

Add green peas and red bell pepper to traditional carrot and cabbage coleslaw for a more lively and colorful salad. Cider vinegar offers a lighter, tart dressing, a refreshing change from the usual mayonnaise-based versions. *(See photo insert.)*

In a medium bowl, stir together all the ingredients, tossing to coat. Let stand for 15 minutes so the flavors blend. For peak flavor and crispness, serve within an hour of preparation.

PER SERVING: Calories **70** • Total Fat **2.5 g** • Saturated Fat **0.0 g** • Trans Fat **0.0 g**
Polyunsaturated Fat **0.5 g** • Monounsaturated Fat **1.5 g** • Cholesterol **0 mg**
Sodium **19 mg** • Carbohydrates **11 g** • Fiber **3 g** • Sugars **8 g** • Protein **2 g**
DIETARY EXCHANGES: 1 vegetable, ½ other carbohydrate, ½ fat

Ginger-Mint Jícama Salad

SERVES 4
½ cup per serving

PREP TIME
10 minutes

STANDING TIME
15 minutes

Jícama (HIH-kah-mah) is a fiber-rich root vegetable indigenous to Mexico with a texture similar to that of a potato, a firm pear, or even a crisp apple. It's crunchy, it's juicy, and it's great as the main attraction in coleslaws or salads or tossed with mixed greens. *(See photo insert.)*

- 8 ounces jícama, peeled and cut into matchstick-size strips (about 1½ cups total)
- ⅓ cup diced red onion
- ¼ cup chopped fresh mint
- 1 teaspoon grated lemon zest
- 3 tablespoons fresh lemon juice
- 2½ tablespoons sugar
- 2 teaspoons grated orange zest
- 1 to 2 teaspoons grated peeled gingerroot

In a medium bowl, stir together all the ingredients. Let stand for 15 minutes so the flavors blend.

SHOP & STORE: If you bought more gingerroot than you need, freeze the unpeeled pieces in an airtight freezer container.

TIPS, TRICKS & TIMESAVERS: To peel gingerroot easily, use a paring knife or vegetable peeler. To make matchstick-size strips of vegetables, such as jícama, with ease, use a julienne peeler, which is similar to a potato peeler but has more space between the blades. Simply glide the julienne peeler over the vegetables to create thin uniform strips and then cut those strips to the desired length.

PER SERVING: Calories 65 • Total Fat **0.0 g** • Saturated Fat **0.0 g** • Trans Fat **0.0 g**
Polyunsaturated Fat **0.0 g** • Monounsaturated Fat **0.0 g** • Cholesterol **0 mg**
Sodium **6 mg** • Carbohydrates **16 g** • Fiber **4 g** • Sugars **10 g** • Protein **1 g**
DIETARY EXCHANGES: ½ starch, ½ other carbohydrate

SERVES 4
½ cup fruit and
2 tablespoons
dressing per serving

PREP TIME
10 minutes

DRESSING

½ **cup fat-free vanilla yogurt**

1 **tablespoon fresh orange juice**

1½ **teaspoons fresh lemon juice**

1 **teaspoon sugar**

½ **teaspoon curry powder**

SALAD

1 **medium mango, peeled and cubed**

½ **cup blueberries**

1 **medium kiwifruit, peeled and cut into 8 wedges**

Mango-Blueberry Salad with Creamy Citrus Dressing

This salad makes a perfect choice for a light brunch. Spooning the dressing onto the plate rather than over the fruit showcases the freshness of the fruit and makes for an attractive presentation. The curry flavor is relatively mild; you can even use the dressing as a topping for fruit at breakfast time.

1. In a small bowl, whisk together the dressing ingredients. Spoon equal amounts onto the center of salad plates. Using the back of a spoon, spread the dressing into a circle about 4 inches in diameter.

2. Arrange the mango, blueberries, and kiwifruit on the dressing.

PER SERVING: Calories **106** • Total Fat **0.5 g** • Saturated Fat **0.0 g** • Trans Fat **0.0 g** Polyunsaturated Fat **0.0 g** • Monounsaturated Fat **0.0 g** • Cholesterol **1 mg** Sodium **23 mg** • Carbohydrates **25 g** • Fiber **2 g** • Sugars **21 g** • Protein **3 g** DIETARY EXCHANGES: 1½ fruit

Cucumber, Radish, and Barley Salad

SERVES 4
1½ cups per serving

PREP TIME
15 minutes

COOKING TIME
15 minutes

With a chewy texture from barley and a peppery bite from watercress and radishes, this salad has plenty of attitude to go around. The tangy, citrusy dressing, with its strong notes of oregano, holds up well against this greens and grains salad.

1. Prepare the barley using the package directions, omitting the salt. Transfer to a colander. Rinse with cold water. Drain well.

2. In a large salad bowl, stir together the salad ingredients.

3. In a small bowl, whisk together the dressing ingredients. Pour over the salad, tossing gently to coat.

SHOP & STORE: Watercress, a member of the mustard family, has small, dark green leaves and a peppery taste. It can be stored for up to five days in the refrigerator, either in a plastic bag or stems down in a glass of water.

TIPS, TRICKS & TIMESAVERS: To easily shred small foods, such as radishes, use a box grater or rasp grater.

PER SERVING: Calories 216 • Total Fat 8.0 g • Saturated Fat 1.0 g • Trans Fat 0.0 g
Polyunsaturated Fat 1.0 g • Monounsaturated Fat 5.0 g • Cholesterol 0 mg
Sodium 99 mg • Carbohydrates 34 g • Fiber 5 g • Sugars 4 g • Protein 5 g
DIETARY EXCHANGES: 2 starch, 1 vegetable, 1 fat

SALAD

1 cup uncooked quick-cooking barley

1 medium cucumber, peeled, seeded, and chopped

1 bunch watercress, stems discarded and leaves torn into pieces

1 cup shredded unpeeled radishes

½ cup sliced green onions

DRESSING

3 tablespoons fresh lemon juice

2 tablespoons chopped fresh oregano

2 tablespoons fresh orange juice

2 tablespoons extra-virgin olive oil

1 teaspoon sugar

½ teaspoon pepper

⅛ teaspoon salt

SERVES 4
½ cup per serving

PREP TIME
10 minutes

COOKING TIME
20 minutes

⅓ cup uncooked
  amaranth

3 small tomatillos, papery
  husks discarded, diced

½ medium cucumber,
  peeled, seeded, and
  diced

½ cup chopped fresh
  cilantro

1 medium poblano
  pepper, seeds and ribs
  discarded, diced (see
  Cook's Tip, page 261)

2 medium green onions,
  finely chopped

2 tablespoons extra-virgin
  olive oil

1 teaspoon grated lime
  zest

1 tablespoon fresh lime
  juice

1 teaspoon cider vinegar

1 medium garlic clove,
  minced

⅛ teaspoon salt

Tomatillo-Amaranth Salad

Amaranth (AM-ah-ranth), an ancient whole grain, has a mild, sweet, and nutty flavor; it has a "sticky" texture, so it's not as fluffy as most other whole grains. It's high in protein, fiber, calcium, and potassium, among other important nutrients, making it a great grain to try in salads and as a hot cereal.

1. Prepare the amaranth using the package directions, omitting the salt and margarine. Transfer to a fine-mesh sieve. Rinse with cold water. Drain well.

2. Meanwhile, in a medium bowl, stir together the remaining ingredients except the salt.

3. Stir the cooled amaranth and salt into the tomatillo mixture.

PER SERVING: Calories 146 • Total Fat 8.5 g • Saturated Fat 1.0 g • Trans Fat 0.0 g
Polyunsaturated Fat 1.5 g • Monounsaturated Fat 5.0 g • Cholesterol 0 mg
Sodium 79 mg • Carbohydrates 16 g • Fiber 3 g • Sugars 3 g • Protein 3 g
DIETARY EXCHANGES: ½ starch, 1 vegetable, 1½ fat

Warm Amaranth Salad with Feta and Currants

SERVES 4
1¼ cups per serving

PREP TIME
5 minutes

COOKING TIME
15 minutes

STANDING TIME
2 minutes

The leaves of the amaranth flower are cultivated in East Asia to be eaten as a vegetable. The amaranth grain, or seed of the flower, is gluten-free and loaded with vitamins and minerals. It provides a healthy vegetarian option and has a consistency similar to creamy polenta.

1. In a large saucepan, bring the broth and amaranth to a boil, covered, over high heat. Reduce the heat and simmer, covered, for 8 to 10 minutes, or until the liquid is fully absorbed, stirring once halfway through. Remove from the heat. Fluff with a fork.

2. Meanwhile, in a medium bowl, whisk together the oil and vinegar until well combined.

3. Stir the currants and green onion into the cooked amaranth. Let stand, covered, for 2 minutes.

4. Add the greens to the oil mixture, tossing well. Transfer to plates. Spoon the amaranth over the salads. Sprinkle with the feta and pepper.

1 cup fat-free, low-sodium vegetable broth

⅓ cup uncooked amaranth

1 tablespoon extra-virgin olive oil

1 tablespoon red wine vinegar

¼ cup dried currants or raisins

1 medium green onion, thinly sliced

4 cups tightly packed mixed field greens or spring greens

½ ounce fat-free feta cheese

¼ teaspoon freshly ground pepper, or to taste

PER SERVING: Calories 134 • Total Fat 4.5 g • Saturated Fat 0.5 g • Trans Fat 0.0 g
Polyunsaturated Fat 1.0 g • Monounsaturated Fat 2.5 g • Cholesterol 0 mg
Sodium 78 mg • Carbohydrates 20 g • Fiber 3 g • Sugars 7 g • Protein 5 g
DIETARY EXCHANGES: 1 starch, ½ fruit, 1 fat

Grilled Salmon on Pasta and Greens

SERVES 4
3 ounces fish and
2 cups salad
per serving

PREP TIME
15 minutes

COOKING TIME
20 minutes

COOLING TIME
15 minutes

Cooking spray

1 teaspoon paprika
(smoked preferred)

½ teaspoon ground cumin

¼ teaspoon salt and
¼ teaspoon salt,
divided use

¼ teaspoon pepper

4 salmon fillets with skin
(about 5 ounces each),
rinsed and patted dry

2 ounces dried whole-
grain rotini

⅔ cup white balsamic
vinegar

1 teaspoon grated orange
zest

¼ cup fresh orange juice

5 ounces spring greens

2 medium oranges, peeled
and sectioned

1 medium red bell pepper,
cut into thin strips

½ cup sliced red onion

1 teaspoon vanilla extract
(optional)

This entrée salad is layered with colors—red, green, orange, and coral—that match the brightness of the citrus flavors. The slight chill from the white balsamic vinegar and citrus dressing nicely complements the paprika- and cumin-covered fish.

1. Lightly spray a grill pan with cooking spray.

2. In a small bowl, stir together the paprika, cumin, ¼ teaspoon salt, and the pepper. Sprinkle over the flesh side of the fish. Using your fingertips, gently press the mixture so it adheres to the fish.

3. Heat the grill pan over medium-high heat. Place the fish with the skin side down in the pan. Cook for 6 minutes. Turn over. Cook for 2 minutes, or until the desired doneness. Transfer the fish to a plate with the skin side down. Let cool.

4. Meanwhile, in a medium saucepan, prepare the pasta using the package directions, omitting the salt. Transfer to a colander. Rinse with cold water. Drain well. Set aside.

5. In the same saucepan, stir together the vinegar and orange juice. Bring to a boil over medium-high heat. Boil for 3 minutes, or until the liquid is reduced by about half (to ½ cup). Pour into a shallow bowl and transfer to the freezer for 5 minutes to cool quickly.

6. Put the spring greens on salad plates. Top with the pasta, orange sections, bell pepper, and onion.

7. Stir the orange zest, vanilla, and the remaining ¼ teaspoon salt into the cooled vinegar mixture. Spoon over the salads. Top with the fish.

PER SERVING: Calories **276** • Total Fat **6.0 g** • Saturated Fat **1.0 g** • Trans Fat **0.0 g** • Polyunsaturated Fat **1.0 g** • Monounsaturated Fat **1.5 g** • Cholesterol **53 mg** • Sodium **403 mg** • Carbohydrates **30 g** • Fiber **5 g** • Sugars **15 g** • Protein **27 g** • DIETARY EXCHANGES: ½ starch, 1 fruit, 1 vegetable, 3 lean meat

Warm Sesame-Ginger Salmon Salad

SERVES 4
3 ounces fish and
1¼ cups salad
per serving

PREP TIME
10 minutes

COOKING TIME
10 minutes

A bed of mixed greens creates an inviting place for sweet and savory baked fish to rest. Enjoy this Asian-influenced salad with a side of mandarin oranges.

1. Preheat the oven to 375°F.

2. Put the fish in a shallow glass baking dish or pan.

3. In a small bowl, whisk together the soy sauce, brown sugar, sherry, gingerroot, and oil. Spoon 3 tablespoons of the soy sauce mixture over the fish. Set aside the remaining soy sauce mixture.

4. Bake the fish for 10 to 12 minutes, or until the desired doneness.

5. Meanwhile, in a large bowl, toss together the salad greens, carrot, cucumber, and 2 tablespoons cilantro. Pour the reserved soy sauce mixture over the salad, tossing to coat. Transfer the salad to plates. Top each serving with a fish fillet. Garnish with the sesame seeds and the remaining 2 tablespoons cilantro.

COOK'S TIP: For a prettier presentation, score the surface of the unpeeled cucumber before slicing. Stand it upright. Pull a fork from top to bottom all the way around the cucumber. This will cause the slices to have a "frilly" look.

COOK'S TIP: If you have extra time, cover and refrigerate the fish in the soy sauce mixture for up to 2 hours before baking. The marinating will give the fish a deeper infusion of umami flavor.

4 salmon fillets (about 4 ounces each), rinsed and patted dry

2 tablespoons soy sauce (lowest sodium available)

1 tablespoon firmly packed light brown sugar

1 tablespoon dry sherry

2 teaspoons finely grated peeled gingerroot

2 teaspoons toasted sesame oil

4 cups tightly packed mixed baby salad greens or spring greens

1 large carrot, very thinly sliced diagonally

1 small pickling, or Kirby, cucumber, thinly sliced

2 tablespoons chopped fresh cilantro and 2 tablespoons chopped fresh cilantro, divided use

2 teaspoons sesame seeds, dry-roasted

PER SERVING: Calories 220 • Total Fat 8.5 g • Saturated Fat 1.5 g • Trans Fat 0.0 g
Polyunsaturated Fat 2.5 g • Monounsaturated Fat 3.0 g • Cholesterol 53 mg
Sodium 312 mg • Carbohydrates 9 g • Fiber 2 g • Sugars 6 g • Protein 26 g
DIETARY EXCHANGES: 1 vegetable, ½ other carbohydrate, 3 lean meat

SERVES 4
2 cups per serving

PREP TIME
15 minutes

COOKING TIME
20 minutes

DRESSING

½ cup loosely packed
  fresh basil

2 tablespoons sliced
  green onions

2 tablespoons white wine
  vinegar

2 tablespoons water

1 teaspoon Dijon mustard
  (lowest sodium
  available)

1 teaspoon extra-virgin
  olive oil

SALAD

1 1-pound tuna steak,
  about 1 inch thick,
  rinsed, patted dry, and
  cut into 4 pieces

4 small red potatoes,
  quartered

4 ounces green beans,
  trimmed (about 1 cup)

4 cups mixed salad greens

1 medium orange or
  yellow bell pepper,
  coarsely chopped

1 large tomato, cut into
  ½-inch wedges

¼ cup sliced green onions

* * *

1 teaspoon olive oil

Seven-Layer Salade Niçoise with Basil Vinaigrette

Based on the well-known salad from the south of France, our version breaks from tradition by layering the ingredients in the style of America's popular seven-layer salad and topping them off with seared tuna steaks. The basil dressing does double duty as a marinade for the fish and a salad dressing.

1. In a food processor or blender, process the dressing ingredients until smooth. Brush 1 tablespoon of the dressing over both sides of the fish. Cover and refrigerate the fish and the remaining dressing until needed, or up to 3 hours.

2. Put the potatoes in a medium saucepan. Pour in enough water to cover the potatoes. Bring to a boil over medium-high heat. Reduce the heat and simmer for 5 minutes. Stir in the green beans. Cook for 3 to 4 minutes, or until the potatoes and green beans are tender. Transfer to a colander. Rinse with cold water to cool slightly. Drain well.

3. Meanwhile, arrange the salad greens in a 9-inch square glass baking dish or on a large platter. Layer over the greens as follows: the bell pepper, tomato, potato mixture, and green onions. Drizzle with the reserved dressing. (The salad can be made to this point up to 3 hours in advance. Cover and refrigerate until serving time.)

4. Heat a large skillet over medium-high heat. Add the remaining 1 teaspoon oil, swirling to coat the bottom. Cook the fish for 3 minutes, or until the desired doneness, turning once halfway through. Place the tuna steaks on the salad.

PER SERVING: Calories 207 • Total Fat 3.5 g • Saturated Fat 0.5 g • Trans Fat 0.0 g
Polyunsaturated Fat 0.5 g • Monounsaturated Fat 2.0 g • Cholesterol 44 mg
Sodium 105 mg • Carbohydrates 13 g • Fiber 4 g • Sugars 4 g • Protein 31 g
DIETARY EXCHANGES: ½ starch, 2 vegetable, 3 lean meat

Blueberry-Walnut Chicken Salad

SERVES 4
1¼ cups per serving

PREP TIME
10 minutes

Want a fresh update on chicken salad? Try our version, which has a creamy yogurt-based dressing speckled with ginger and lemon zest and is topped with fruit and walnut accents. It's a great use for Sunday's leftover roasted chicken or turkey!

1. In a medium bowl, whisk together the dressing ingredients. Add the chicken, stirring to coat.

2. Put the greens in a large salad bowl. Spoon the chicken mixture onto the greens. Top with the blueberries, celery, green onions, and cherries. Just before serving, sprinkle with the walnuts.

COOK'S TIP: To make 2 cups of shredded chicken breast, put 1 pound of boneless, skinless chicken breasts, all visible fat discarded, in a large skillet or saucepan. Pour in water to cover. Bring to a boil over medium-high heat. Reduce the heat and simmer for 8 to 10 minutes, or until the chicken is no longer pink in the center. Drain well. Transfer the chicken to a flat surface. Using two forks, shred the chicken. Let it cool for at least 10 minutes before stirring it together with the dressing.

PER SERVING: Calories 302 • Total Fat 8.5 g • Saturated Fat 1.5 g • Trans Fat 0.0 g
Polyunsaturated Fat 4.5 g • Monounsaturated Fat 2.0 g • Cholesterol 60 mg
Sodium 260 mg • Carbohydrates 29 g • Fiber 5 g • Sugars 19 g • Protein 27 g
DIETARY EXCHANGES: 1½ fruit, 1 vegetable, 3½ lean meat

DRESSING

½ cup fat-free plain yogurt

1 tablespoon minced peeled gingerroot

1 teaspoon grated lemon zest

1 tablespoon fresh lemon juice

1 teaspoon sugar

¼ teaspoon salt

¼ teaspoon pepper

SALAD

2 cups shredded, cooked skinless chicken breast, cooked without salt, all visible fat discarded

6 cups mixed baby salad greens

1½ cups blueberries

½ cup sliced celery

½ cup sliced green onions

½ cup dried tart cherries

¼ cup chopped walnuts, dry-roasted

SERVES 4
1 tuna burger,
1 cup greens, and
½ cup avocado
mixture per serving

PREP TIME
20 minutes

COOKING TIME
5 minutes

DRESSING

2 tablespoons fresh lime juice

2 tablespoons water

1 tablespoon plus 1 teaspoon rice vinegar

2½ teaspoons honey

2 teaspoons soy sauce (lowest sodium available)

2 teaspoons toasted sesame oil

2 teaspoons canola or corn oil

¼ teaspoon crushed red pepper flakes

(continued)

Thai Tuna Burger and Mango-Avocado Salad with Soy-Lime Vinaigrette

This tuna burger is made partly with soft tofu, which helps keep the burger moist and flavorful. It tops an avocado, mango, and red onion salad dressed with an Asian-inspired vinaigrette. There's so much goodness going on, you surely won't miss the bun for this burger!

1. In a small bowl, whisk together the dressing ingredients. Set aside.

2. In a medium bowl, using your hands or a spoon, combine the tuna, tofu, green onions, basil, gingerroot, and the remaining 1 teaspoon soy sauce. Shape into 4 burgers, each about 3 to 4 inches in diameter. Transfer to a large plate.

3. Lightly spray a medium skillet with cooking spray. Heat over medium heat. Cook the burgers for 2 minutes on each side, or until the fish is the desired doneness.

4. Meanwhile, in a large bowl, toss together the salad greens, avocado, mango, onion, and dressing. Transfer to plates. Top each salad with a burger. Serve immediately.

SHOP & STORE: Thai basil has a thin green leaf with a purplish cast, and its flavor is spicy and licoricelike. If you can't find it in your grocery store, look for it in Asian markets or specialty grocery stores, as well as at your local farmers' market. If it's not available, you can substitute sweet Italian basil, but the flavor will be different.

PER SERVING: Calories **231** • Total Fat **11.0 g** • Saturated Fat **1.5 g** • Trans Fat **0.0 g** Polyunsaturated Fat **2.5 g** • Monounsaturated Fat **6.0 g** • Cholesterol **22 mg** Sodium **150 mg** • Carbohydrates **17 g** • Fiber **5 g** • Sugars **11 g** • Protein **18 g** DIETARY EXCHANGES: 1 fruit, 1 vegetable, 2 lean meat, 1 fat

* * *

1 8-ounce tuna fillet, rinsed, patted dry, and finely chopped

3 ounces light soft tofu, drained and patted dry

3 tablespoons sliced green onions

2 tablespoons finely chopped Thai basil

1 teaspoon finely chopped peeled gingerroot

1 teaspoon soy sauce (lowest sodium available)

Cooking spray

4 cups tightly packed mixed salad greens

1 cup diced avocado

1 cup diced mango

¼ cup thinly sliced red onion

SERVES 4
3 ounces chicken,
2 cups salad, and
1 tablespoon
dressing per serving

PREP TIME
20 minutes

COOKING TIME
15 minutes

Ancho Chicken and Black Bean Salad with Cilantro-Lime Dressing

Ancho powder, made from dried poblano peppers, provides this chicken with a rich, sweet, peppery flavor without an overpowering heat. Plenty of lime zest, lime juice, and cilantro add just the right amount of zing to the dressing to complete this Southwestern-style main dish salad.

Cooking spray

6 cups tightly packed torn or sliced romaine

1 cup canned no-salt-added black beans, rinsed and drained

1 cup corn kernels, cut from 2 medium ears of corn, husks and silk discarded

1 medium red bell pepper, cut lengthwise into short, thin strips

1 medium garlic clove

½ cup tightly packed fresh cilantro, stems discarded

¼ cup light mayonnaise

2 tablespoons extra-virgin olive oil

2 teaspoons finely shredded lime zest

1 tablespoon fresh lime juice

1 teaspoon ancho powder or chipotle powder

(continued)

1. Lightly spray the grill rack with cooking spray. Preheat the grill on medium or use a grill pan.

2. In a large bowl, stir together the romaine, beans, corn, and bell pepper. Cover and refrigerate.

3. With the motor running, drop the garlic through the feed tube of a food processor. Process until finely chopped. Add the cilantro. Process until finely chopped. Add the mayonnaise, oil, and lime juice. Process until smooth. Cover and refrigerate.

4. In a small bowl, stir together the ancho powder, cumin, and salt. Sprinkle over the chicken. Using your fingertips, gently press the mixture so it adheres to the chicken. Lightly spray with cooking spray.

5. Grill the chicken for 8 to 10 minutes, or until no longer pink in the center, turning once halfway through. Transfer to a cutting board. Cut crosswise into ½-inch slices.

6. Toss the salad and transfer to plates. Arrange the chicken on the salad. Drizzle with the dressing. Sprinkle with the lime zest.

> **TIPS, TRICKS & TIMESAVERS:** To easily remove corn kernels from the cob, place one end of the corn cob in the hole in the center of a tube pan or Bundt pan. As you carefully cut downward along the cob, the corn kernels will fall into the pan.

1 teaspoon ground cumin

1/8 teaspoon salt

4 boneless, skinless chicken breast halves (about 4 ounces each), all visible fat discarded

PER SERVING: Calories **349** • Total Fat **14.5 g** • Saturated Fat **2.0 g** • Trans Fat **0.0 g**
Polyunsaturated Fat **4.0 g** • Monounsaturated Fat **7.0 g** • Cholesterol **78 mg**
Sodium **351 mg** • Carbohydrates **26 g** • Fiber **6 g** • Sugars **7 g** • Protein **31 g**
DIETARY EXCHANGES: 1½ starch, 1 vegetable, 3½ lean meat, ½ fat

Herbed Chicken Salad with Swiss

Thick, juicy tomato slices along with a thin layer of Swiss are topped with a mound of richly Italian-herbed chicken salad in our nod to the classic Caprese salad.

2 medium tomatoes, cut into 8 slices total

4 thin slices low-fat Swiss cheese, halved diagonally

2 cups diced cooked skinless chicken breast, cooked without salt, all visible fat discarded

¼ cup chopped fresh basil

2 tablespoons finely chopped red onion

2 tablespoons chopped fresh Italian (flat-leaf) parsley

1 tablespoon fresh lemon juice

1 tablespoon extra-virgin olive oil

2 medium garlic cloves, minced

½ teaspoon salt

¼ teaspoon pepper

1. On plates, arrange the tomato and cheese slices in a fan shape, alternating the tomato and cheese and slightly overlapping the slices.

2. In a medium bowl, stir together the remaining ingredients. Spoon over the tomato and cheese. Serve immediately for peak flavor.

HEALTHY SWAP: If cooked chicken is not available, you can use chicken tenders, which cook more quickly than chicken breast halves. In a large nonstick skillet, heat 1 teaspoon canola oil over medium heat, swirling to coat the bottom. Cook the chicken for 5 minutes on each side, or until no longer pink in the center. Transfer to a cutting board to cool slightly. Dice the chicken and proceed as directed.

PER SERVING: Calories 197 • Total Fat 6.5 g • Saturated Fat 1.5 g • Trans Fat 0.0 g
Polyunsaturated Fat 1.0 g • Monounsaturated Fat 3.5 g • Cholesterol 62 mg
Sodium 505 mg • Carbohydrates 5 g • Fiber 1 g • Sugars 3 g • Protein 28 g
DIETARY EXCHANGES: 1 vegetable, 4 lean meat

Orange-Poached Chicken Salad

Looking for a new way to cook an old standby? Try poaching chicken on slices of fresh orange, allowing the citrus to permeate the chicken while it cooks. A splash of citrusy dressing adds even more fruity flavor to this main-dish salad.

1. In a small bowl, stir together the cumin, pepper, and red pepper flakes. Sprinkle over the smooth side of the chicken.

2. Pour the water into a large nonstick skillet. Place the orange slices in the skillet. Cover each orange slice with a chicken breast half. Bring to a boil over medium-high heat. Reduce the heat and simmer, covered, for 8 to 10 minutes, or until the chicken is no longer pink in the center. Transfer the chicken to a plate. Let stand for 10 minutes to cool slightly.

3. Meanwhile, in a small bowl, whisk together the orange zest, orange juice, lemon zest, lemon juice, sugar, oil, and salt.

4. Arrange the salad greens and onion on plates. Top with the chicken. Spoon the dressing over all.

PER SERVING: Calories **205** • Total Fat **5.5 g** • Saturated Fat **1.0 g** • Trans Fat **0.0 g**
Polyunsaturated Fat **1.0 g** • Monounsaturated Fat **2.5 g** • Cholesterol **73 mg**
Sodium **299 mg** • Carbohydrates **13 g** • Fiber **2 g** • Sugars **9 g** • Protein **26 g**
DIETARY EXCHANGES: 1 vegetable, ½ other carbohydrate, 3 lean meat

---

SERVES 4
3 ounces chicken,
1½ cups salad, and
1½ tablespoons
dressing per serving

PREP TIME
5 minutes

COOKING TIME
15 minutes

STANDING TIME
10 minutes

¼ teaspoon ground cumin

¼ teaspoon pepper

⅛ teaspoon crushed red pepper flakes

4 boneless, skinless chicken breast halves (about 4 ounces each), all visible fat discarded

½ cup water

1 medium orange, cut crosswise into four slices (rounds)

1 teaspoon grated orange zest

3 tablespoons fresh orange juice

1 teaspoon grated lemon zest

3 tablespoons fresh lemon juice

2 tablespoons sugar

2 teaspoons canola oil

¼ teaspoon salt

6 cups mixed salad greens

½ cup diced red onion

SERVES 4
1½ cups per serving

PREP TIME
10 minutes

COOKING TIME
15 minutes

Turkey and Green Bean Pasta Salad with Feta

Dig into a hearty salad of moist turkey breast, tender-crisp green beans, and penne pasta dressed with a basil-rosemary vinaigrette. Enjoy this one-dish meal with a crusty whole-grain roll.

3 quarts water

4 ounces dried whole-grain penne

3 ounces green beans, trimmed and broken into 1-inch pieces

2 cups diced cooked skinless turkey or chicken breast, cooked without salt, all visible fat discarded

2 tablespoons chopped fresh basil

2 tablespoons white balsamic vinegar

2 tablespoons canola or corn oil

2 teaspoons chopped fresh rosemary

4 ounces crumbled low-fat feta cheese

1. In a large saucepan, bring the water to a boil over high heat. Stir in the pasta. Boil for 6 minutes.

2. Stir in the green beans. Boil for 5 minutes, or until tender-crisp. Immediately transfer to a colander and rinse with cold water. Drain well. Transfer to a serving bowl.

3. Stir in the remaining ingredients except the feta. Gently stir in the feta.

PER SERVING: Calories 326 • Total Fat **11.5 g** • Saturated Fat **3.0 g** • Trans Fat **0.0 g**
Polyunsaturated Fat **3.0 g** • Monounsaturated Fat **5.5 g** • Cholesterol **70 mg**
Sodium **417 mg** • Carbohydrates **25 g** • Fiber **4 g** • Sugars **3 g** • Protein **30 g**
DIETARY EXCHANGES: 1½ starch, 4 lean meat

Ginger Beef and Snow Pea Salad

Looking for a quick and easy summertime salad? If so, try this: a grilled steak thinly sliced over crisp veggies and topped with a cool, refreshing, and tangy dressing made with fresh lime and ginger.

1. Lightly spray the grill rack with cooking spray. Preheat the grill on medium high. Or lightly spray a grill pan and heat over medium-high heat.

2. Sprinkle the salt and pepper over both sides of the beef.

3. Grill the beef for 4 to 5 minutes on each side for medium rare, or until the desired doneness. Transfer the beef to a cutting board and let stand for 10 minutes to cool.

4. Meanwhile, in a medium bowl, whisk together the lime juice, sugar, vinegar, water, gingerroot, salt, and red pepper flakes.

5. Put the spring greens on salad plates. Arrange the snow peas and bell pepper on the greens. Sprinkle with ¼ cup cilantro.

6. Thinly slice the beef across the grain. Top the salads with the beef. Spoon the dressing over the salads. Sprinkle with the remaining ¼ cup cilantro.

> **TIPS, TRICKS & TIMESAVERS:** To get more juice out of a lime or other citrus fruit, warm it briefly in your hands or microwave on 100 percent power (high) for 10 seconds before juicing it.

PER SERVING: Calories **211** • Total Fat **4.5 g** • Saturated Fat **2.0 g** • Trans Fat **0.0 g**
Polyunsaturated Fat **0.5 g** • Monounsaturated Fat **2.0 g** • Cholesterol **56 mg**
Sodium **362 mg** • Carbohydrates **17 g** • Fiber **3 g** • Sugars **12 g** • Protein **26 g**
DIETARY EXCHANGES: 1 vegetable, ½ other carbohydrate, 3 lean meat

SERVES 4
3 ounces beef,
2 cups salad, and
2 tablespoons
dressing per serving

PREP TIME
10 minutes

COOKING TIME
15 minutes

STANDING TIME
10 minutes

Cooking spray

¼ teaspoon salt

¼ teaspoon pepper

1 pound boneless top sirloin steak, all visible fat discarded

⅓ cup fresh lime juice

3 tablespoons sugar

1 tablespoon plain rice vinegar

1 tablespoon water

2 teaspoons grated peeled gingerroot

¼ teaspoon salt

⅛ teaspoon crushed red pepper flakes

6 cups mixed spring greens

3 ounces snow peas, trimmed and cut into thirds diagonally

½ medium red bell pepper, cut into strips

¼ cup chopped cilantro and ¼ cup chopped cilantro, divided use

DRESSING

⅓ cup loosely packed
    assorted fresh herbs
    such as basil, dillweed,
    chives, tarragon, and
    chervil

¼ cup low-fat buttermilk

¼ cup fat-free plain Greek
    yogurt

1 small garlic clove

¼ teaspoon pepper

⅛ teaspoon salt

* * *

1 teaspoon canola or
    corn oil

(continued)

All-American Chopped Steak Salad with Creamy Herb Dressing

This hearty entrée salad, featuring some American favorites like meat and cheese, uses all chopped ingredients to allow the flavors to mingle. The salad is coated with fresh, aromatic herbs bathed in a creamy dressing.

1. In a food processor or blender, process the dressing ingredients until bright green and smooth.

2. In a medium nonstick skillet, heat the oil over medium-high heat, swirling to coat the bottom. Cook the beef for 3 minutes, or until browned on both sides, turning once halfway through. Reduce the heat to medium. Cook for 2 minutes, or until the desired doneness. Transfer to a cutting board. Let stand for 10 minutes. Cut the beef into thin slices. Coarsely chop the slices.

3. Meanwhile, put the romaine in a large salad bowl. Arrange the remaining salad ingredients except the Cheddar on the romaine. Top the salad with the beef. Sprinkle with the Cheddar. Serve the salad with the dressing.

PER SERVING: Calories **225** • Total Fat **6.0 g** • Saturated Fat **2.0 g** • Trans Fat **0.0 g**
Polyunsaturated Fat **0.5 g** • Monounsaturated Fat **3.0 g** • Cholesterol **59 mg**
Sodium **293 mg** • Carbohydrates **10 g** • Fiber **3 g** • Sugars **5 g** • Protein **32 g**
DIETARY EXCHANGES: 2 vegetable, 3½ lean meat

SALAD

1 1-pound boneless top sirloin steak, about 1 inch thick, all visible fat discarded

4 cups chopped romaine

1½ cups peeled and chopped cucumber

1¼ cups chopped tomato

1 cup chopped button mushrooms

½ cup chopped red onion

2 ounces fat-free sharp Cheddar cheese, finely chopped or shredded

PREP TIME
5 minutes

COOKING TIME
10 minutes

STANDING TIME
5 minutes

Romaine Roll-ups with Mediterranean Beef

To create these roll-ups, blend ground beef with plum tomatoes, Italian-style herbs, garlic, and red pepper flakes and wrap the mixture in crisp romaine leaves. You can pick them up to eat them or serve them as a "stuffed lettuce" salad with knives and forks. Fennel seeds, basil, and oregano provide a savory departure from the Asian flavors of the more familiar lettuce wrap.

1 teaspoon canola or corn oil

12 ounces extra-lean ground beef

¼ teaspoon crushed red pepper flakes

4 medium plum (Roma) tomatoes, diced

1½ teaspoons sugar

2 medium garlic cloves, minced

¼ teaspoon dried fennel seeds

2 tablespoons chopped fresh basil

2 teaspoons chopped fresh oregano

⅜ teaspoon salt

8 medium to large romaine leaves

¼ cup shredded or grated Parmesan cheese

1. In a large nonstick skillet, heat the oil over medium-high heat, swirling to coat the bottom. Cook the beef and red pepper flakes for 4 minutes, or until the beef is browned on the outside and no longer pink in the center, stirring frequently to turn and break up the beef.

2. Stir in the tomatoes, sugar, garlic, and fennel seeds. Reduce the heat to medium. Cook for 2 minutes, or until the tomatoes are just soft, stirring frequently. Remove from the heat.

3. Stir in the basil and oregano. Let stand for 5 minutes so the flavors blend and the mixture cools slightly. Sprinkle with the salt.

4. Spoon ⅓ cup of the beef mixture down the center of each romaine leaf. Sprinkle with the Parmesan. Fold the edges of the leaves toward the center so they overlap slightly.

PER SERVING: Calories **173** • Total Fat **7.0 g** • Saturated Fat **2.5 g** • Trans Fat **0.5 g** • Polyunsaturated Fat **1.0 g** • Monounsaturated Fat **3.0 g** • Cholesterol **50 mg** • Sodium **373 mg** • Carbohydrates **7 g** • Fiber **2 g** • Sugars **4 g** • Protein **22 g** • DIETARY EXCHANGES: 1 vegetable, 3 lean meat

Rosemary Steak and Arugula Salad with Pomegranate Dressing

SERVES 4
3 ounces beef and 1 cup salad per serving

PREP TIME
5 minutes

COOKING TIME
10 to 15 minutes

STANDING TIME
5 minutes

As a tart twist on traditional semisweet balsamic vinaigrette, this recipe uses pomegranate molasses to brighten up steak salad. *(See photo insert.)*

1. In a small bowl, stir together the rosemary, garlic, salt, and ½ teaspoon pepper. Sprinkle over the top of the beef.

2. In a large nonstick skillet or grill pan, cook the beef over medium heat for 3 to 4 minutes on each side, or until the internal temperature registers 130°F on an instant-read thermometer, for medium rare. Transfer the beef to a cutting board. Let stand for 5 minutes. The temperature will rise about 5 degrees.

3. Meanwhile, in a large bowl, whisk together the oil, molasses, and the remaining ¼ teaspoon pepper. Add the arugula and pomegranate seeds, tossing to coat. Transfer the salad to plates.

4. Cut the beef diagonally across the grain into thin slices. Serve the beef on the salad.

1 tablespoon minced fresh rosemary

2 medium garlic cloves, minced

½ teaspoon salt

½ teaspoon freshly ground pepper and ¼ teaspoon freshly ground pepper, divided use

1 1-pound boneless top sirloin steak, about ¾ inch thick, all visible fat discarded

1½ tablespoons extra-virgin olive oil

2 teaspoons pomegranate molasses

6 cups loosely packed arugula or baby arugula

½ cup pomegranate seeds, or arils

HEALTHY SWAP: You can find pomegranate molasses in the ethnic aisles of most supermarkets and in specialty grocery stores. Or, for this recipe, whisk together 1½ teaspoons 100% pomegranate juice, ½ teaspoon Dijon mustard (lowest sodium available), and a pinch of sugar (optional).

PER SERVING: Calories **224** • Total Fat **10.0 g** • Saturated Fat **2.5 g** • Trans Fat **0.0 g**
Polyunsaturated Fat **1.0 g** • Monounsaturated Fat **6.0 g** • Cholesterol **56 mg**
Sodium **349 mg** • Carbohydrates **9 g** • Fiber **2 g** • Sugars **6 g** • Protein **25 g**
DIETARY EXCHANGES: ½ fruit, 3 lean meat

SERVES 4
3 ounces pork,
1½ cups salad, and
1 tablespoon
dressing per serving

PREP TIME
15 minutes

COOKING TIME
10 minutes

STANDING TIME
3 minutes

1 teaspoon ground cumin

1 teaspoon pepper

¼ teaspoon salt and
¼ teaspoon salt,
divided use

4 boneless center-cut
pork chops (about
4 ounces each), all
visible fat discarded

1 teaspoon canola or corn
oil and 2 tablespoons
canola or corn oil,
divided use

* * *

8 ounces shredded
romaine

1 medium unpeeled
cucumber, diced

(continued)

Cumin Pork on Shredded Romaine with Anaheim Peppers

This crisp salad is brimming with authentic Mexican ingredients, including tomatillo, mild chiles, lime, and cilantro. The citrus-based vinaigrette lightly coats the salad, allowing the seasoned seared pork and the freshness of the vegetables to shine through.

1. In a small bowl, stir together the cumin, pepper, and ¼ teaspoon salt. Sprinkle over both sides of the pork. Using your fingertips, gently press the mixture so it adheres to the pork.

2. In a large nonstick skillet, heat 1 teaspoon oil over medium-high heat, swirling to coat the bottom. Cook the pork for 4 minutes on each side, or until slightly pink in the center. Transfer to a cutting board. Let stand for 3 minutes, or until the desired doneness. Cut into thin slices.

3. Meanwhile, in the order listed, arrange the romaine, cucumber, Anaheim peppers, onion, and tomatillo on plates. Dollop with the sour cream. Top with the pork.

4. In a small bowl, whisk together the lime juice and the remaining 2 tablespoons oil and ¼ teaspoon salt. Drizzle the mixture over the salads. Sprinkle with the cilantro. Serve with the lime wedges.

COOK'S TIP ON ANAHEIM PEPPERS: First brought to the Anaheim, California, area by farmer Emilio Ortega, these mild chiles originated in New Mexico. They are also known as California, Magdalena, or Ortega chiles. The New Mexican variety tends to be hotter than those grown in California.

PER SERVING: Calories **296** • Total Fat **14.5 g** • Saturated Fat **2.5 g** • Trans Fat **0.0 g** • Polyunsaturated Fat **3.5 g** • Monounsaturated Fat **7.5 g** • Cholesterol **65 mg** • Sodium **380 mg** • Carbohydrates **15 g** • Fiber **4 g** • Sugars **6 g** • Protein **27 g**
DIETARY EXCHANGES: 2 vegetable, ½ starch, 3 lean meat, 1 fat

2 medium Anaheim peppers, seeds and ribs discarded, cut crosswise into thin rounds (see Cook's Tip, page 261)

½ cup diced onion

1 medium tomatillo, papery husk discarded, diced

½ cup fat-free sour cream

2 tablespoons fresh lime juice

½ cup chopped fresh cilantro

1 medium lime, cut into 4 wedges

SERVES 6
½ cup vegetables,
1 cup greens, and
2 tablespoons
dressing per serving

PREP TIME
10 minutes

COOKING TIME
25 minutes

Grilled Summer Veggie Salad with Hummus Dressing

Smoky grilled summer vegetables and crisp salad greens get the royal treatment with this creamy dressing made from puréed chickpeas and seasoned with cumin, honey, green onions, and lemon juice. The crowning touch is a sprinkle of chickpeas and pumpkin seeds.

Cooking spray

1 small or ½ large red bell pepper

DRESSING

½ cup no-salt-added canned chickpeas, rinsed and drained

¼ cup unsweetened soy milk or ¼ cup fat-free milk

2 tablespoons chopped green onions (green part only)

2 tablespoons tahini (sesame seed paste)

2 tablespoons cider vinegar

1½ tablespoons fresh lemon juice

1 teaspoon Dijon mustard (lowest sodium available)

1 teaspoon honey

½ teaspoon ground cumin

1 medium garlic clove, crushed

⅛ teaspoon salt

(continued)

1. Lightly spray the grill rack with cooking spray. Preheat the grill on medium high. Put the bell pepper on the grill and close the lid. Grill for 15 minutes, or until the bell pepper skin is blistered and charred, turning frequently. Transfer to a paper bag. Close the bag. Set aside.

2. Meanwhile, in a food processor or blender, process the dressing ingredients for 1 minute, or until smooth and creamy. If the dressing seems too thick, stir in 1 or 2 tablespoons of water. Set aside.

3. Lightly brush both sides of the eggplant, zucchini, summer squash, and mushroom with the oil. Grill for 5 minutes on each side, or until the vegetables are tender and cooked through. Transfer to a cutting board and chop into ½-inch pieces.

4. In a large bowl, gently toss together the vegetables and basil.

5. Remove the bell pepper from the bag. Discard the skin, seeds, and ribs. Chop the flesh into ½-inch pieces. Stir into the eggplant mixture.

6. Put the salad greens on plates. Top with the eggplant mixture. Sprinkle with the remaining ¾ cup chickpeas and the pumpkin seeds. Drizzle with the dressing.

TIPS, TRICKS & TIMESAVERS: To make this recipe do double duty, grill and chop extra vegetables. Toss them with additional basil. Cover and refrigerate for up to one week. Stir together with whole-grain pasta, brown rice, or quinoa for a quick dinner, or use as a side dish to accompany grilled chicken or fish.

COOK'S TIP: The hummus dressing may thicken while in the refrigerator. To thin it out, just add 1 tablespoon of water at a time, whisking vigorously until the dressing is the desired consistency.

PER SERVING: Calories **182** • Total Fat **8.5 g** • Saturated Fat **1.0 g** • Trans Fat **0.0 g**
Polyunsaturated Fat **3.0 g** • Monounsaturated Fat **3.5 g** • Cholesterol **0 mg**
Sodium **103 mg** • Carbohydrates **21 g** • Fiber **7 g** • Sugars **5 g** • Protein **8 g**
DIETARY EXCHANGES: 1 starch, 1 vegetable, ½ lean meat, 1 fat

* * *

1 small eggplant, peeled and cut crosswise into ½-inch rounds

1 small zucchini, cut lengthwise into ½-inch slices

1 small yellow summer squash, cut lengthwise into ½-inch slices

1 small portobello mushroom cap, stem discarded

1 tablespoon canola or corn oil

¼ cup shredded fresh basil

6 cups tightly packed mixed salad greens

¾ cup no-salt-added canned chickpeas, rinsed and drained

¼ cup raw unsalted shelled pumpkin seeds

SERVES 4
1½ cups per serving

PREP TIME
10 minutes

COOKING TIME
15 minutes

Dilled Barley-Pasta Salad

Accented with the crunch of cucumber and suffused with the delicate flavor of dillweed, this pasta salad steps up a nutritious notch by using a whole-grain variety and adding a second whole grain—barley. As a time-saver, the pasta and barley cook together so you can get this wholesome meal on the table that much faster.

3 ounces dried whole-grain rotini

⅓ cup uncooked quick-cooking barley

½ 15.5-ounce can no-salt-added chickpeas, rinsed and drained

½ 14-ounce can quartered artichoke hearts, drained and coarsely chopped

½ medium cucumber, peeled if desired, chopped

6 large black olives, coarsely chopped

4 very thin slices fat-free Swiss cheese, cut into ½-inch squares

½ cup diced red onion

¼ cup chopped fresh dillweed

3 tablespoons cider vinegar

2 tablespoons canola or corn oil

2 medium garlic cloves, minced

1 teaspoon Dijon mustard (lowest sodium available)

⅛ teaspoon salt

1. Prepare the pasta and barley using the pasta package directions, omitting the salt. Transfer to a colander. Rinse with cold water. Drain well.

2. Meanwhile, in a large bowl, stir together the remaining ingredients except the salt.

3. Stir the pasta mixture into the chickpea mixture. Stir in the salt.

PER SERVING: Calories 302 • Total Fat 9.0 g • Saturated Fat 0.5 g • Trans Fat 0.0 g Polyunsaturated Fat 2.5 g • Monounsaturated Fat 5.0 g • Cholesterol 5 mg Sodium 581 mg • Carbohydrates 43 g • Fiber 7 g • Sugars 4 g • Protein 13 g DIETARY EXCHANGES: 2½ starch, 1 vegetable, 1 lean meat, 1 fat

Bulgur-Lentil Salad with Goat Cheese

SERVES 4
1 cup per serving

PREP TIME
10 minutes

COOKING TIME
30 to 35 minutes

Unlike dried beans, dried lentils are quick to prepare because they require no soaking time, so they can be easily included in your weeknight cooking repertoire. They are also a good source of protein and an ideal main ingredient for a vegetarian main dish.

1. In a large saucepan, bring the water and lentils to a boil over high heat. Reduce the heat and simmer, covered, for 15 minutes.

2. Stir in the bulgur. Cook, covered, for 12 to 14 minutes, or until the lentils are just tender. Transfer the mixture to a fine-mesh sieve. Rinse with cold water to cool. Drain well. Transfer to a serving bowl.

3. Stir in the remaining ingredients except the romaine.

4. Place the romaine leaves on plates. Top with the salad.

PER SERVING: Calories 259 • Total Fat 9.5 g • Saturated Fat 2.0 g • Trans Fat 0.0 g
Polyunsaturated Fat 2.0 g • Monounsaturated Fat 5.0 g • Cholesterol 5 mg
Sodium 343 mg • Carbohydrates 33 g • Fiber 8 g • Sugars 3 g • Protein 13 g
DIETARY EXCHANGES: 2 starch, 1 lean meat, 1 fat

3 cups water

½ cup dried lentils, sorted for stones and shriveled lentils, rinsed, and drained

½ cup uncooked instant, or fine-grain, bulgur

1 medium tomato, diced

½ medium unpeeled cucumber, diced

½ cup chopped fresh mint

1½ ounces soft goat cheese, low-fat blue cheese, or fat-free feta, crumbled

2 tablespoons fresh lemon juice

2 tablespoons canola or corn oil

½ teaspoon salt

4 large romaine leaves

PREP TIME
10 minutes

COOKING TIME
15 minutes

COOLING TIME
10 minutes

STANDING TIME
10 minutes

Panzanella Salad

Grab a fork and sit down to savor every morsel of this salad that abounds with the rustic flavors of Italy, courtesy of garlic, onion, basil, and olives. Rather than enjoying a piece of warm bread alongside your entrée, try a salad that includes toasted bread right *in* the meal to bring this dish together.

2 tablespoons extra-virgin olive oil

2 tablespoons red wine vinegar

2 medium garlic cloves, minced

½ teaspoon pepper

2 ounces multigrain Italian bread (lowest sodium available), cut into 1-inch cubes (about 2 cups total)

1 15.5-ounce can no-salt-added Great Northern or navy beans, rinsed and drained

1½ cups grape tomatoes, halved

1 cup loosely packed baby spinach

4 very thin slices fat-free Swiss cheese, torn into bite-size pieces

8 kalamata olives, coarsely chopped

¼ cup diced red onion

¼ cup chopped fresh basil

1. Preheat the oven to 350°F.

2. In a small bowl, whisk together the oil, vinegar, garlic, and pepper. Set aside.

3. On a large baking sheet, arrange the bread cubes in a single layer. Bake for 10 to 12 minutes, or until golden. Set aside to cool completely, about 10 minutes.

4. Meanwhile, in a large bowl, stir together the remaining ingredients. Stir in the bread cubes. Pour the dressing over the salad, tossing gently to coat well. Let stand for 10 minutes so the flavors blend.

PER SERVING: Calories **274** • Total Fat **10.0 g** • Saturated Fat **1.0 g** • Trans Fat **0.0 g** • Polyunsaturated Fat **1.5 g** • Monounsaturated Fat **6.5 g** • Cholesterol **2 mg** • Sodium **436 mg** • Carbohydrates **33 g** • Fiber **9 g** • Sugars **5 g** • Protein **13 g**
DIETARY EXCHANGES: 1½ starch, 2 vegetable, 1 lean meat, 1 fat

Creamy Dijon Vinaigrette

SERVES 4
2 tablespoons
per serving

PREP TIME
5 minutes

This tangy salad dressing is a fresh, healthy alternative to the bottled varieties, and it takes only a few minutes to whip together. Use it on dark, leafy greens or drizzled over grilled fish, chicken, or pork—even over steamed or roasted vegetables.

In a food processor or blender, process all the ingredients until smooth. Serve the same day for peak flavor.

PER SERVING: Calories 77 • Total Fat **5.5 g** • Saturated Fat **0.5 g** • Trans Fat **0.0 g** • Polyunsaturated Fat **1.5 g** • Monounsaturated Fat **3.5 g** • Cholesterol **4 mg** • Sodium **133 mg** • Carbohydrates **5 g** • Fiber **0 g** • Sugars **2 g** • Protein **2 g**
DIETARY EXCHANGES: ½ other carbohydrate, 1 fat

⅓ cup fat-free sour cream

3 tablespoons fat-free milk

2 tablespoons diced onion

2 tablespoons fresh basil

1½ tablespoons canola or corn oil

2 teaspoons cider vinegar

1½ teaspoons Dijon mustard (lowest sodium available)

1 medium garlic clove, minced

⅛ teaspoon salt

¼ cup fresh parsley

3 small pimiento-stuffed green olives

2½ tablespoons extra-virgin olive oil

2 tablespoons dry white wine (regular or nonalcoholic)

½ teaspoon grated lemon zest

1½ tablespoons fresh lemon juice

1 tablespoon fresh oregano

1 medium garlic clove, minced

½ teaspoon fresh rosemary

⅛ teaspoon salt

Italian Vinaigrette

In just a few minutes, you can have an herb-infused dressing that will bring new freshness to any salad. With such lively flavors, a little goes a long way.

In a food processor or blender, process all the ingredients until smooth. Serve immediately for peak flavor.

COOK'S TIP: Be sure to use a dry white wine, such as a Chardonnay, Sauvignon Blanc, or Pinot Grigio, to make this dressing. Avoid using sweeter whites, such as Riesling or Moscato.

PER SERVING: Calories 88 • Total Fat 9.0 g • Saturated Fat 1.0 g • Trans Fat 0.0 g Polyunsaturated Fat 1.0 g • Monounsaturated Fat 6.5 g • Cholesterol 0 mg Sodium 138 mg • Carbohydrates 1 g • Fiber 0 g • Sugars 0 g • Protein 0 g DIETARY EXCHANGES: 2 fat

Raspberry-Blackberry Dressing

SERVES 8
2 tablespoons
per serving

PREP TIME
5 minutes

Bursting with fresh berry flavor, this zingy dressing is a natural for green salads, but you also can use it as a sauce for melon and other fruits. For an even fruitier taste, try lemon or lime juice instead of the vinegar.

½ cup raspberries

½ cup blackberries

¼ cup 100% cranberry juice

2½ tablespoons sugar

2½ tablespoons red wine vinegar

1 tablespoon canola or corn oil

¼ teaspoon almond extract

⅛ teaspoon salt

In a food processor or blender, process all the ingredients until smooth. Place a fine-mesh sieve over a small bowl. Drain the fruit mixture, using a rubber spatula to press out any juices. Discard the seeds. (For a poppy-seed-like, crunchy texture, skip the straining step.) Cover and refrigerate for up to three days.

PER SERVING: Calories **42** • Total Fat **2.0 g** • Saturated Fat **0.0 g** • Trans Fat **0.0 g** Polyunsaturated Fat **0.5 g** • Monounsaturated Fat **1.0 g** • Cholesterol **0 mg** Sodium **37 mg** • Carbohydrates **7 g** • Fiber **1 g** • Sugars **6 g** • Protein **0 g** DIETARY EXCHANGES: ½ other carbohydrate, ½ fat

SEAFOOD

Blackened Fish with Crisp Kale and Creamy Lemon Sauce

SERVES 4
3 ounces fish
and 2 heaping
tablespoons sauce
per serving

PREP TIME
5 minutes

COOKING TIME
20 minutes

A tangy, creamy, lemony sauce adds coolness to this smoky, peppery whitefish, while baked kale adds crispness to the meal.

1. Preheat the oven to 400°F. Lightly spray a 13 × 9 × 2-inch baking dish and a rimmed baking sheet with cooking spray.

2. Arrange the fish in a single layer in the baking dish. Arrange the kale in a single layer on the baking sheet.

3. In a small bowl, stir together 1 tablespoon thyme, the paprika, pepper, salt, and cayenne. Sprinkle over both sides of the fish. Place the fish on the center rack of the oven and the kale on the top rack. Bake the fish and the kale for 8 to 10 minutes, or until the fish flakes easily when tested with a fork and the kale stems are tender and the leaves are crisp and slightly browned.

4. Meanwhile, in a small bowl, whisk together the yogurt, lemon zest, lemon juice, and the remaining 1 tablespoon thyme.

5. Just before serving, top each fillet with the yogurt mixture. Serve with the lemon wedges.

Olive oil cooking spray

4 firm white fish fillets, such as whitefish, halibut, or walleyed pike (about 4 ounces each), rinsed and patted dry

8 large curly kale leaves, any large stems discarded

1 tablespoon chopped fresh thyme and 1 tablespoon chopped fresh thyme, divided use

1 teaspoon paprika (smoked preferred)

½ teaspoon freshly ground pepper

¼ teaspoon salt

¼ teaspoon cayenne

½ cup fat-free plain Greek yogurt

1½ teaspoons grated lemon zest

1 teaspoon fresh lemon juice

1 medium lemon, cut into 4 wedges

COOK'S TIP: Use curly kale for this dish because it bakes well, browning slightly on the edges and softening in the middle. Don't use flat-leaf, or Tuscan, kale, which is great when used raw in salads but can overbake and develop a bitter taste.

PER SERVING: Calories 143 • Total Fat 2.5 g • Saturated Fat 0.5 g • Trans Fat 0.0 g
Polyunsaturated Fat 0.5 g • Monounsaturated Fat 0.5 g • Cholesterol 57 mg
Sodium 228 mg • Carbohydrates 5 g • Fiber 1 g • Sugars 1 g • Protein 26 g
DIETARY EXCHANGES: 1 vegetable, 3 lean meat

SERVES 4
3 ounces fish
and scant
1½ tablespoons
sauce per serving

PREP TIME
5 minutes

COOKING TIME
15 minutes

Cod and Cherry Tomatoes with Spinach-Herb Sauce

High-heat roasting is the key to this quick meal. The intense heat sears the fish while the short roasting time preserves the color and shape of the tomatoes. You make the sauce while the fish and tomatoes are cooking, saving some time.

Olive oil cooking spray

4 cod fillets (about
    4 ounces each), about
    1 inch thick, rinsed
    and patted dry

1½ cups cherry tomatoes,
    halved

⅛ teaspoon salt

⅛ teaspoon pepper

SAUCE

1 cup tightly packed baby
    spinach

⅓ cup tightly packed
    assorted fresh herbs
    such as basil, dillweed,
    tarragon, chives, and
    cilantro

1 teaspoon chopped
    walnuts, dry-roasted

1 medium garlic clove

¼ cup fat-free, low-
    sodium chicken broth

1 tablespoon shredded
    or grated Parmesan
    cheese

1. Preheat the oven to 450°F. Line a small rimmed baking sheet with aluminum foil. Lightly spray the foil with cooking spray.

2. Arrange the fish and tomatoes in a single layer on the baking sheet. Lightly sprinkle the salt and pepper over the fish. Lightly spray the fish and tomatoes with cooking spray.

3. Bake for 8 to 10 minutes, or until the fish flakes easily when tested with a fork and the tomatoes are slightly soft. Transfer the fish to plates. Set aside the tomatoes. Set aside 2 tablespoons of the cooking juices.

4. Meanwhile, in a food processor or blender, process the spinach, herbs, walnuts, and garlic until finely chopped. With the motor running, slowly pour in the broth through the feed tube. Process until almost smooth.

5. Transfer the spinach mixture to a small saucepan. Stir in the Parmesan and reserved cooking juices. Cook over medium heat for 1 minute, or until heated through, stirring constantly. Spoon the sauce over the fish. Serve the tomatoes on the side.

COOK'S TIP: Dry-roasting the nuts intensifies their flavor.

PER SERVING: Calories **125** • Total Fat **2.0 g** • Saturated Fat **0.5 g** • Trans Fat **0.0 g**
Polyunsaturated Fat **0.5 g** • Monounsaturated Fat **0.5 g** • Cholesterol **50 mg**
Sodium **173 mg** • Carbohydrates **5 g** • Fiber **1 g** • Sugars **3 g** • Protein **22 g**
DIETARY EXCHANGES: 1 vegetable, 3 lean meat

Chard-Wrapped Cod with Balsamic Glaze

A lightning-fast balsamic glaze sweetens cod fillets that are encased within bitter greens.

1. Arrange the chard on a large microwaveable plate. Microwave on 100 percent power (high) for 15 to 20 seconds, or until the leaves are just softened.

2. Sprinkle the salt and pepper over the fish. Wrap each fillet in a chard leaf, enclosing as much of the fish as possible.

3. In a large skillet, heat the oil over medium heat. Carefully place the wrapped fish in the skillet with the seam side down. Cook for 3 to 4 minutes on each side, or until the fish flakes easily when tested with a fork and the chard is tender. Transfer to serving plates.

4. In the same skillet, cook the garlic for 30 seconds, or until fragrant, stirring constantly. Stir in the vinegar and mustard. Cook for 1 minute, or until the mixture is reduced by half (to about 2 tablespoons) and slightly thickened, stirring occasionally. Drizzle the glaze over the fish.

PER SERVING: Calories **142** • Total Fat **4.5 g** • Saturated Fat **0.5 g** • Trans Fat **0.0 g** Polyunsaturated Fat **0.5 g** • Monounsaturated Fat **2.5 g** • Cholesterol **49 mg** Sodium **266 mg** • Carbohydrates **4 g** • Fiber **0 g** • Sugars **4 g** • Protein **21 g** DIETARY EXCHANGES: 3 lean meat

SERVES 4
3 ounces fish and 1½ teaspoons glaze per serving

PREP TIME
5 minutes

COOKING TIME
10 minutes

4 large Swiss chard leaves, tough stems discarded

¼ teaspoon salt

¼ teaspoon freshly ground pepper

4 cod or scrod fillets (about 4 ounces each), rinsed and patted dry

1 tablespoon olive oil

1 medium garlic clove, minced

¼ cup balsamic vinegar

1 teaspoon Dijon mustard (lowest sodium available)

Nutty Baked Flounder

A light lemony sauce and nutty coating enhance mild flounder, a rich source of vitamin D. The two-ingredient coating is extremely easy to make and the sauce is just as quick, so this is a go-to recipe when you're in the mood for flavorful, fast fish.

Cooking spray

4 flounder or other mild fish fillets (about 4 ounces each), rinsed and patted dry

¼ cup plus 2 tablespoons slivered almonds, dry-roasted and very finely chopped

SAUCE

3 tablespoons light tub margarine, melted

2 teaspoons fresh lemon juice

1½ teaspoons Worcestershire sauce (lowest sodium available)

⅛ teaspoon salt

¼ teaspoon pepper

1. Preheat the oven to 450°F. Line a baking sheet with aluminum foil. Lightly spray the foil with cooking spray.

2. Put the fish on the baking sheet. Lightly spray both sides of the fish with cooking spray. Sprinkle the almonds over both sides of the fish. Using your fingertips, gently press the almonds so they adhere to the fish. Bake for 10 minutes, or until the fish flakes easily when tested with a fork.

3. Meanwhile, in a small bowl, whisk together the sauce ingredients.

4. Transfer the fish to plates. Spoon the sauce over the fish.

PER SERVING: Calories **162** • Total Fat **11.0 g** • Saturated Fat **1.0 g** • Trans Fat **0.0 g** • Polyunsaturated Fat **2.5 g** • Monounsaturated Fat **5.5 g** • Cholesterol **44 mg** • Sodium **433 mg** • Carbohydrates **3 g** • Fiber **1 g** • Sugars **1 g** • Protein **14 g**
DIETARY EXCHANGES: 2 lean meat, 1 fat

Grouper with Tarragon-Lemon Sour Cream Sauce

SERVES 4
3 ounces fish and
2 tablespoons sauce
per serving

PREP TIME
5 minutes

COOKING TIME
10 minutes

Tarragon is often paired with lemon to give dishes a well-balanced taste. It has a flavor that's similar to anise or fennel, which is somewhat sweet with a faint hint of licorice. For this recipe, the winning combination is whisked together with sour cream to create a sauce that's just perfect for a hearty fish.

1. Lightly spray the grill rack with cooking spray. Preheat the grill on medium high.

2. In a small bowl, whisk together the sauce ingredients. Set aside.

3. Rub the fish on both sides with the cut side of the garlic halves. Sprinkle with the pepper and salt. Lightly spray both sides of the fish with cooking spray.

4. Grill for 3 minutes on each side, or until the fish flakes easily when tested with a fork.

5. Spoon the sauce over the fish. Drizzle the oil over the sauce. Serve with the lemon wedges.

Cooking spray

SAUCE

½ cup fat-free sour cream

2 teaspoons chopped fresh tarragon

1 medium garlic clove, minced

½ teaspoon grated lemon zest

¼ teaspoon salt

* * *

4 grouper or other firm fish fillets (about 4 ounces each), rinsed and patted dry

1 medium garlic clove, halved crosswise

½ teaspoon pepper

¼ teaspoon salt

2 teaspoons extra-virgin olive oil

1 medium lemon, cut into 4 wedges

COOK'S TIP ON TARRAGON: Use leftover tarragon in a mixed salad dressed with a lemony vinaigrette.

PER SERVING: Calories 158 • Total Fat 3.5 g • Saturated Fat 0.5 g • Trans Fat 0.0 g
Polyunsaturated Fat 0.5 g • Monounsaturated Fat 2.0 g • Cholesterol 47 mg
Sodium 376 mg • Carbohydrates 6 g • Fiber 0 g • Sugars 2 g • Protein 24 g
DIETARY EXCHANGES: ½ other carbohydrate, 3 lean meat

SERVES 4
3 ounces fish and
½ cup vegetables
per serving

PREP TIME
15 minutes

COOKING TIME
15 minutes

8 ounces asparagus
   spears, trimmed and
   cut diagonally into
   2-inch pieces

1 large carrot, cut into
   matchstick-size strips

1 medium leek (white
   and light green
   parts only), halved
   lengthwise, each half
   cut lengthwise into
   ⅜-inch strips

4 halibut steaks (about
   4 ounces each), about
   1 inch thick, rinsed
   and patted dry

¼ teaspoon salt

¼ teaspoon pepper

4 fresh sprigs of tarragon,
   about 4 inches long

2 tablespoons sliced
   chives

2 teaspoons olive oil

Herbed Halibut and Spring Vegetables en Papillote

Baking food in a parchment packet is a French technique known as *en papillote*—it's easy and yields delectable results. For this recipe, a halibut fillet and a sprig of fresh tarragon are baked on a bed of spring vegetables in each packet. As the packets bake, the delicate juices from the fish and vegetables mingle to create a mouthwatering flavor. *(See photo insert.)*

1. Preheat the oven to 425°F. Cut eight 15-inch-long sheets of cooking parchment or aluminum foil. Set aside.

2. Place the asparagus in the center of four of the parchment sheets. Place the carrot and leek on the asparagus. Place the fish on the vegetables. Sprinkle with the salt and pepper. Place a tarragon sprig on each piece of fish. Sprinkle with the chives. Drizzle with the oil. Place one of the remaining four sheets of parchment over the fish. Fold the edges toward the center. Holding the tops together, fold several times to seal securely. Transfer the packets to a large rimmed baking sheet. (The packets can be made up to 6 hours in advance. Cover and refrigerate until baking time.)

3. Bake for 10 minutes. Using the tines of a fork, carefully open a packet away from you (to prevent steam burns). If the fish flakes easily when tested with a fork, carefully open the remaining packets and serve. If the fish isn't cooked enough, reclose the open packet and bake all the packets for 1 to 2 minutes. Serve the fish and vegetables in the packets.

PER SERVING: Calories 156 • Total Fat **4.0 g** • Saturated Fat **0.5 g** • Trans Fat **0.0 g** Polyunsaturated Fat **0.5 g** • Monounsaturated Fat **2.0 g** • Cholesterol **56 mg** Sodium **241 mg** • Carbohydrates **7 g** • Fiber **2 g** • Sugars **3 g** • Protein **23 g** DIETARY EXCHANGES: 1 vegetable, 3 lean meat

Grilled Halibut with Green Onion and Avocado Salsa

SERVES 4
3 ounces fish and
½ cup salsa
per serving

PREP TIME
5 minutes

COOKING TIME
10 minutes

Grilled halibut goes from good to great with an outstandingly fresh salsa made from avocado, cucumber, and tomato.

1. Lightly spray the grill rack with cooking spray. Preheat the grill on medium high.

2. In a medium bowl, gently stir together the salsa ingredients. Set aside.

3. Sprinkle the fish on both sides with the pepper. Lightly spray both sides of the fish with cooking spray.

4. Brush both sides of the green onions with the oil.

5. Grill the fish and green onions for 3 minutes on each side, or until the fish flakes easily when tested with a fork and the green onions are richly browned. Transfer the fish to a platter and the green onions to a cutting board.

6. Quickly chop the green onions. Stir into the salsa.

7. Squeeze the lime wedges over the fish. Spoon the salsa over the fish.

Cooking spray

SALSA

1 medium avocado, diced

½ cup peeled and diced cucumber

½ cup grape tomatoes, quartered

1 tablespoon cider vinegar

¼ teaspoon salt

* * *

4 halibut steaks or other firm fish fillets (about 4 ounces each), rinsed and patted dry

½ teaspoon pepper

4 medium green onions

2 teaspoons canola or corn oil

1 medium lime, cut into 4 wedges

PER SERVING: Calories **227** • Total Fat **11.5 g** • Saturated Fat **1.5 g** • Trans Fat **0.0 g**
Polyunsaturated Fat **2.0 g** • Monounsaturated Fat **7.0 g** • Cholesterol **56 mg**
Sodium **234 mg** • Carbohydrates **9 g** • Fiber **5 g** • Sugars **3 g** • Protein **23 g**
DIETARY EXCHANGES: 2 vegetable, 3 lean meat, ½ fat

SERVES 4
3 ounces fish and
1 tablespoon sauce
per serving

PREP TIME
5 minutes

COOKING TIME
15 minutes

Cooking spray

**4 salmon fillets with skin
(about 5 ounces each),
rinsed and patted dry**

SAUCE

**1 teaspoon grated orange
zest**

**2 tablespoons fresh
orange juice**

2 tablespoons honey

**1½ tablespoons soy
sauce (lowest sodium
available)**

**1 tablespoon white
balsamic vinegar**

**1 medium jalapeño, seeds
and ribs discarded,
finely chopped (see
Cook's Tip, page 261)**

* * *

⅛ teaspoon salt

Orange-Honey Salmon

This tangy salmon dish is a delicious way to get in half your omega-3s for the week, along with a hefty dose of vitamin D. It's not only super healthy but also super simple to make.

1. Preheat the broiler. Line a baking sheet with aluminum foil. Lightly spray the foil with cooking spray.

2. Put the fish on the baking sheet with the skin side down.

3. In a small saucepan, whisk together the sauce ingredients. Spoon 1 teaspoon sauce over each fillet.

4. Broil the fish about 6 inches from the heat for 8 minutes, or until the desired doneness.

5. Meanwhile, bring the remaining sauce to a boil over medium-high heat. Boil for 1 to 2 minutes, or until reduced by 1½ tablespoons (to about ¼ cup).

6. Transfer the fish to a serving plate. Spoon the sauce over the fish. Sprinkle with the salt.

PER SERVING: Calories **218** • Total Fat **6.0 g** • Saturated Fat **1.0 g** • Trans Fat **0.0 g**
Polyunsaturated Fat **1.0 g** • Monounsaturated Fat **2.0 g** • Cholesterol **62 mg**
Sodium **323 mg** • Carbohydrates **11 g** • Fiber **0 g** • Sugars **11 g** • Protein **28 g**
DIETARY EXCHANGES: 1 other carbohydrate, 2 lean meat

Broiled Salmon over Garden-Fresh Corn and Bell Peppers

SERVES 4
3 ounces fish and
½ cup corn mixture
per serving

PREP TIME
10 minutes

COOKING TIME
15 minutes

Celebrate summer with a dish that marries seasonal local corn, bell peppers, and garden-grown basil and mint with the rich taste of salmon. Serve this dish with brown rice, whole-wheat couscous, or quinoa, and dinner is ready! *(See photo insert.)*

1. Preheat the broiler. Line a baking sheet with aluminum foil. Lightly spray the foil with cooking spray.

2. Put the fish on the baking sheet. Sprinkle 1 tablespoon basil, 1 teaspoon mint, ⅛ teaspoon salt, and ⅛ teaspoon pepper over the top of the fish. Lightly spray with cooking spray.

3. In a large nonstick skillet, heat the oil over medium heat, swirling to coat the bottom. Cook the onion for 1 minute, stirring frequently. Stir in the bell peppers. Cook for 1 minute, stirring frequently. Stir in the corn. Cook for 5 to 6 minutes, or until the onion is soft and the vegetables are tender-crisp, stirring occasionally. Remove from the heat.

4. Stir in the remaining 3 tablespoons basil, 1 teaspoon mint, ⅛ teaspoon salt, and ⅛ teaspoon pepper.

5. Meanwhile, broil the fish about 4 to 6 inches from the heat for 5 to 8 minutes, or until the desired doneness.

6. Transfer the onion mixture to plates. Top with the fish.

COOK'S TIP: Look for packages of sweet baby bell peppers in red, orange, and yellow so you'll have an assortment of colors for this recipe.

Cooking spray

4 salmon fillets (about 4 ounces each), about 1 inch thick, rinsed and patted dry

1 tablespoon chopped fresh basil and 3 tablespoons chopped fresh basil, divided use

1 teaspoon chopped fresh mint and 1 teaspoon chopped fresh mint, divided use

⅛ teaspoon salt and ⅛ teaspoon salt, divided use

⅛ teaspoon pepper and ⅛ teaspoon pepper, divided use

2 teaspoons olive oil

½ cup coarsely chopped red onion

¾ cup chopped bell peppers

2 cups corn kernels, cut from 3 or 4 medium ears of corn, husks and silk discarded

PER SERVING: Calories 245 • Total Fat 8.5 g • Saturated Fat 1.5 g • Trans Fat 0.0 g
Polyunsaturated Fat 1.5 g • Monounsaturated Fat 3.5 g • Cholesterol 53 mg
Sodium 245 mg • Carbohydrates 17 g • Fiber 2 g • Sugars 6 g • Protein 27 g
DIETARY EXCHANGES: 1 starch, 3 lean meat

SERVES 4
3 ounces fish and
2/3 cup pasta
per serving

PREP TIME
5 minutes

COOKING TIME
25 minutes

Wine-Poached Salmon with Spinach and Whole-Grain Linguine

Poaching, a healthful cooking technique, keeps you from overcooking fish and infuses salmon with subtle flavors. Leeks and white wine add a provincial French appeal to this dish.

½ teaspoon salt

¼ teaspoon freshly ground pepper

4 salmon fillets (about 4 ounces each), rinsed and patted dry

2 teaspoons olive oil

1 cup thinly sliced leeks (white part only)

½ cup dry white wine (regular or nonalcoholic)

½ cup water

4 ounces dried whole-grain linguine

4 cups tightly packed baby spinach

⅓ cup fat-free plain Greek yogurt

1½ tablespoons chopped fresh dillweed

1. Sprinkle the salt and pepper over both sides of the fish.

2. In a large skillet, heat the oil over medium heat, swirling to coat the bottom. Cook the leeks for 2 minutes, or until softened, stirring occasionally. Push them to the outer edges of the skillet.

3. Cook the fish in the center of the skillet for 2 minutes. Turn over. Pour in the wine and water. Reduce the heat and simmer, covered, for 5 to 6 minutes, or until the fish is the desired doneness.

4. Meanwhile, prepare the pasta using the package directions, omitting the salt. Set aside 2 tablespoons of the cooking water. Drain the pasta well in a colander. Transfer to a bowl. Stir in the reserved cooking water.

5. In a large microwaveable bowl, microwave the spinach on 100 percent power (high) for 20 seconds, or until slightly wilted. Stir into the pasta. Transfer to plates.

6. Using a slotted spatula, top the pasta mixture with the fish and leeks. Set aside 3 tablespoons of the poaching liquid.

7. In a medium bowl, whisk together the yogurt and reserved poaching liquid. Whisk in the dillweed. Spoon the sauce over the fish, leeks, and pasta.

PER SERVING: Calories 320 • Total Fat 8.5 g • Saturated Fat 1.5 g • Trans Fat 0.0 g Polyunsaturated Fat 1.5 g • Monounsaturated Fat 3.5 g • Cholesterol 53 mg Sodium 415 mg • Carbohydrates 26 g • Fiber 4 g • Sugars 3 g • Protein 30 g DIETARY EXCHANGES: 1½ starch, 1 vegetable, 3 lean meat

Lemon-Baked Tilapia with Dijon Topping

Cooking these tilapia fillets on lemon slices prevents the fish from drying out, imparts a delicate citrus flavor, and makes for a pleasing presentation.

SERVES 4
3 ounces fish and
1 tablespoon
topping per serving

PREP TIME
5 minutes

COOKING TIME
20 minutes

1. Preheat the oven to 375°F. Line a baking sheet with aluminum foil.

2. Arrange the lemon slices on the baking sheet in 4 rows of 2 slices each. Place a fish fillet on each row of lemon slices.

3. In a small bowl, stir together the paprika, pepper, and ⅛ teaspoon salt. Sprinkle over the top of the fish.

4. Bake for 15 minutes, or until the fish flakes easily when tested with a fork.

5. Meanwhile, in the same small bowl, stir together the topping ingredients.

6. Using a slotted spatula, transfer the fillets (on the lemon slices if desired) to plates. Spoon the topping over the fish.

1 medium lemon, cut into 8 slices

4 tilapia fillets (about 4 ounces each), rinsed and patted dry

½ teaspoon paprika

¼ teaspoon pepper

⅛ teaspoon salt

TOPPING

¼ cup light tub margarine

2 tablespoons finely chopped green onions

1 tablespoon chopped fresh Italian (flat-leaf) parsley

1 teaspoon fresh thyme

1 teaspoon Dijon mustard (lowest sodium available)

½ teaspoon finely chopped fresh rosemary

⅛ teaspoon salt

PER SERVING: Calories 154 • Total Fat **6.5 g** • Saturated Fat **0.5 g** • Trans Fat **0.0 g**
Polyunsaturated Fat **1.5 g** • Monounsaturated Fat **3.0 g** • Cholesterol **57 mg**
Sodium **322 mg** • Carbohydrates **1 g** • Fiber **0 g** • Sugars **0 g** • Protein **23 g**
DIETARY EXCHANGES: 3 lean meat

⅓ cup fresh orange juice

2 tablespoons fresh lime juice

1 tablespoon soy sauce (lowest sodium available)

1 medium garlic clove, minced

½ teaspoon ground cumin

½ teaspoon paprika

¼ teaspoon pepper

4 tilapia fillets (about 4 ounces each), rinsed and patted dry

2 tablespoons chopped fresh parsley

Citrus-Soy Tilapia

While the fish cooks, the liquid in the pan reduces to an intensely flavored citrusy glaze. Serve the tilapia over brown rice and with a side salad of baby arugula.

1. In a large nonstick skillet, stir together the orange juice, lime juice, soy sauce, garlic, cumin, paprika, and pepper. Bring to a boil over medium-high heat. Add the fish. Return to a boil. Reduce the heat and simmer for 5 to 6 minutes, or until the fish flakes easily when tested with a fork and the liquid is slightly thickened and reduced to a glaze, turning the fish once halfway through.

2. Just before serving, sprinkle with the parsley.

COOK'S TIP: You'll want the liquid in the pan to be at a high simmer or gentle boil while the fish cooks. It needs to bubble enough for the liquid to cook down to a glaze. If the liquid is reducing faster than the fish is cooking, reduce the heat. Alternatively, increase the heat if the fish is nearly done and the glaze looks too runny.

PER SERVING: Calories **127** • Total Fat **2.0 g** • Saturated Fat **0.5 g** • Trans Fat **0.0 g**
Polyunsaturated Fat **0.5 g** • Monounsaturated Fat **0.5 g** • Cholesterol **57 mg**
Sodium **159 mg** • Carbohydrates **4 g** • Fiber **0 g** • Sugars **3 g** • Protein **23 g**
DIETARY EXCHANGES: 3 lean meat

Tomato-Basil Tilapia

Serve these delicate fillets smothered with fresh tomatoes, basil, garlic, and lemon over brown rice or whole-grain spaghetti. While the fish is cooking, put together a simple dark green leafy salad, steam a head of broccoli, or make Broccolini with Toasted Walnuts (page 219) to serve alongside.

1. Preheat the oven to 375°F. Line a baking sheet with aluminum foil. Lightly spray the foil with cooking spray.

2. Put the fish on the baking sheet. Spoon 1 tablespoon lemon juice over the fish. Sprinkle the pepper and 1/8 teaspoon salt over the fish. Bake for 15 minutes, or until the fish flakes easily when tested with a fork.

3. Meanwhile, in a small bowl, stir together the topping ingredients. Spoon over the fish.

PER SERVING: Calories 154 • Total Fat 5.5 g • Saturated Fat 1.0 g • Trans Fat 0.0 g
Polyunsaturated Fat 1.0 g • Monounsaturated Fat 3.0 g • Cholesterol 3 mg
Sodium 281 mg • Carbohydrates 4 g • Fiber 1 g • Sugars 2 g • Protein 24 g
DIETARY EXCHANGES: 3 lean meat

SERVES 4
3 ounces fish and
1/2 cup tomato
mixture per serving

PREP TIME
10 minutes

COOKING TIME
20 minutes

Cooking spray

4 tilapia or other mild fish fillets (about 4 ounces each), rinsed and patted dry

1 tablespoon fresh lemon juice

1/2 teaspoon pepper

1/8 teaspoon salt

TOPPING

2 medium tomatoes, diced

1/4 cup chopped fresh basil

1 tablespoon extra-virgin olive oil

1/2 teaspoon grated lemon zest

1 tablespoon fresh lemon juice

1 medium garlic clove, minced

1/4 teaspoon salt

SERVES 4
3 ounces fish and
2 tablespoons sauce
per serving

PREP TIME
5 minutes

COOKING TIME
10 minutes

Braised Trout with Blueberry-Maple Sauce

The subtle sweetness of blueberries, plus a shot of more pronounced sweetness from maple syrup, is the perfect complement to trout fillets.

1 cup blueberries

1 tablespoon pure maple syrup

½ teaspoon grated lemon zest

1½ teaspoons fresh lemon juice

⅛ teaspoon pepper and ¼ teaspoon pepper, divided use

⅛ teaspoon salt

¾ cup fat-free, low-sodium vegetable broth

¼ cup chopped fresh parsley and chopped fresh parsley to taste, divided use

4 trout fillets (about 4 ounces each), rinsed and patted dry

1. In a small saucepan, stir together the blueberries, maple syrup, lemon zest, lemon juice, ⅛ teaspoon pepper, and salt. Bring to a boil over medium-high heat. Reduce the heat and simmer for 8 to 10 minutes, or until the sauce is slightly thickened, stirring occasionally. As the blueberries cook, using the back of a spoon, gently press some to break them open, leaving a few unbroken.

2. Meanwhile, in a large skillet, bring the broth, ¼ cup parsley, and the remaining ¼ teaspoon pepper to a boil over high heat. Add the fish. Return to a boil. Reduce the heat and simmer for 5 to 6 minutes, or until the fish flakes easily when tested with a fork, turning once halfway through. Using a slotted spatula, transfer the fish to plates. Spoon the sauce over the fish. Sprinkle with the remaining parsley to taste.

PER SERVING: Calories 173 • Total Fat 4.0 g • Saturated Fat 1.0 g • Trans Fat 0.0 g
Polyunsaturated Fat 1.5 g • Monounsaturated Fat 1.5 g • Cholesterol 67 mg
Sodium 115 mg • Carbohydrates 9 g • Fiber 1 g • Sugars 7 g • Protein 24 g
DIETARY EXCHANGES: ½ fruit, 3 lean meat

Sautéed Trout with Herb Vinaigrette

SERVES 4
3 ounces fish
and 2 teaspoons
vinaigrette
per serving

PREP TIME
5 minutes

COOKING TIME
10 minutes

With only a few ingredients and a few minutes, you can put this super-fast sautéed fish dish on the table. The perfect pairing of equal parts of fresh herb and vinegar keeps this entrée as simple as can be and, best of all, simply delicious.

1. Sprinkle half the salt and pepper over the top of the fish.

2. In a large nonstick skillet, heat the oil over medium-high heat, swirling to coat the bottom. Place the fish in the skillet with the seasoned side down. Sprinkle the remaining half of the salt and pepper over the fish. Cook for 5 to 6 minutes, or until the fish flakes easily when tested with a fork, turning once halfway through. Transfer to a platter. Cover to keep warm.

3. Pour the vinegar into the skillet. Using a rubber scraper or wooden spoon, stir, scraping to dislodge any browned bits. Work quickly, as the vinegar will bubble and begin to evaporate. Stir in the chives. Spoon the vinaigrette over the fish.

¼ teaspoon salt

¼ teaspoon pepper

4 trout fillets (about 4 ounces each), rinsed and patted dry

1 tablespoon olive oil

2 tablespoons sherry vinegar, champagne vinegar, or plain rice vinegar

2 tablespoons chopped fresh chives, parsley, or chervil

HEALTHY SWAP: If you don't have any of the types of vinegars or herbs listed on hand, you can substitute any kind of mild vinegar or fresh herb you have available.

PER SERVING: Calories **166** • Total Fat **7.5 g** • Saturated Fat **1.5 g** • Trans Fat **0.0 g**
Polyunsaturated Fat **2.0 g** • Monounsaturated Fat **4.0 g** • Cholesterol **67 mg**
Sodium **181 mg** • Carbohydrates **0 g** • Fiber **0 g** • Sugars **0 g** • Protein **23 g**
DIETARY EXCHANGES: 3 lean meat

Tuna Kebabs with Asian Dipping Sauce

Grilled tuna is the ideal foil for this Asian sauce that boasts a perfect balance of flavors—a smidgen of sweet, a speck of spice, a touch of tang, and a note of nuttiness from the sesame oil.

1. Soak four 12-inch wooden skewers for at least 10 minutes in cold water to keep them from charring, or use metal skewers.

2. Meanwhile, in a small bowl, whisk together the sauce ingredients. Set aside.

3. Lightly spray the grill rack with cooking spray. Preheat the grill on medium high. Or lightly spray a grill pan and heat over medium-high heat.

4. On each skewer, thread, in order, 1 tuna cube, 2 snow peas, 1 green onion, and 1 bell pepper square. Repeat this pattern twice on each skewer. Lightly brush the kebabs with the canola oil. Sprinkle the pepper over the kebabs.

5. Grill the kebabs for 2 minutes on each side, or until the tuna is the desired doneness. Serve the kebabs with the sauce.

SHOP & STORE: Look for snow peas that are light green, with smooth, firm skins and small seeds. Avoid any that are cracked or wilted, or showing signs of decay. Any extra snow peas can be added raw to salads or cooked in a stir-fry; they are a rich source of vitamin C and iron.

SAUCE

2 tablespoons sugar

1 tablespoon plus 2 teaspoons soy sauce (lowest sodium available)

1 tablespoon fresh lime juice

1 tablespoon cider vinegar

2 teaspoons toasted sesame oil

⅛ teaspoon crushed red pepper flakes

⅛ teaspoon salt

✳ ✳ ✳

Cooking spray

1 pound tuna steak, cut into 12 1-inch cubes

24 medium snow peas, trimmed

12 medium green onions, each cut to 6 inches long and folded in half

1 medium red or yellow bell pepper, cut into 12 1-inch squares

1 tablespoon canola or corn oil

½ teaspoon pepper

PER SERVING: Calories **254** • Total Fat **6.5 g** • Saturated Fat **1.0 g** • Trans Fat **0.0 g**
Polyunsaturated Fat **2.0 g** • Monounsaturated Fat **3.5 g** • Cholesterol **44 mg**
Sodium **304 mg** • Carbohydrates **17 g** • Fiber **4 g** • Sugars **12 g** • Protein **29 g**
DIETARY EXCHANGES: 2 vegetable, ½ other carbohydrate, 3 lean meat

Tuna Steaks with Gremolata

Basic gremolata is a mixture of parsley, lemon zest, and garlic. We livened up ours even more, adding a splash of lemon juice, a hint of rosemary, and a bit of red onion to punch up the flavor of these seared tuna steaks.

1. In a small bowl, stir together the topping ingredients. Set aside.

2. In a large nonstick skillet, heat the canola oil over medium-high heat, swirling to coat the bottom. Sprinkle the pepper and salt over both sides of the fish. Cook the fish for 1½ minutes on each side, or to the desired doneness.

3. Spoon the topping over the fish. Serve with the lemon wedges.

PER SERVING: Calories **172** • Total Fat **5.0 g** • Saturated Fat **1.0 g** • Trans Fat **0.0 g**
Polyunsaturated Fat **1.0 g** • Monounsaturated Fat **3.5 g** • Cholesterol **44 mg**
Sodium **273 mg** • Carbohydrates **2 g** • Fiber **1 g** • Sugars **1 g** • Protein **28 g**
DIETARY EXCHANGES: 3 lean meat

SERVES 4
3 ounces fish and 2 tablespoons topping per serving

PREP TIME
10 minutes

COOKING TIME
5 minutes

TOPPING

⅓ cup chopped fresh Italian (flat-leaf) parsley

3 tablespoons finely chopped red onion

2 teaspoons grated lemon zest

1 tablespoon fresh lemon juice

1 tablespoon extra-virgin olive oil

1 medium garlic clove, minced

½ teaspoon chopped fresh rosemary

⅛ teaspoon salt

* * *

1 teaspoon canola or corn oil

½ teaspoon coarsely ground pepper

¼ teaspoon salt

4 tuna steaks (about 4 ounces each), about 1 inch thick, rinsed and patted dry

1 medium lemon, cut into 4 wedges (optional)

⅓ cup fat-free sour cream

2 to 3 teaspoons fat-free
milk or water

1 teaspoon grated peeled
horseradish and
2 teaspoons grated
peeled horseradish,
divided use

⅛ teaspoon salt,
⅛ teaspoon salt,
and ¼ teaspoon salt,
divided use

⅛ teaspoon pepper,
¼ teaspoon pepper,
and ⅛ teaspoon
pepper, or to taste
(all coarsely ground),
divided use

1 teaspoon toasted
sesame oil and
1 teaspoon toasted
sesame oil, divided
use

4 cups sliced bok choy
(4 to 6 medium
leaves with stalks, cut
crosswise into ¼-inch
strips)

(continued)

Pan-Seared Tuna Steaks on Bok Choy

Horseradish and jalapeños add a spicy kick to the fish and bok choy. Quickly searing the tuna keeps it succulent and tender and also helps get dinner on the table in a hurry. Each serving of bok choy boasts a generous dose of vitamin C and calcium.

1. In a small bowl, whisk together the sour cream, milk, 1 teaspoon horseradish, ⅛ teaspoon salt, and ⅛ teaspoon pepper. Set aside.

2. In a large nonstick skillet, heat 1 teaspoon oil over medium-high heat, swirling to coat the bottom. Cook the bok choy for 4 minutes, or until tender-crisp, stirring frequently.

3. Stir in the garlic. Cook for 15 seconds, stirring constantly.

4. Transfer the bok choy mixture to a serving platter. Sprinkle with ⅛ teaspoon salt and the remaining 2 teaspoons horseradish. Cover to keep warm.

5. Sprinkle ¼ teaspoon pepper and the remaining ¼ teaspoon salt over both sides of the fish.

6. In the same skillet, heat the remaining 1 teaspoon oil, swirling to coat the bottom. Cook the fish for 1½ minutes on each side, or until the desired doneness.

7. Arrange the fish on the bok choy. Sprinkle with the jalapeño. Spoon the sauce over the fish and bok choy. Sprinkle with the remaining ⅛ teaspoon pepper.

PER SERVING: Calories 179 • Total Fat 3.0 g • Saturated Fat 0.5 g • Trans Fat 0.0 g Polyunsaturated Fat 1.0 g • Monounsaturated Fat 1.0 g • Cholesterol 48 mg Sodium 406 mg • Carbohydrates 6 g • Fiber 1 g • Sugars 3 g • Protein 30 g DIETARY EXCHANGES: ½ other carbohydrate, 3 lean meat

1 medium garlic clove, minced

4 tuna steaks (about 4 ounces each), rinsed and patted dry

1 medium jalapeño, seeds left in if desired and ribs discarded, finely chopped (see Cook's Tip, page 261)

SERVES 4
3 ounces mussels
and ¾ cup spaghetti
mixture per serving

4 ounces whole-grain thin spaghetti

2 tablespoons olive oil

6 medium garlic cloves, minced

2 cups halved red and yellow cherry tomatoes

½ cup fat-free, low-sodium chicken broth

1 teaspoon crushed red pepper flakes, or to taste

1 pound fresh debearded and rinsed medium mussels

½ cup chopped fresh Italian (flat-leaf) parsley

Mussels Fra Diavolo with Thin Spaghetti

Fra Diavolo means "Brother Devil" in Italian. It was the nickname of a soldier who fought the French during the invasion of Naples. The term is often used in Italian-American cooking to describe dishes such as this that feature spicier tomato-based sauces.

1. Prepare the pasta using the package directions, omitting the salt. Drain well in a colander. Set aside.

2. Meanwhile, in a large deep skillet, heat the oil over medium heat, swirling to coat the bottom. Cook the garlic for 1 minute, stirring constantly. Stir in the tomatoes. Cook for 3 minutes, stirring once halfway through.

3. Stir in the broth and red pepper flakes. Cook for 5 minutes, or until the mixture is reduced and slightly thickened.

4. Stir in the mussels. Simmer, covered, for 5 to 7 minutes, or until the mussels open wide (discard any mussels that do not open during cooking).

5. Transfer the pasta to shallow bowls. Spoon the mussel mixture over the pasta. Sprinkle with the parsley.

SHOP & STORE: When buying mussels, look for those with moist, shiny, and closed shells. Mussels are best cooked and eaten as soon as possible after purchasing. Farmed mussels are usually debearded before they are sold.

PER SERVING: Calories **267** • Total Fat **10.0 g** • Saturated Fat **1.5 g** • Trans Fat **0.0 g**
Polyunsaturated Fat **1.5 g** • Monounsaturated Fat **5.5 g** • Cholesterol **24 mg**
Sodium **269 mg** • Carbohydrates **32 g** • Fiber **5 g** • Sugars **4 g** • Protein **16 g**
DIETARY EXCHANGES: 1½ starch, 1 vegetable, 2 lean meat, ½ fat

Pan-Seared Scallops with Watercress and Pistachios

SERVES 4
2 ounces scallops
per serving

PREP TIME
10 minutes

COOKING TIME
10 minutes

A garlicky orange sauce complements the sweetness of the caramelized scallops and the bite from the watercress. Pistachios top off the dish and add an unexpected crunch.

1. In a large skillet, heat 2 teaspoons oil over medium heat, swirling to coat the bottom. Sprinkle the pepper and salt over the scallops. Cook the scallops in a single layer for 2 minutes on each side, or until browned and opaque in the center. Transfer to a plate. Cover to keep warm.

2. In the same skillet, still over medium heat, heat the remaining 2 teaspoons oil, swirling to coat the bottom. Cook the onion for 1 minute, stirring constantly. Stir in the garlic. Cook for 30 seconds, or until fragrant.

3. Pour in the orange juice. Increase the heat to medium high. Simmer for 2 minutes, or until the liquid is reduced by half (to about ⅓ cup).

4. Transfer the scallops to warmed serving plates. Top with the watercress. Drizzle the orange sauce over the scallops and watercress. Sprinkle with the orange zest and pistachios.

2 teaspoons olive oil and 2 teaspoons olive oil, divided use

¼ teaspoon freshly ground pepper

⅛ teaspoon salt

12 ounces sea scallops, rinsed and patted dry

¼ cup finely chopped red onion

2 medium garlic cloves, minced

¼ teaspoon finely grated orange zest

⅔ cup fresh orange juice

1½ cups torn watercress or baby arugula

3 tablespoons shelled, dry-roasted, unsalted pistachios, chopped

TIPS, TRICKS & TIMESAVERS: One easy way to juice an orange or other citrus fruit is to use a reamer. Cut the fruit in half, then push the pointed end of the reamer into the center of the fruit. Holding them over a bowl or measuring cup, twist the reamer and the fruit in opposite directions while pressing them together.

PER SERVING: Calories **158** • Total Fat **7.5 g** • Saturated Fat **1.0 g** • Trans Fat **0.0 g**
Polyunsaturated Fat **1.5 g** • Monounsaturated Fat **4.5 g** • Cholesterol **20 mg**
Sodium **413 mg** • Carbohydrates **10 g** • Fiber **1 g** • Sugars **4 g** • Protein **12 g**
DIETARY EXCHANGES: ½ fruit, 2 lean meat

Rotini with Shrimp and Broccoli

You'll love this dish not only for its nutty and cheesy flavors but also for the convenience it offers. Cooking the pasta, shrimp, and broccoli in one pan saves time before and after dinner by cutting down on cooking *and* cleanup time.

6 cups water

4 ounces dried whole-grain rotini

2 cups broccoli florets

10 ounces raw medium shrimp, peeled, rinsed, and patted dry

¼ cup chopped fresh parsley

¼ cup pine nuts, dry-roasted

3 tablespoons fat-free evaporated milk

2 tablespoons light tub margarine

2 medium garlic cloves, minced

¼ teaspoon salt

½ ounce Parmesan cheese, shredded or grated

1. In a large saucepan, bring the water to a boil over high heat. Cook the pasta for 6 minutes, or until tender. Stir in the broccoli and shrimp. Return to a boil. Cook for 2 to 3 minutes, or until the shrimp are pink on the outside. Drain well in a colander. Return the pasta mixture to the pan.

2. Stir in the remaining ingredients except the Parmesan. Transfer to shallow bowls. Sprinkle with the Parmesan.

TIPS, TRICKS & TIMESAVERS: To save time, purchase easy-peel shrimp, which are deveined with the shell split open along one side. To peel, just run your finger along the inside of the shell and slip it off.

PER SERVING: Calories 251 • Total Fat 8.5 g • Saturated Fat 1.5 g • Trans Fat 0.0 g
Polyunsaturated Fat 2.5 g • Monounsaturated Fat 3.0 g • Cholesterol 92 mg
Sodium 441 mg • Carbohydrates 28 g • Fiber 5 g • Sugars 4 g • Protein 19 g
DIETARY EXCHANGES: 1½ starch, 1 vegetable, 2 lean meat

Sugar Snap Threads and Yellow Rice with Shrimp

SERVES 4
1¼ cups per serving

PREP TIME
10 minutes

COOKING TIME
15 minutes

Turmeric gives the brown rice a bright yellow color to match the bright flavors of the lemon and cilantro, while edamame and nuts add crunch to this versatile dish. To serve it chilled or at room temperature, rinse the cooked rice with cold water before draining to cool it quickly. *(See photo insert.)*

¾ cup uncooked instant brown rice

⅛ teaspoon ground turmeric

8 ounces cooked medium shrimp, peeled, rinsed, and patted dry

½ cup sugar snap peas, trimmed and very thinly sliced diagonally

½ cup shelled edamame

½ cup chopped fresh cilantro

¼ cup shelled, dry-roasted, unsalted pistachios or slivered almonds, dry-roasted

2 tablespoons canola or corn oil

1 tablespoon grated lemon zest

1 to 2 tablespoons fresh lemon juice

½ teaspoon salt

1. Prepare the rice using the package directions, omitting the salt and margarine and adding the turmeric. Transfer the rice to a fine-mesh sieve. Drain well. Transfer the rice to a large bowl.

2. Stir in the remaining ingredients.

TIPS, TRICKS & TIMESAVERS: There's no need to heat the oven if you don't have dry-roasted nuts on hand. Put the nuts in a single layer in a small skillet. Dry-roast over medium heat for about 4 minutes, or until just fragrant, stirring frequently.

PER SERVING: Calories **240** • Total Fat **12.0 g** • Saturated Fat **1.0 g** • Trans Fat **0.0 g**
Polyunsaturated Fat **3.0 g** • Monounsaturated Fat **6.5 g** • Cholesterol **72 mg**
Sodium **424 mg** • Carbohydrates **19 g** • Fiber **3 g** • Sugars **2 g** • Protein **14 g**
DIETARY EXCHANGES: 1½ starch, 1½ lean meat, 1 fat

POULTRY

Chicken Diable

Diable means "devil" in French. The balsamic vinegar and cracked black pepper give this chicken dish a devilishly tangy bite.

1. Sprinkle the salt and ¼ teaspoon pepper over both sides of the chicken.

2. In a large nonstick skillet, heat the oil over medium-high heat, swirling to coat the bottom. Cook the chicken for 4 minutes. Turn over. Cook for 2 to 4 minutes, or until no longer pink in the center. Transfer the chicken to a platter. Cover to keep warm.

3. In the same skillet, cook the shallot for 1 to 2 minutes, or until tender, stirring constantly.

4. Stir in the tomato, vinegar, tomato paste, and remaining ½ teaspoon pepper, scraping to dislodge any browned bits. Bring to a gentle boil. Boil for 2 to 3 minutes, or until most of the liquid is evaporated, stirring occasionally.

5. Pour in the broth. Return to a boil and boil for 3 to 4 minutes, or until reduced by half (to about ¼ cup). Stir in the chives. Spoon the sauce over the chicken.

TIPS, TRICKS & TIMESAVERS: To flatten a chicken breast, place it with the smooth side up between two pieces of plastic wrap. Using the smooth side of a meat mallet or a heavy pan, lightly flatten the breast to the desired thickness, being careful not to tear the meat.

SERVES 4
3 ounces chicken and 2½ tablespoons sauce per serving

PREP TIME
5 minutes

COOKING TIME
15 minutes

¼ teaspoon salt

¼ teaspoon pepper and ½ teaspoon pepper (cracked), divided use

4 boneless, skinless chicken breast halves (about 4 ounces each), all visible fat discarded, flattened to ¼-inch thickness

1 tablespoon olive oil

¼ cup finely chopped shallot

½ cup chopped tomato

¼ cup balsamic vinegar

1 tablespoon no-salt-added tomato paste

½ cup fat-free, low-sodium chicken broth

1 tablespoon chopped fresh chives

PER SERVING: Calories 182 • Total Fat **6.5 g** • Saturated Fat **1.0 g** • Trans Fat **0.0 g**
Polyunsaturated Fat **1.0 g** • Monounsaturated Fat **3.5 g** • Cholesterol **73 mg**
Sodium **294 mg** • Carbohydrates **6 g** • Fiber **1 g** • Sugars **4 g** • Protein **25 g**
DIETARY EXCHANGES: 1 vegetable, 3 lean meat

SERVES 4
3 ounces chicken
and ½ cup salsa
per serving

PREP TIME
10 minutes

COOKING TIME
10 minutes

1 medium unpeeled red
apple, such as Jonathan
or Gala, diced

⅓ cup diced red bell
pepper

⅓ cup diced red onion

¼ cup chopped fresh
cilantro

1 medium jalapeño, seeds
and ribs discarded,
minced (see Cook's Tip,
page 261)

2 to 3 tablespoons fresh
lime juice

1 teaspoon sugar

1 teaspoon grated orange
zest

1½ teaspoons paprika
(smoked preferred)

1 teaspoon ground cumin

1 teaspoon onion powder

¼ teaspoon salt

4 boneless, skinless
chicken breast halves
(about 4 ounces each),
all visible fat discarded,
flattened to ¼-inch
thickness

1 tablespoon olive oil

1 medium lime, cut into
4 wedges

Cumin Chicken with Apple-Chile Salsa

Splashed with citrus juice, apple and jalapeño come alive in this sweet-heat salsa. This fruit-based condiment accentuates the smoky, earthy flavor from the paprika-cumin rub on the chicken. *(See photo insert.)*

1. In a medium bowl, stir together the apple, bell pepper, onion, cilantro, jalapeño, lime juice, sugar, and orange zest. Set aside.

2. In a small bowl, stir together the paprika, cumin, onion powder, and salt. Brush the chicken on both sides with the oil. Sprinkle the paprika mixture over both sides of the chicken. Using your fingertips, gently press the mixture so it adheres to the chicken.

3. Heat a large skillet over medium-high heat. Cook the chicken for 4 minutes. Turn over and cook for 2 to 4 minutes, or until no longer pink in the center. Just before serving, squeeze the lime wedges over the chicken. Spoon the salsa over the chicken.

PER SERVING: Calories **209** • Total Fat **6.5 g** • Saturated Fat **1.0 g** • Trans Fat **0.0 g** Polyunsaturated Fat **1.0 g** • Monounsaturated Fat **3.5 g** • Cholesterol **73 mg** Sodium **281 mg** • Carbohydrates **13 g** • Fiber **2 g** • Sugars **8 g** • Protein **25 g**
DIETARY EXCHANGES: 1 fruit, 3 lean meat

Grilled Lemon-Tarragon Chicken

This recipe for citrus-and-herb-infused chicken will let you have dinner on the table in short order. Grilling the lemon counters the fruit's usual tartness with a sweetness, thanks to the caramelization, while the crushed charred tarragon adds a smoky flavor.

SERVES 4
3 ounces chicken
per serving

PREP TIME
10 minutes

MARINATING TIME
10 minutes

COOKING TIME
20 minutes

1. Lightly spray the grill rack with cooking spray. Preheat the grill on medium.

2. In a small cup, stir together the lemon juice and oil.

3. In a separate small cup, stir together 2 tablespoons chopped tarragon, the garlic, pepper, and salt.

4. Place the chicken in a shallow glass baking dish. Brush the lemon juice mixture over both sides of the chicken. Sprinkle the tarragon mixture over both sides of the chicken. Using your fingertips, gently press the tarragon mixture so it adheres to the chicken. Cover and refrigerate for 10 minutes.

5. Meanwhile, soak the tarragon sprigs in water for 10 minutes.

6. Grill the chicken for 8 to 10 minutes, or until no longer pink in the center, turning once halfway through.

7. Place the lemon slices in a cooler area of the grill. Grill for 1 to 2 minutes on each side, or until slightly charred. Arrange the lemon slices on a serving platter.

8. Place the tarragon sprigs crosswise in a cooler area of the grill. Grill for 1 to 2 minutes, or until charred, watching very carefully so the sprigs don't burn.

9. Place the chicken on the lemons. Crumble the charred tarragon over the chicken.

Cooking spray

1 tablespoon fresh lemon juice

1 teaspoon extra-virgin olive oil

2 tablespoons chopped fresh tarragon and 8 sprigs of fresh tarragon, about 5 inches long, divided use

2 large garlic cloves, minced

¼ teaspoon pepper

⅛ teaspoon salt

4 boneless, skinless chicken breast halves (about 4 ounces each), all visible fat discarded

8 lemon slices, about ¼ inch thick

PER SERVING: Calories 146 • Total Fat 4.0 g • Saturated Fat 1.0 g • Trans Fat 0.0 g
Polyunsaturated Fat 0.5 g • Monounsaturated Fat 1.5 g • Cholesterol 73 mg
Sodium 205 mg • Carbohydrates 1 g • Fiber 0 g • Sugars 0 g • Protein 24 g
DIETARY EXCHANGES: 3 lean meat

Cooking spray

4 boneless, skinless chicken breast halves (about 4 ounces each), all visible fat discarded, flattened to ½-inch thickness

1½ teaspoons grated orange zest

¼ cup fresh orange juice and 1 tablespoon fresh orange juice, divided use

2 teaspoons canola or corn oil

½ teaspoon ground cumin

¼ teaspoon ground cardamom

¼ teaspoon salt

⅛ teaspoon cayenne (optional)

1 teaspoon cornstarch

2 tablespoons finely chopped fresh mint

Indian-Spiced Chicken

Let your taste buds enjoy cuisine from a faraway land by experiencing the flavors of two spices popular in Indian food. Cumin adds an earthy, nutty, and slightly pungent flavor, while spicy-sweet cardamom pairs extremely well with the orange-flavored chicken.

1. Preheat the oven to 425°F. Lightly spray an 11 × 7 × 2-inch glass baking dish with cooking spray. Arrange the chicken with the smooth side up in the dish.

2. In a small bowl, whisk together the orange zest, ¼ cup orange juice, and the oil. Spoon over the chicken.

3. In a separate small bowl, stir together the cumin, cardamom, salt, and cayenne. Sprinkle over the chicken.

4. Bake for 18 minutes, or until the chicken is no longer pink in the center. Transfer to a serving plate. Set aside the baking dish.

5. Put the cornstarch in a small bowl. Add the remaining 1 tablespoon orange juice, whisking to dissolve. Stir into the drippings in the baking dish, scraping to dislodge any browned bits. Return the baking dish to the oven for 3 minutes, or until the mixture is slightly thickened. Remove from the oven.

6. Return the chicken to the baking dish, turning to coat well. Just before serving, sprinkle the chicken with the mint.

PER SERVING: Calories 165 • Total Fat 5.5 g • Saturated Fat 1.0 g • Trans Fat 0.0 g
Polyunsaturated Fat 1.0 g • Monounsaturated Fat 2.5 g • Cholesterol 73 mg
Sodium 279 mg • Carbohydrates 3 g • Fiber 0 g • Sugars 2 g • Protein 24 g
DIETARY EXCHANGES: 3 lean meat

Shallot and Sage Chicken Breasts

SERVES 4
3 ounces chicken
per serving

PREP TIME
5 minutes

COOKING TIME
30 minutes

Shallots, which offer a mild, oniony taste, combined with a trio of aromatic herbs form a flavor medley that makes this dish sing. The entrée requires so little work that you'll want to make it again and again.

1. Preheat the oven to 425°F. Lightly spray a shallow 9-inch glass pie pan with cooking spray.

2. Put the chicken in the pan.

3. In a small bowl, stir together the shallots, parsley, sage, thyme, salt, and pepper. Sprinkle over the chicken. Spoon the oil over the chicken. Bake for 18 to 20 minutes, or until the chicken is no longer pink in the center.

Cooking spray

4 boneless, skinless chicken breast halves (about 4 ounces each), all visible fat discarded

2 medium shallots, finely chopped

2 tablespoons chopped fresh Italian (flat-leaf) parsley

1 tablespoon finely chopped fresh sage

1½ teaspoons fresh thyme

¼ teaspoon salt

¼ teaspoon pepper

1 tablespoon plus 1 teaspoon olive oil

PER SERVING: Calories 177 • Total Fat **7.5 g** • Saturated Fat **1.5 g** • Trans Fat **0.0 g** Polyunsaturated Fat **1.0 g** • Monounsaturated Fat **4.0 g** • Cholesterol **73 mg** Sodium **279 mg** • Carbohydrates **2 g** • Fiber **0 g** • Sugars **0 g** • Protein **24 g** DIETARY EXCHANGES: 3 lean meat

Rosemary-Peach Chicken Kebabs with Orange Glaze

End your day on a sweet note with these chicken-and-peach kebabs brushed with a honeyed citrus glaze. Serve Poblano-Lentil Pilaf (page 230) and asparagus on the side. (*See photo insert.*)

Cooking spray

1 pound boneless, skinless chicken breasts, all visible fat discarded, cut into 16 1½-inch pieces

2 large ripe but firm peaches, cut into 16 1-inch wedges

1 large green bell pepper, cut into 16 1½-inch squares

¼ teaspoon pepper

⅛ teaspoon salt

GLAZE

¾ teaspoon grated orange zest

3 tablespoons fresh orange juice

1 tablespoon chopped fresh rosemary

1½ teaspoons honey

1½ teaspoons canola or corn oil

1. Lightly spray the grill rack with cooking spray. Preheat the grill on medium.

2. Meanwhile, thread the chicken, peaches, and bell pepper alternately onto four 14- to 16-inch metal skewers. Sprinkle the pepper and salt over the kebabs.

3. In a small bowl, whisk together the glaze ingredients. Set aside half the glaze (about 2 tablespoons). Brush both sides of the kebabs with the remaining glaze.

4. Grill the kebabs for 6 to 8 minutes, or until the chicken is no longer pink in the center and the vegetables are almost tender, turning once halfway through and brushing with the reserved 2 tablespoons of glaze, using a clean basting brush. Reduce the heat or move the kebabs to a cooler area of the grill if they are cooking too fast.

COOK'S TIP: Ripe but firm peaches are important for this recipe. The direct heat softens and sweetens the fruit, even if it's not quite at its prime.

HEALTHY SWAP: You can replace the peaches with other stone fruits, such as nectarines and plums.

PER SERVING: Calories **202** • Total Fat **5.0 g** • Saturated Fat **1.0 g** • Trans Fat **0.0 g** Polyunsaturated Fat **1.0 g** • Monounsaturated Fat **2.0 g** • Cholesterol **73 mg** Sodium **206 mg** • Carbohydrates **14 g** • Fiber **2 g** • Sugars **11 g** • Protein **25 g** DIETARY EXCHANGES: 1 fruit, 3 lean meat

Buffalo Chicken with Slaw

SERVES 6
3 ounces chicken and 1 cup slaw per serving

PREP TIME
15 minutes

COOKING TIME
10 minutes

With our recipe you can enjoy the flavors of Buffalo chicken wings without the fat. The secret is to go skinless! The tangy, cooling slaw is a more satisfying replacement for the ho-hum celery sticks and blue cheese dressing that usually accompany wings.

1. In a large bowl, stir together the cabbage, carrots, and celery.

2. In a small bowl, whisk together the buttermilk, yogurt, blue cheese, vinegar, sugar, and pepper. Pour over the cabbage mixture, stirring to coat. Set aside, stirring occasionally until serving time.

3. In a large nonstick skillet, heat the oil over medium-high heat, swirling to coat the bottom. Cook the chicken for 5 to 6 minutes, or until lightly browned on the outside and no longer pink in the center, stirring occasionally. Add the sauce, stirring to coat the chicken. Serve with the slaw.

COOK'S TIP: The longer the slaw stands, the more tender the cabbage becomes. Be sure to shred the cabbage or chop it finely so it can wilt slightly and not be too raw.

6 cups shredded green cabbage

1 cup shredded carrots

½ cup thinly sliced celery

½ cup low-fat buttermilk

¼ cup fat-free plain Greek yogurt

¼ cup crumbled low-fat blue cheese

1 tablespoon cider vinegar

1 teaspoon sugar

¼ teaspoon pepper

1 teaspoon canola or corn oil

1½ pounds boneless, skinless chicken breasts, all visible fat discarded, cut into 4 × ½-inch strips

2 tablespoons Buffalo wing sauce (lowest sodium available)

PER SERVING: Calories 200 • Total Fat 5.5 g • Saturated Fat 2.0 g • Trans Fat 0.0 g
Polyunsaturated Fat 1.0 g • Monounsaturated Fat 2.0 g • Cholesterol 78 mg
Sodium 392 mg • Carbohydrates 9 g • Fiber 3 g • Sugars 5 g • Protein 28 g
DIETARY EXCHANGES: 1 vegetable, 3 lean meat

SERVES 4
1½ cups per serving

PREP TIME
10 minutes

COOKING TIME
15 minutes

4 ounces dried whole-grain rotini

1 teaspoon olive oil and 2 teaspoons extra-virgin olive oil, divided use

12 ounces boneless, skinless chicken breasts, all visible fat discarded, cut into bite-size pieces

3 medium garlic cloves, minced

12 kalamata olives, coarsely chopped

3 ounces baby spinach or spring greens

¼ cup chopped fresh basil

2 tablespoons shredded or grated Parmesan cheese and 2 tablespoons shredded or grated Parmesan cheese, divided use

Chicken with Kalamatas and Pasta

Escape to the Greek Isles with this chicken dish that spotlights Mediterranean ingredients, including garlic, kalamata olives, spinach, and basil.

1. Prepare the pasta using the package directions, omitting the salt. Drain well in a colander.

2. Meanwhile, in a large nonstick skillet, heat 1 teaspoon oil over medium-high heat, swirling to coat the bottom. Cook the chicken for 3 minutes, or until no longer pink in the center, stirring frequently. Stir in the garlic. Cook for 15 seconds, stirring constantly.

3. Stir in the olives, spinach, basil, 2 tablespoons Parmesan, and the remaining 2 teaspoons oil. Cook for 30 seconds, or until the spinach has wilted slightly, stirring to combine. Remove from the heat. Sprinkle with the remaining 2 tablespoons Parmesan.

PER SERVING: Calories 289 • Total Fat 11.0 g • Saturated Fat 2.0 g • Trans Fat 0.0 g
Polyunsaturated Fat 1.5 g • Monounsaturated Fat 6.0 g • Cholesterol 58 mg
Sodium 384 mg • Carbohydrates 24 g • Fiber 4 g • Sugars 1 g • Protein 25 g
DIETARY EXCHANGES: 1½ starch, 3 lean meat

Country Thyme Chicken Strips

Whole-wheat panko forms a slightly darker and crunchier crust around these chicken strips than would ordinary bread crumbs, giving these tenders an appetizing appearance and a crisp coating.

1. In a shallow bowl, stir together the panko, dillweed, thyme, paprika, and pepper.

2. Pour the buttermilk into a medium bowl. Add the chicken, turning to coat. Dip the chicken in the panko mixture, turning to coat and gently shaking off any excess. Using your fingertips, gently press the panko mixture so it adheres to the chicken. Transfer to a plate. Discard any remaining panko mixture.

3. In a large nonstick skillet, heat the oil over medium-high heat, swirling to coat the bottom. Put the chicken in the skillet. Reduce the heat to medium. Sprinkle the chicken with 1/8 teaspoon salt. Cook for 6 minutes, or until browned. Turn over. Cook for 5 minutes, or until no longer pink in the center. Transfer to a platter.

4. Sprinkle the chicken with the remaining 1/8 teaspoon salt. Let stand for 3 minutes so the flavors blend.

> **COOK'S TIP ON PANKO:** Japanese bread crumbs, known as panko, have less sodium than traditional bread crumbs, making them a heart-healthy choice.

SERVES 4
3 ounces chicken
per serving

PREP TIME
10 minutes

COOKING TIME
15 minutes

STANDING TIME
3 minutes

¾ cup whole-wheat panko (Japanese-style bread crumbs)

1 tablespoon chopped fresh dillweed

1½ teaspoons fresh thyme

1 teaspoon paprika

¼ teaspoon pepper

½ cup low-fat buttermilk

1 pound chicken breast tenders, all visible fat discarded

2 tablespoons canola or corn oil

⅛ teaspoon salt and ⅛ teaspoon salt, divided use

PER SERVING: Calories 259 • Total Fat **10.5 g** • Saturated Fat **1.5 g** • Trans Fat **0.0 g**
Polyunsaturated Fat **2.5 g** • Monounsaturated Fat **5.5 g** • Cholesterol **74 mg**
Sodium **327 mg** • Carbohydrates **13 g** • Fiber **2 g** • Sugars **2 g** • Protein **28 g**
DIETARY EXCHANGES: 1 starch, 3 lean meat

12 teaspoons canola or corn oil

1 pound boneless, skinless chicken breasts, all visible fat discarded, cut into bite-size pieces

6 medium garlic cloves, minced

¼ to ½ teaspoon crushed red pepper flakes

1 medium red bell pepper, cut lengthwise into 2 × ¼-inch strips

1 medium orange or green bell pepper, cut lengthwise into 2 × ¼-inch strips

¼ cup fat-free, low-sodium chicken broth

1 tablespoon capers, drained

2 teaspoons white wine vinegar

Skillet Chicken Scampi with Bell Peppers

This recipe has all the garlicky goodness of the classic shrimp dish, but forgoes the butter in favor of a tangy finish with vinegar and capers. Serve it over whole-grain linguine if you like.

1. In a large nonstick skillet, heat the oil over medium heat, swirling to coat the bottom. Cook the chicken, garlic, and red pepper flakes for 5 to 6 minutes, or until the chicken is no longer pink in the center. Transfer to a plate.

2. In the same skillet, cook the bell peppers and broth for 4 to 5 minutes, or until the bell peppers are tender-crisp, stirring occasionally. Return the chicken and any accumulated juices to the skillet. Stir in the capers and vinegar. Bring to a boil, still over medium heat. Boil gently for 2 to 3 minutes, or until the liquid is reduced by half (to about 3 tablespoons).

TIPS, TRICKS & TIMESAVERS: To mince garlic easily and quickly, use a garlic press. You don't even need to peel the cloves first, as the peel will remain in the press.

PER SERVING: Calories 177 • Total Fat 5.5 g • Saturated Fat 1.0 g • Trans Fat 0.0 g
Polyunsaturated Fat 1.0 g • Monounsaturated Fat 2.5 g • Cholesterol 73 mg
Sodium 202 mg • Carbohydrates 5 g • Fiber 1 g • Sugars 2 g • Protein 25 g
DIETARY EXCHANGES: 1 vegetable, 3 lean meat

Chicken and Sweet Potato Curry

SERVES 4
1¼ cups per serving

PREP TIME
10 minutes

COOKING TIME
25 minutes

This stewlike curry features chunks of chicken thigh flanked by an array of vegetables, including orange sweet potato, green bell pepper, and red Swiss chard. Serve this curry on its own or try it over brown rice topped with a dollop of fat-free plain yogurt.

1. Lightly spray a large skillet with cooking spray. Heat over medium-high heat. Cook the chicken for 3 to 5 minutes, or until browned, turning once halfway through (the chicken won't be done at this point). Transfer to a plate.

2. Reduce the heat to medium. Cook the onion for 1 minute, stirring occasionally.

3. Stir in the sweet potato, bell pepper, and garlic. Cook for 1 minute, stirring occasionally. Stir in the chicken and remaining ingredients except the cilantro.

4. Increase the heat to medium high and bring to a boil. Reduce the heat and simmer, partially covered, for 15 minutes, or until the vegetables are tender and the chicken is no longer pink in the center, stirring occasionally. Just before serving, sprinkle the curry with the cilantro.

SHOP & STORE: Any type of chard can be used in this recipe—from red Swiss to rainbow or even the common green (with white stems). All types are rich in potassium and vitamins A and C. Look for chard with firm stems and unblemished leaves.

PER SERVING: Calories **267** • Total Fat **8.0 g** • Saturated Fat **4.0 g** • Trans Fat **0.0 g** Polyunsaturated Fat **1.0 g** • Monounsaturated Fat **1.5 g** • Cholesterol **73 mg** Sodium **358 mg** • Carbohydrates **21 g** • Fiber **4 g** • Sugars **8 g** • Protein **27 g** DIETARY EXCHANGES: 1 starch, 1 vegetable, 3 lean meat

Cooking spray

1 pound boneless, skinless chicken thighs, all visible fat discarded, cut into 1-inch pieces

1 large onion, halved, cut into ½-inch wedges

1 6-ounce orange sweet potato, quartered lengthwise, cut crosswise into ½-inch slices (about 1¼ cups)

1 medium green bell pepper, cut into 1-inch squares

2 large garlic cloves, minced

1 13.5- to 13.75-ounce can lite coconut milk

6 ounces red Swiss chard, tough stems discarded, thinly sliced

1 tablespoon curry powder

⅛ teaspoon salt

Dash of cayenne, or to taste

3 tablespoons chopped fresh cilantro

SERVES 4
1²/₃ cups per serving

PREP TIME
10 minutes

COOKING TIME
25 minutes

1 pound boneless,
   skinless chicken
   thighs, all visible fat
   discarded, cut into
   1-inch pieces

1 tablespoon salt-free
   Creole or Cajun
   seasoning blend

½ teaspoon salt

1 tablespoon canola or
   corn oil

2 medium bell peppers,
   diced (1 red and
   1 green preferred)

1 cup chopped onion

3 medium garlic cloves,
   minced

2 tablespoons all-purpose
   flour

1½ cups fat-free, low-
   sodium chicken broth

1 8.8-ounce microwave-
   able pouch brown rice
   (about 2 cups)

2 cups chopped tomatoes

¼ cup chopped fresh
   parsley

Chicken Gumbo

Our spicy gumbo tastes as if it's been simmering for hours, but it really takes just minutes before it's ready to serve. Enjoy this taste of southern cooking with cornbread or a crusty whole-grain roll to sop up all the goodness this gumbo has to offer.

1. In a large bowl, combine the chicken, seasoning blend, and salt, stirring to coat.

2. In a large saucepan, heat the oil over medium heat, swirling to coat the bottom. Cook the chicken for 5 minutes, or until no longer pink on the outside (the chicken won't be done at this point), stirring frequently.

3. Stir in the bell peppers, onion, and garlic. Cook for 5 minutes, stirring occasionally.

4. Stir in the flour. Cook for 1 minute.

5. Increase the heat to high. Stir in the broth and bring to a boil. Reduce the heat and simmer for 10 minutes, or until the chicken is no longer pink in the center and the vegetables are tender.

6. Meanwhile, prepare the rice using the package directions.

7. Stir the rice and tomatoes into the chicken mixture. Cook for 2 minutes, or until heated through. Ladle into shallow bowls. Sprinkle with the parsley.

COOK'S TIP: If you're cooking this ahead of time, don't add the rice until you reheat the gumbo or it will absorb all the liquid.

PER SERVING: Calories 343 • Total Fat 11.5 g • Saturated Fat 2.0 g • Trans Fat 0.0 g
Polyunsaturated Fat 3.0 g • Monounsaturated Fat 5.5 g • Cholesterol 106 mg
Sodium 398 mg • Carbohydrates 31 g • Fiber 4 g • Sugars 6 g • Protein 24 g
DIETARY EXCHANGES: 1½ starch, 2 vegetable, 2½ lean meat, 1 fat

Turkey Tenderloin with Grapefruit Sauce

SERVES 4
3 ounces turkey and
2 tablespoons sauce
per serving

PREP TIME
5 minutes

COOKING TIME
30 minutes

STANDING TIME
5 minutes

There's no rule that says turkey is only for Thanksgiving or that a citrus-based sauce can't take the place of a savory gravy. Either Sweet Orange-Roasted Root Vegetables (page 247) or Roasted Parsnips and Carrots (page 235) makes for a convenient side.

1. Preheat the oven to 425°F. Lightly spray an 11 × 7 × 2-inch glass baking dish with cooking spray. Set aside.

2. In a small bowl, stir together the chili powder, cinnamon, cumin, salt, and red pepper flakes. Sprinkle over both sides of the turkey. Using your fingertips, gently press the mixture so it adheres to the turkey.

3. In a medium nonstick skillet, heat the oil over medium-high heat, swirling to coat the bottom. Cook the turkey for 2½ minutes on each side. Transfer to the baking dish.

4. Pour the water into the skillet. Bring to a boil, still over medium-high heat, scraping to dislodge any browned bits. Pour over the turkey.

5. Bake for 22 minutes, or until the turkey registers 160°F on an instant-read thermometer. Remove from the oven. Don't turn off the oven. Transfer the turkey to a cutting board, leaving the liquid in the baking dish. Let the turkey stand for 5 minutes, or until it registers 165°F.

6. Meanwhile, add the remaining ingredients to the liquid in the baking dish, stirring well and scraping to dislodge any browned bits. Bake the mixture for 3 minutes.

7. Thinly slice the turkey diagonally across the grain. Arrange the slices on a serving platter. Spoon the sauce over the turkey or serve it on the side.

Cooking spray
1 teaspoon chili powder
½ teaspoon ground cinnamon
¼ teaspoon ground cumin
¼ teaspoon salt
⅛ teaspoon crushed red pepper flakes
1 1-pound turkey tenderloin, all visible fat discarded
1 teaspoon canola or corn oil
¼ cup water
½ teaspoon grated grapefruit zest (see Cook's Tip on page 40)
½ cup fresh grapefruit juice
1 tablespoon plus 1 teaspoon white balsamic vinegar
2 teaspoons sugar

PER SERVING: Calories 162 • Total Fat 2.0 g • Saturated Fat 0.5 g • Trans Fat 0.0 g
Polyunsaturated Fat 0.5 g • Monounsaturated Fat 1.0 g • Cholesterol 70 mg
Sodium 215 mg • Carbohydrates 6 g • Fiber 1 g • Sugars 5 g • Protein 28 g
DIETARY EXCHANGES: ½ fruit, 3 lean meat

Turkey Cutlets with Cranberry-Pineapple Relish

Cranberries are an expected accompaniment to turkey, but you're sure to find surprises in this side with a burst of citrus, a bite from red pepper flakes, and a tang from pineapple—it's a dish you'll relish!

RELISH

¾ cup diced pineapple

⅓ cup cranberries, finely chopped

¼ cup finely chopped red onion

2 teaspoons sugar

2 teaspoons white balsamic vinegar

1 teaspoon grated orange zest

⅛ teaspoon crushed red pepper flakes (optional)

* * *

2 teaspoons fresh thyme

1½ teaspoons chopped fresh rosemary

½ teaspoon pepper

¼ teaspoon salt

1 pound turkey cutlets, flattened to ¼-inch thickness, all visible fat discarded

2 teaspoons olive oil

1. In a small bowl, stir together the relish ingredients.

2. In a small bowl, stir together the thyme, rosemary, pepper, and salt. Sprinkle over both sides of the turkey. Using your fingertips, gently press the mixture so it adheres to the turkey.

3. In a large nonstick skillet, heat the oil over medium-high heat, swirling to coat the bottom. Cook the turkey for 4 minutes on each side, or until no longer pink in the center. Serve the turkey with the relish.

SHOP & STORE: Buy extra packages of fresh cranberries when they're in season, freeze them, and use them throughout the year to add fiber, vitamin C, and flavor.

PER SERVING: Calories **182** • Total Fat **3.0 g** • Saturated Fat **0.5 g** • Trans Fat **0.0 g** • Polyunsaturated Fat **0.5 g** • Monounsaturated Fat **2.0 g** • Cholesterol **70 mg** • Sodium **203 mg** • Carbohydrates **9 g** • Fiber **1 g** • Sugars **7 g** • Protein **28 g**
DIETARY EXCHANGES: ½ fruit, 3 lean meat

Spicy Turkey Cutlets and Olives

SERVES 4
3 ounces turkey and
3 tablespoons sauce
per serving

PREP TIME
5 minutes

COOKING TIME
10 minutes

Cutlets cook so quickly, you can have turkey any night of the week. In this zesty entrée, tomato sauce is livened up with spicy chipotle powder and tangy olives. Barley "Risotto" with Sautéed Mushrooms and Garlic (page 214) or Broccolini with Toasted Walnuts (page 219) are good choices for side dishes.

1. Sprinkle the chipotle powder and pepper over both sides of the turkey. Using your fingertips, gently press the seasonings so they adhere to the turkey.

2. In a large nonstick skillet, heat 1 teaspoon canola oil over medium-high heat, swirling to coat the bottom. Cook half the turkey cutlets for 1½ minutes on each side, or until no longer pink in the center. Transfer to a plate. Cover to keep warm. Repeat with the remaining 1 teaspoon canola oil and cutlets.

3. In the same skillet, stir together the tomato sauce, olives, green onions, and vinegar. Bring to a boil, still over medium-high heat. Boil for 1 minute, or until the mixture is reduced by one-fourth (to about ¾ cup), stirring occasionally. Spoon the sauce over the turkey. Drizzle with the olive oil. Sprinkle with the basil.

HEALTHY SWAP: If you can't find turkey cutlets, substitute 1 pound of boneless, skinless chicken breasts flattened to a thickness of ⅛ inch.

¼ to ½ teaspoon chipotle powder

⅛ teaspoon pepper

1 pound thinly sliced turkey cutlets, all visible fat discarded

1 teaspoon canola or corn oil and 1 teaspoon canola or corn oil, divided use

1 8-ounce can no-salt-added tomato sauce

14 medium pimiento-stuffed green olives, coarsely chopped

¼ cup finely chopped green onions

2 teaspoons red wine vinegar

1 tablespoon plus 1 teaspoon extra-virgin olive oil

2 tablespoons chopped fresh basil

PER SERVING: Calories 221 • Total Fat 9.5 g • Saturated Fat 1.5 g • Trans Fat 0.0 g
Polyunsaturated Fat 1.5 g • Monounsaturated Fat 6.0 g • Cholesterol 70 mg
Sodium 358 mg • Carbohydrates 5 g • Fiber 1 g • Sugars 3 g • Protein 29 g
DIETARY EXCHANGES: 1 vegetable, 3 lean meat

¼ teaspoon salt

¼ teaspoon pepper

1 pound skinless turkey breast fillets, all visible fat discarded, flattened to ¼-inch thickness

1 tablespoon olive oil

2 medium garlic cloves, minced

1 cup fat-free, low-sodium chicken broth

1 tablespoon balsamic vinegar

1 cup halved seedless red grapes (about 6 ounces)

1 tablespoon honey

2 tablespoons chopped fresh parsley

Turkey Véronique

Véronique refers to dishes that are garnished with seedless white grapes. Our sauce uses the red variety instead for a touch of color. The sweet-tartness of grapes complements a mild protein such as turkey, chicken, or fish.

1. Sprinkle the salt and pepper over both sides of the turkey.

2. In a large nonstick skillet, heat the oil over medium-high heat, swirling to coat the bottom. Cook the turkey for 6 to 8 minutes, or until no longer pink in the center, turning once halfway through. Transfer to a platter. Cover to keep warm.

3. In the same skillet, cook the garlic for 30 seconds, stirring constantly.

4. Stir in the broth and vinegar, scraping to dislodge any browned bits. Bring to a boil. Boil for 6 to 7 minutes, or until the liquid is reduced by half (to about ½ cup).

5. Stir in the grapes and honey. Simmer for 2 to 3 minutes, or until the liquid is syrupy and the grapes are heated through, stirring occasionally. Spoon the sauce over the turkey. Sprinkle with the parsley.

SHOP & STORE: Choose grapes that are plump, free of wrinkles, and firmly attached to their stems. Loosely wrap the unwashed grapes in a paper towel. Transfer them to an airtight container or resealable plastic bag and refrigerate. They will keep for up to two weeks.

PER SERVING: Calories 207 • Total Fat **4.0 g** • Saturated Fat **0.5 g** • Trans Fat **0.0 g**
Polyunsaturated Fat **0.5 g** • Monounsaturated Fat **3.0 g** • Cholesterol **70 mg**
Sodium **220 mg** • Carbohydrates **13 g** • Fiber **1 g** • Sugars **11 g** • Protein **29 g**
DIETARY EXCHANGES: 1 fruit, 3 lean meat

Turkey Lula Kebabs with Yogurt Sauce

SERVES 4
3 ounces turkey and
2 tablespoons sauce
per serving

PREP TIME
15 minutes

COOKING TIME
20 minutes

Lula kebabs are a Middle Eastern specialty typically made with highly seasoned ground lamb and served with a creamy, tangy yogurt sauce. We use ground turkey breast instead, which provides a leaner but still flavorful meal. Serve these kebabs with Grilled Summer Veggie Salad with Hummus Dressing (page 108).

1. Soak four 8-inch wooden skewers for at least 10 minutes in cold water to keep them from charring, or use metal skewers.

2. Meanwhile, lightly spray the grill or a baking sheet with cooking spray. Preheat the grill on medium or preheat the broiler.

3. In a large bowl, using your hands or a spoon, combine all the ingredients for the kebabs except the turkey. Add the turkey. Using wet hands (to keep the turkey mixture from sticking), shape the mixture into eight 4 × 1½-inch logs. Thread the logs onto the skewers.

4. Grill the kebabs for 16 to 18 minutes, turning occasionally, or broil them about 4 inches from the heat for 10 to 12 minutes, turning once halfway through, or until they register 160°F on an instant-read thermometer and are no longer pink in the center.

5. Meanwhile, in a small bowl, stir together the sauce ingredients. Serve with the kebabs.

COOK'S TIP: If you prefer not to use skewers, you can shape the turkey mixture into 8 patties about ¾ inch thick. Follow the cooking instructions as directed above.

Cooking spray

KEBABS

¼ cup minced onion

¼ cup chopped fresh parsley

1 tablespoon soy sauce (lowest sodium available)

1 teaspoon chopped fresh mint

1 medium garlic clove, minced

½ teaspoon ground coriander

½ teaspoon pepper

¼ teaspoon ground cumin

1 pound ground skinless turkey breast

SAUCE

⅓ cup fat-free plain Greek yogurt

¼ cup peeled, seeded, and finely chopped cucumber

1 teaspoon chopped fresh mint

Dash of pepper

PER SERVING: Calories 148 • Total Fat 1.0 g • Saturated Fat 0.5 g • Trans Fat 0.0 g
Polyunsaturated Fat 0.0 g • Monounsaturated Fat 0.0 g • Cholesterol 70 mg
Sodium 164 mg • Carbohydrates 3 g • Fiber 1 g • Sugars 2 g • Protein 30 g
DIETARY EXCHANGES: 3½ lean meat

Turkey Patties with Mushroom Gravy

These herbed patties smothered in mushroom gravy are sure to make your list of comfort foods and may even conjure up fond food memories of Thanksgiving dinner. Sage is a natural complement to turkey and often used in holiday stuffing or dressing.

12 ounces ground skinless turkey breast

2 ounces low-fat turkey breakfast sausage (not the smoked variety), casings discarded

½ cup diced onion and ½ cup diced onion, divided use

1½ tablespoons chopped fresh sage

¼ teaspoon salt and ⅛ teaspoon salt, divided use

¼ teaspoon pepper

1 teaspoon canola or corn oil and 1 teaspoon canola or corn oil, divided use

8 ounces sliced button mushrooms

1 medium garlic clove, minced

½ cup fat-free milk

1 teaspoon cornstarch

1 packet (1 teaspoon) salt-free instant chicken bouillon (optional)

1 tablespoon light tub margarine

1. In a medium bowl, using your hands or a spoon, combine the ground turkey, sausage, ½ cup onion, the sage, ¼ teaspoon salt, and the pepper. Shape into 4 patties, each about ½ inch thick.

2. In a large nonstick skillet, heat 1 teaspoon oil over medium heat, swirling to coat the bottom. Cook the patties for 4 minutes on each side, or until no longer pink in the center. Transfer to a plate. Cover to keep warm.

3. Heat the remaining 1 teaspoon oil over medium heat, swirling to coat the bottom. Cook the remaining ½ cup onion for 2 minutes. Stir in the mushrooms and garlic. Cook for 3 minutes, or until the onion is lightly browned on the edges, stirring occasionally.

4. Meanwhile, in a small bowl, whisk together the milk, cornstarch, and bouillon until the cornstarch is dissolved. Stir into the onion mixture. Bring to a boil, still over medium heat. Boil for 1 minute, or until slightly thickened.

5. Add the margarine and remaining ⅛ teaspoon salt, stirring until well blended.

6. Just before serving, spoon the gravy over the patties.

PER SERVING: Calories **204** • Total Fat **7.0 g** • Saturated Fat **1.0 g** • Trans Fat **0.0 g** • Polyunsaturated Fat **2.0 g** • Monounsaturated Fat **3.0 g** • Cholesterol **76 mg** • Sodium **386 mg** • Carbohydrates **9 g** • Fiber **1 g** • Sugars **4 g** • Protein **26 g**
DIETARY EXCHANGES: 1 vegetable, 3 lean meat

Italian Turkey Sausage on Bulgur

With plenty of protein and fiber, this stick-to-your-ribs dish is both hearty *and* healthy—what a winning combination! Serve with Salad Greens with Blue Cheese and Italian Herb Vinaigrette (page 81) or Baby Spinach and Tomato Salad with Warm Olive Vinaigrette (page 83).

(page 81)

(page 83)

SERVES 4
1 cup per serving

PREP TIME
10 minutes

COOKING TIME
15 minutes

½ cup instant, or fine-grain, bulgur

6 ounces sweet Italian turkey sausage, casings discarded

1½ cups diced onion

8 ounces sliced button mushrooms

½ cup thinly sliced carrot

⅓ cup chopped fresh Italian (flat-leaf) parsley

¼ cup pine nuts, dry-roasted

⅛ teaspoon salt

1. Prepare the bulgur using the package directions, omitting the salt. Transfer to a medium bowl. Fluff with a fork. Set aside.

2. Meanwhile, in a large nonstick skillet, cook the sausage for 2 minutes over medium-high heat, stirring frequently to turn and break up the sausage. Stir in the onion, mushrooms, and carrot. Cook for 8 minutes, or until the sausage is browned on the outside and no longer pink in the center and the vegetables are beginning to brown. Remove from the heat.

3. Stir in the bulgur, parsley, and pine nuts. Sprinkle with the salt.

HEALTHY SWAP: You can substitute 2 cups of cooked brown rice for the cooked bulgur.

PER SERVING: Calories 211 • Total Fat 8.5 g • Saturated Fat 2.0 g • Trans Fat 0.0 g
Polyunsaturated Fat 3.0 g • Monounsaturated Fat 3.0 g • Cholesterol 36 mg
Sodium 400 mg • Carbohydrates 24 g • Fiber 6 g • Sugars 5 g • Protein 13 g
DIETARY EXCHANGES: 1 starch, 2 vegetable, 1 lean meat, 1 fat

MEATS

Filets Mignons with Blackberry-Soy Reduction

SERVES 4
3 ounces beef and
2 tablespoons sauce
per serving

PREP TIME
5 minutes

COOKING TIME
15 minutes

Whether it's a special occasion or any ordinary weeknight that you need to get dinner done on demand, this recipe will fit the bill. Meltingly tender steaks are cooked to perfection and topped with a sauce featuring balsamic vinegar, blackberries, and fresh tarragon.

½ teaspoon paprika

½ teaspoon pepper

¼ teaspoon salt

4 filets mignons without bacon (about 4 ounces each), all visible fat discarded

3 tablespoons white balsamic vinegar

1 tablespoon plus 1 teaspoon soy sauce (lowest sodium available)

1½ teaspoons sugar

1 teaspoon canola or corn oil

1 cup blackberries

1 tablespoon plus 1 teaspoon finely chopped fresh tarragon, or to taste

1. In a small bowl, stir together the paprika, pepper, and salt. Sprinkle over both sides of the beef. Using your fingertips, gently press the mixture so it adheres to the beef.

2. In the same small bowl, whisk together the vinegar, soy sauce, and sugar. Set aside.

3. In a large nonstick skillet, heat the oil over medium-high heat, swirling to coat the bottom. Cook the beef for 3 minutes on each side, or until richly browned. Reduce the heat to medium. Cook for 2 minutes on each side, or to the desired doneness. Transfer to a plate. Cover to keep warm.

4. Increase the heat to medium high. Bring the vinegar mixture to a boil, scraping to dislodge any browned bits. Gently stir in the blackberries. Cook for 2 minutes, or until the liquid has thickened and the blackberries are just soft.

5. Spoon the sauce over the beef. Sprinkle with the tarragon.

PER SERVING: Calories 192 • Total Fat **6.5 g** • Saturated Fat **2.5 g** • Trans Fat **0.0 g**
Polyunsaturated Fat **0.5 g** • Monounsaturated Fat **3.5 g** • Cholesterol **53 mg**
Sodium **330 mg** • Carbohydrates **8 g** • Fiber **2 g** • Sugars **5 g** • Protein **25 g**
DIETARY EXCHANGES: ½ fruit, 3 lean meat

SERVES 4
3 ounces beef and
½ cup pico de gallo
per serving

PREP TIME
10 minutes

COOKING TIME
10 minutes

STANDING TIME
10 minutes

Cooking spray

PICO DE GALLO

1½ cups seeded and chopped tomatoes

½ cup chopped fresh cilantro

⅓ cup chopped red onion

1 small serrano pepper, seeds and ribs discarded, minced (see Cook's Tip, page 261)

1 tablespoon fresh lime juice

* * *

1½ teaspoons ancho or chipotle powder

1 teaspoon ground cumin

½ teaspoon salt

1 1-pound flank steak, all visible fat discarded

Chile-Spiced Flank Steak with Pico de Gallo

This Mexican-spiced steak and chunky salsa pack plenty of heat, but if you want to really kick it up a level, use some of the seeds from the serrano. Add brown rice and a spinach salad with raw jícama and orange sections to round out your meal. To end on a sweet note, serve Broiled Vanilla Peaches Topped with Meringue (page 298).

1. Preheat the broiler. Line a broiler pan with aluminum foil. Lightly spray the foil and a broiler rack with cooking spray.

2. In a medium bowl, stir together the pico de gallo ingredients. Set aside.

3. In a small bowl, stir together the ancho powder, cumin, and salt. Sprinkle over both sides of the beef. Using your fingertips, gently press the mixture so it adheres to the beef. Broil the beef about 4 inches from the heat for 3 minutes on each side for medium rare, or until the desired doneness.

4. Transfer the beef to a cutting board. Let stand under a tented piece of aluminum foil for 8 to 10 minutes before thinly slicing diagonally across the grain. Serve topped with the pico de gallo.

HEALTHY SWAP: If large ripe tomatoes are out of season, choose juicy cherry or grape tomatoes instead.

PER SERVING: Calories **185** • Total Fat **7.0 g** • Saturated Fat **3.0 g** • Trans Fat **0.0 g** • Polyunsaturated Fat **0.5 g** • Monounsaturated Fat **3.5 g** • Cholesterol **48 mg** • Sodium **355 mg** • Carbohydrates **5 g** • Fiber **2 g** • Sugars **3 g** • Protein **25 g**
DIETARY EXCHANGES: 1 vegetable, 3 lean meat

Espresso-Rubbed Flank Steak with Hot Tomato Relish

SERVES 4
3 ounces beef and ½ cup relish per serving

PREP TIME
10 minutes

COOKING TIME
25 minutes

STANDING TIME
5 minutes

This boldly flavored, coffee-crusted steak won't keep you up at night, but it might have your taste buds dancing until the wee hours. While this steak is grilling, put together a cooling cucumber salad with Italian Vinaigrette (page 114) and pop some baking or sweet potatoes, such as Ginger-Honey Sweet Potatoes (page 245), in the microwave.

1. Lightly spray the grill rack with cooking spray. Preheat the grill on medium.

2. In a small bowl, stir together the espresso powder, chili powder, cumin, oregano, garlic powder, and ⅛ teaspoon salt. Sprinkle over both sides of the beef. Using your fingertips, gently press the mixture so it adheres to the beef.

3. Grill the beef for 15 to 17 minutes for medium, or until the desired doneness, turning once halfway through. Transfer to a cutting board. Let stand for 5 minutes before thinly slicing diagonally across the grain.

4. Meanwhile, in a large nonstick skillet, heat the oil over medium heat, swirling to coat the bottom. Cook the tomatoes and onion for 5 to 6 minutes, or until the vegetables are soft, stirring occasionally. Stir in the parsley, vinegar, pepper, and the remaining ⅛ teaspoon salt. Serve the relish with the beef.

Cooking spray

2 teaspoons instant espresso powder

½ teaspoon chili powder

½ teaspoon ground cumin

½ teaspoon dried oregano, crumbled

¼ teaspoon garlic powder

⅛ teaspoon salt and ⅛ teaspoon salt, divided use

1 1-pound flank steak, all visible fat discarded

2 teaspoons olive oil

2 cups halved pear or grape tomatoes (a combination of red and yellow preferred)

½ cup slivered red onion

2 tablespoons chopped fresh parsley

2 teaspoons malt vinegar

¼ teaspoon pepper

PER SERVING: Calories 216 • Total Fat 9.0 g • Saturated Fat 3.5 g • Trans Fat 0.0 g
Polyunsaturated Fat 0.5 g • Monounsaturated Fat 5.0 g • Cholesterol 48 mg
Sodium 205 mg • Carbohydrates 8 g • Fiber 2 g • Sugars 4 g • Protein 25 g
DIETARY EXCHANGES: 1 vegetable, 3 lean meat

Sirloin with Roasted Potatoes and Green Beans

High-heat roasting comes to the rescue in getting this family favorite to the table in a hurry. The vegetables get a head start on roasting when they're placed on a sizzling hot baking sheet. (*See photo insert.*)

12 ounces unpeeled red potatoes, thinly sliced (¼- to ⅜-inch slices)

8 ounces green beans, trimmed

1 medium onion, sliced

2 teaspoons olive oil and 1 teaspoon olive oil, divided use

1 tablespoon fresh thyme and 1 tablespoon fresh thyme, divided use

1 large garlic clove, minced, and 1 large garlic clove, minced, divided use

¼ teaspoon pepper and ¼ teaspoon pepper, divided use

⅛ teaspoon salt and ⅛ teaspoon salt, divided use

Cooking spray

1 1-pound boneless top sirloin steak, about 1 inch thick, all visible fat discarded, cut into 4 pieces

1. Place a large heavy rimmed baking sheet on the center rack in the oven. Preheat the oven with the baking sheet to 475°F.

2. Meanwhile, in a large bowl, stir together the potatoes, green beans, onion, and 2 teaspoons oil. Stir in 1 tablespoon thyme, 1 minced garlic clove, ¼ teaspoon pepper, and ⅛ teaspoon salt.

3. Remove the baking sheet from the oven and immediately spray it with cooking spray. Arrange the vegetables in a single layer, as much as possible, on the hot baking sheet. Return to the oven.

4. Roast for 15 minutes, or until the potatoes are beginning to brown and the green beans are almost tender.

5. Meanwhile, in a small bowl, stir together the remaining 1 tablespoon thyme, ¼ teaspoon pepper, and ⅛ teaspoon salt. Rub one side of the beef with the remaining minced garlic clove. Sprinkle the same side with the thyme mixture. Using your fingertips, gently press the garlic and seasonings so they adhere to the beef.

6. In a large nonstick skillet, heat the remaining 1 teaspoon oil over medium-high heat, swirling to coat the bottom. Cook the beef for 3 to 4 minutes, or until browned on one side. Remove from the heat.

7. Transfer the pieces of beef with the browned sides up to the baking sheet, arranging the vegetables around them.

8. Roast the beef and vegetables for 3 to 4 minutes, or until the beef is the desired doneness and the vegetables are tender. If the vegetables need more oven time, transfer the beef to plates, arrange the vegetables in a single layer, and roast for 5 minutes.

TIPS, TRICKS & TIMESAVERS: There's no need to chop fresh thyme because the leaves are so small. Simply pull your fingers down the stem and the leaves will detach.

PER SERVING: Calories **279** • Total Fat **8.0 g** • Saturated Fat **2.5 g** • Trans Fat **0.0 g**
Polyunsaturated Fat **1.0 g** • Monounsaturated Fat **5.0 g** • Cholesterol **60 mg**
Sodium **223 mg** • Carbohydrates **23 g** • Fiber **4 g** • Sugars **5 g** • Protein **29 g**
DIETARY EXCHANGES: 1 starch, 1 vegetable, 1 lean meat

SERVES 4
3 ounces beef and
¼ cup tomato
mixture per serving

PREP TIME
10 minutes

COOKING TIME
20 minutes

STANDING TIME
5 minutes

1 medium tomato, diced

¾ cup light beer (regular or nonalcoholic)

1½ tablespoons Worcestershire sauce (lowest sodium available)

2 teaspoons sugar

1 teaspoon olive oil and 1 teaspoon olive oil, divided use

1 1-pound boneless sirloin steak, all visible fat discarded

½ teaspoon pepper

1 medium green bell pepper, diced

½ cup diced onion

2 medium garlic cloves, minced

¼ cup chopped fresh parsley and 1 tablespoon chopped fresh Italian (flat-leaf) parsley, divided use

½ teaspoon salt

Sirloin Steak with Fresh Tomato-Beer Reduction

This hearty meat dish is delicious on its own, but if you're looking for meat *and* potatoes tonight, try it with a serving of our Potato-Veggie Bake (page 236).

1. In a medium bowl, stir together the tomato, beer, Worcestershire sauce, and sugar. Set aside.

2. In a large nonstick skillet, heat 1 teaspoon oil over medium-high heat, swirling to coat the bottom. Sprinkle both sides of the beef with the pepper. Cook the beef for 4 minutes on each side for medium rare, or until the desired doneness. Transfer to a cutting board. Let stand for 5 minutes. Thinly slice diagonally across the grain.

3. Meanwhile, in the same skillet, still over medium-high heat, heat the remaining 1 teaspoon oil, swirling to coat the bottom. Cook the bell pepper and onion for 3 minutes, or until the bell pepper is tender-crisp and the onion is soft, stirring frequently. Stir in the garlic. Cook for 15 seconds, stirring constantly.

4. Stir in the tomato mixture. Bring to a boil. Boil for 6 minutes, or until reduced to 1 cup and thickened. Remove from the heat.

5. Stir in ¼ cup parsley and the salt.

6. Serve the beef topped with the tomato mixture. Sprinkle with the remaining 1 tablespoon parsley.

PER SERVING: Calories 203 • Total Fat 5.0 g • Saturated Fat 1.5 g • Trans Fat 0.0 g
Polyunsaturated Fat 0.5 g • Monounsaturated Fat 3.0 g • Cholesterol 56 mg
Sodium 359 mg • Carbohydrates 10 g • Fiber 2 g • Sugars 6 g • Protein 25 g
DIETARY EXCHANGES: 1 vegetable, 3 lean meat

Peppered Sirloin with Steakhouse Onions

Enjoy these sweet caramelized onions over a well-seasoned, juicy steak. Combining salt-free beef bouillon with the onion boosts the beefy flavor of this dish without adding sodium.

1. Sprinkle the grilling blend over both sides of the beef. Using your fingertips, gently press the seasoning so it adheres to the beef.

2. In a large skillet, heat 1 teaspoon oil over medium-high heat, swirling to coat the bottom. Cook the beef for 4 minutes on each side for medium-rare, or until the desired doneness. Transfer to a cutting board. Let stand for 5 minutes. Thinly slice diagonally across the grain.

3. Meanwhile, in the same skillet, still over medium-high heat, heat the remaining 1 teaspoon oil, swirling to coat the bottom. Cook the onion for 5 minutes, or until richly browned, stirring occasionally. Cook the garlic for 15 seconds, stirring constantly. Stir in ¼ cup water, the bouillon, mustard, and salt. Bring to a boil. Boil for 30 seconds, or until the liquid has evaporated. Remove from the heat.

4. Stir in the remaining ⅓ cup water. Serve the beef topped with the onion mixture.

> **COOK'S TIP:** You can leave the steak whole to be thinly sliced after it's cooked or cut it into four individual pieces before you start.

PER SERVING: Calories **177** • Total Fat **5.0 g** • Saturated Fat **1.5 g** • Trans Fat **0.0 g** Polyunsaturated Fat **1.0 g** • Monounsaturated Fat **3.0 g** • Cholesterol **56 mg** Sodium **357 mg** • Carbohydrates **5 g** • Fiber **1 g** • Sugars **2 g** • Protein **25 g** DIETARY EXCHANGES: 1 vegetable, 3 lean meat

---

SERVES 4
3 ounces beef and 2 tablespoons onion mixture per serving

PREP TIME
15 minutes

COOKING TIME
20 minutes

STANDING TIME
5 minutes

---

2 teaspoons no-salt-added steak grilling blend

1 1-pound boneless sirloin steak, all visible fat discarded

1 teaspoon canola or corn oil and 1 teaspoon canola or corn oil, divided use

1 cup thinly sliced onion

2 medium garlic cloves, minced

¼ cup water and ⅓ cup water, divided use

2 packets (2 teaspoons) salt-free instant beef bouillon

1 teaspoon Dijon mustard (lowest sodium available)

½ teaspoon salt

PREP TIME
10 minutes

CHILLING TIME
5 minutes

COOKING TIME
20 minutes

1 tablespoon olive oil

1 tablespoon balsamic
vinegar

1 tablespoon chopped
fresh oregano

1 teaspoon grated lemon
zest

1 medium garlic clove,
minced

¼ teaspoon salt

¼ teaspoon pepper

1 pound boneless sirloin
steak, all visible fat
discarded, cut into
bite-size pieces

1 cup uncooked whole-
wheat couscous

1 large red bell pepper,
cut into 2 × ¼-inch
strips

Greek Beef and Bell Pepper Skillet

Tender sirloin steak is immersed in Mediterranean flavors, then pan-seared and laid over a bed of fluffy couscous. Serve with a side of crisp romaine salad or Lemon Artichokes (page 212) and Mini Fruited Phyllo Tarts (page 289) for dessert.

1. In a medium shallow glass dish, such as a 9-inch pie pan, whisk together the oil, vinegar, oregano, lemon zest, garlic, salt, and pepper. Add the beef, turning to coat. Cover and refrigerate for 5 minutes, turning occasionally.

2. Meanwhile, prepare the couscous using the package directions, omitting the salt. Fluff with a fork.

3. Heat a large nonstick skillet over medium-high heat. Cook the beef mixture and bell pepper for 5 to 7 minutes for medium rare, or until the beef is the desired doneness, stirring occasionally. Serve the beef mixture over the couscous.

COOK'S TIP: Make sure the skillet is very hot before adding the beef. You want it to sear and not steam. Test the skillet with drops of water. They should sizzle vigorously and dance across the surface when the skillet is heated to the correct temperature.

PER SERVING: Calories 390 • Total Fat 7.5 g • Saturated Fat 2.0 g • Trans Fat 0.0 g Polyunsaturated Fat 1.0 g • Monounsaturated Fat 4.0 g • Cholesterol 56 mg Sodium 184 mg • Carbohydrates 49 g • Fiber 8 g • Sugars 3 g • Protein 33 g DIETARY EXCHANGES: 3 starch, 3 lean meat

Burgers with Chimichurri Sauce

SERVES 4
1 burger per serving

PREP TIME
15 minutes

COOKING TIME
15 minutes

Chimichurri sauce, the "steak sauce" of Argentina, traditionally blends its main ingredients: parsley, olive oil, vinegar, and plenty of garlic. Italian (flat-leaf) parsley offers a stronger, brighter flavor and cilantro provides a tangier taste. Keep the grill on for Maple-Cinnamon Grilled Pears (page 294) to serve for dessert.

1. Lightly spray the grill rack with cooking spray. Preheat the grill on medium. Or lightly spray a grill pan and heat over medium heat.

2. In a medium bowl, using your hands or a spoon, combine the beef, cumin, onion powder, and pepper. Using wet hands (to keep the beef mixture from sticking), shape into 4 patties, each about ¾ inch thick.

3. In a food processor or blender, process the parsley, broth, oil, vinegar, garlic, and red pepper flakes until the parsley is finely chopped and the ingredients are well combined.

4. Grill the burgers for 4 minutes on each side, or until the internal temperature registers 160°F on an instant-read thermometer and the burgers are no longer pink in the center. Spread half the sauce over the bottoms of the sandwich thins. Top with the arugula and onion. Place the burgers on the onion, spreading the remaining sauce over the burgers. Put the tops of the sandwich thins on the burgers.

Cooking spray

1 pound extra-lean ground beef

1 teaspoon ground cumin

1 teaspoon onion powder

½ teaspoon freshly ground pepper

1 cup chopped fresh Italian (flat-leaf) parsley or cilantro

3 tablespoons fat-free, low-sodium vegetable broth

1 tablespoon extra-virgin olive oil

1 tablespoon red wine vinegar

2 medium garlic cloves, minced

¼ teaspoon crushed red pepper flakes

4 whole-grain round sandwich thins (lowest sodium available), lightly toasted if desired

1 cup loosely packed baby arugula or mixed spring greens

4 thin slices red onion

PER SERVING: Calories 324 • Total Fat **12.0 g** • Saturated Fat **3.0 g** • Trans Fat **0.5 g**
Polyunsaturated Fat **1.5 g** • Monounsaturated Fat **6.0 g** • Cholesterol **62 mg**
Sodium **295 mg** • Carbohydrates **24 g** • Fiber **4 g** • Sugars **4 g** • Protein **30 g**
DIETARY EXCHANGES: 1½ starch, 3 lean meat

½ cup diced tomato

2 tablespoons finely chopped fresh parsley

1 medium jalapeño, seeds left in if desired and ribs discarded, finely chopped (see Cook's Tip, page 261)

Cooking spray

1 pound extra-lean ground beef

1 tablespoon plus 1 teaspoon Dijon mustard (lowest sodium available)

1 teaspoon canola or corn oil

1 tablespoon plus 1 teaspoon soy sauce (lowest sodium available)

Stuffed Burgers

Packed between two patties is a hidden punch of flavor, thanks to a spicy tomato mixture inside. Serve these knife-and-fork burgers with Crunchy Coleslaw with Peas (page 84) or use a second burner to prepare Green Rice (page 240) at the same time.

1. In a small bowl, gently stir together the tomato, parsley, and jalapeño.

2. Lightly spray a large plate with cooking spray.

3. Using your hands or a spoon, shape the beef into 8 thin patties, each about ¼ inch thick. Transfer to the plate. Spread the mustard on the tops of the patties. Spoon 1 tablespoon of the tomato mixture onto the mustard on each patty. Place a second beef patty on each tomato-topped patty. Pinch the edges of the beef together to seal well.

4. In a large nonstick skillet, heat the oil over medium-high heat, swirling to coat the bottom. Cook the patties for 5 to 7 minutes on each side, or until the beef is no longer pink in the center. Transfer to plates. Pour the soy sauce on the patties. Top with the remaining tomato mixture.

COOK'S TIP: Lightly spraying the plate with cooking spray makes it easier to remove the thin beef patties that are placed on it.

PER SERVING: Calories 175 • Total Fat 7.5 g • Saturated Fat 2.5 g • Trans Fat 0.5 g Polyunsaturated Fat 1.0 g • Monounsaturated Fat 3.0 g • Cholesterol 62 mg Sodium 322 mg • Carbohydrates 3 g • Fiber 1 g • Sugars 2 g • Protein 25 g DIETARY EXCHANGES: 3 lean meat

Moroccan Squash and Sweet-Spiced Beef

Cardamom, a member of the ginger family, is native to India and is a popular spice in Middle Eastern cuisines. It has a strong, unique, spicy-sweet taste, so go lightly when using it. Less is more in this Moroccan dish!

1. Prepare the bulgur using the package directions, omitting the salt. Stir in ¼ teaspoon salt. Fluff with a fork. Set aside.

2. Meanwhile, in a large nonstick skillet, heat the oil over medium-high heat, swirling to coat the bottom. Cook the beef for 2 minutes, stirring constantly to turn and break up the beef. Stir in the squash, bell pepper, and onion. Cook for 8 minutes, or until the beef is browned on the outside and no longer pink in the center and the onion is tender, stirring frequently.

3. Stir in the remaining ingredients, including the remaining ½ teaspoon salt. Cook for 5 minutes, or until thickened. Remove from the heat. Let stand for 5 minutes so the flavors blend. Serve the beef mixture over the bulgur.

PER SERVING: Calories 346 • Total Fat 13.5 g • Saturated Fat 2.5 g • Trans Fat 0.5 g
Polyunsaturated Fat 4.0 g • Monounsaturated Fat 5.0 g • Cholesterol 47 mg
Sodium 515 mg • Carbohydrates 37 g • Fiber 7 g • Sugars 15 g • Protein 25 g
DIETARY EXCHANGES: 1 starch, 1 fruit, 1 vegetable, 3 lean meat, ½ fat

SERVES 4
1 cup beef mixture and ½ cup bulgur per serving

PREP TIME
15 minutes

COOKING TIME
20 minutes

STANDING TIME
5 minutes

½ cup instant, or fine-grain, bulgur

¼ teaspoon salt and ½ teaspoon salt, divided use

1 teaspoon canola or corn oil

12 ounces extra-lean ground beef

1 medium yellow summer squash, chopped

½ medium green bell pepper, diced

½ cup diced onion

2 medium tomatoes, chopped

⅓ cup raisins

½ cup unsalted shelled sunflower seeds, dry-roasted

1½ to 2 teaspoons sugar

1½ teaspoons ground cinnamon

1 teaspoon grated peeled gingerroot

¼ teaspoon ground cardamom or allspice

SERVES 4
1 tostada per serving

PREP TIME
10 minutes

COOKING TIME
10 minutes

4 6-inch corn tortillas

1 4-ounce can chopped mild green chiles, drained

2 ounces shredded fat-free sharp Cheddar cheese

1 teaspoon canola or corn oil

8 ounces extra-lean ground beef

1 medium jalapeño with seeds and ribs, finely chopped (see Cook's Tip, page 261)

1½ to 2 teaspoons paprika (smoked preferred)

½ teaspoon ground cumin

⅛ teaspoon salt

8 ounces shredded romaine

1 medium tomato, diced

1 cup corn kernels, cut from 2 medium ears of corn, husks and silk discarded

½ cup fat-free sour cream

1 medium lime, cut into 4 wedges

Smoky Tostadas

Here is Mexican "fast food" you can feel good about. Piled with layers of lettuce, tomato, corn, and spicy ground beef, these tostadas require a knife and fork to dig in.

1. Preheat the oven to 350°F.

2. Place the tortillas on a baking sheet. Using the back of a spoon, spread the green chiles over the tortillas. Sprinkle the Cheddar over the chiles.

3. Bake for 5 minutes, or until the Cheddar has melted slightly.

4. Meanwhile, in a medium nonstick skillet, heat the oil over medium-high heat, swirling to coat the bottom. Cook the beef, jalapeño, paprika, and cumin for 5 to 7 minutes, or until the beef is browned on the outside and no longer pink in the center, stirring frequently to turn and break up the beef. Stir in the salt.

5. Transfer the tortillas to plates. Top each tortilla with, in order, the romaine, tomato, corn, sour cream, and the beef mixture. Serve with the lime wedges.

PER SERVING: Calories 233 • Total Fat 5.0 g • Saturated Fat 1.5 g • Trans Fat 0.0 g Polyunsaturated Fat 1.0 g • Monounsaturated Fat 2.0 g • Cholesterol 39 mg Sodium 418 mg • Carbohydrates 26 g • Fiber 4 g • Sugars 5 g • Protein 22 g DIETARY EXCHANGES: 1½ starch, 1 vegetable, 2½ lean meat

Tomato-Basil Stuffed Pork Tenderloin

SERVES 4
3 ounces pork
per serving

PREP TIME
10 minutes

COOKING TIME
20 to 25 minutes

STANDING TIME
3 minutes

This dish looks impressive, but it's simple to prepare. A pork tenderloin is sliced open, filled with fresh tomatoes and basil, cooked on the stovetop, and finished in the oven. This two-step cooking method ensures that the pork is nicely browned on the outside but still moist and tender on the inside. Serve with Smoky Roasted Red Potatoes (page 237) and steamed broccoli.

Cooking spray

1 1-pound pork tenderloin, all visible fat discarded

¼ teaspoon salt

¼ teaspoon pepper

2 small plum (Roma) tomatoes, cut crosswise into ¼-inch slices

⅓ cup loosely packed fresh basil

2 large garlic cloves, minced

1½ teaspoons olive oil

1. Preheat the oven to 425°F. Line a rimmed baking sheet with aluminum foil. Lightly spray the foil with cooking spray.

2. Using a sharp knife, butterfly the pork. Starting at the top of the widest edge, cut the pork almost in half parallel to your work surface (through the middle of the meat), stopping about ½ inch from the opposite edge so the two halves are still joined. Open the split pork like a book. Press the inside firmly with your hand to flatten it slightly.

3. Sprinkle the salt and pepper over the pork. Arrange the tomatoes on the right half, slightly overlapping them. Top with the basil. Fold the left half of the pork over the tomatoes and basil. Securely tie the tenderloin in four places with kitchen twine. Spread the garlic over the outside. Using your fingertips, gently press the garlic so it adheres to the pork.

4. In a large nonstick skillet, heat the oil over medium-high heat, swirling to coat the bottom. Cook the pork for 3 minutes, turning to brown on all sides. Transfer to the baking sheet.

5. Roast the pork for 15 to 20 minutes, or until it registers 145°F on an instant-read thermometer and is slightly pink in the center. Transfer the pork to a cutting board. Let stand for 3 minutes, or until the desired doneness. Discard the twine. Cut crosswise into slices.

PER SERVING: Calories **173** • Total Fat **7.0 g** • Saturated Fat **2.0 g** • Trans Fat **0.0 g**
Polyunsaturated Fat **0.5 g** • Monounsaturated Fat **3.5 g** • Cholesterol **75 mg**
Sodium **199 mg** • Carbohydrates **2 g** • Fiber **1 g** • Sugars **1 g** • Protein **25 g**
DIETARY EXCHANGES: 3 lean meat

Pork Tenderloin with Kickin' Raspberry Sauce

SERVES 4
3 ounces pork and 2 tablespoons sauce per serving

PREP TIME
5 minutes

COOKING TIME
25 minutes

STANDING TIME
3 minutes

Cooking spray

½ teaspoon ground allspice

½ teaspoon pepper

¼ teaspoon salt

1 1-pound pork tenderloin, all visible fat discarded

1 teaspoon canola or corn oil and 1 teaspoon canola or corn oil, divided use

¼ cup finely chopped red onion

1 medium jalapeño with seeds and ribs, finely chopped, and 1 medium jalapeño, seeds and ribs discarded, finely chopped, divided use (see Cook's Tip, page 261)

2 tablespoons balsamic vinegar

(continued)

Kick up your taste buds with fork-tender pork drenched in a raspberry sauce made with balsamic vinegar and jalapeño. You'll love not only this entrée's flavor but also how fast it is to put together—it's oven-ready in 5 minutes!

1. Preheat the oven to 425°F. Lightly spray a baking sheet with cooking spray. Set aside.

2. In a small bowl, stir together the allspice, pepper, and salt. Sprinkle all over the pork. Using your fingertips, gently press the mixture so it adheres to the pork.

3. In a large nonstick skillet, heat 1 teaspoon oil over medium-high heat, swirling to coat the bottom. Cook the pork for 4 minutes, or until richly browned. Turn over. Cook for 2 minutes, or until golden brown. Transfer to the baking sheet.

4. Roast the pork for 15 minutes, or until it registers 145°F on an instant-read thermometer and is slightly pink in the center. Transfer the pork to a cutting board. Let stand for 3 minutes, or until the desired doneness. Cut crosswise into slices.

5. Meanwhile, in the same skillet, still over medium-high heat, heat the remaining 1 teaspoon oil, swirling to coat the bottom. Cook the onion and 1 jalapeño (with seeds and ribs) for 2 minutes, or until the onion is beginning to brown on the edges, stirring occasionally.

6. Stir in the vinegar, soy sauce, and sugar. Cook for 30 seconds, or until slightly thickened.

7. Gently stir in the raspberries. Cook for 30 seconds, or until slightly softened. Remove from the heat.

8. Serve the pork topped with the sauce. For a dressy presentation, pool the raspberry sauce on plates and fan the pork slices on top of the sauce. Sprinkle with the remaining jalapeño (seeds and ribs discarded).

2 tablespoons soy sauce (lowest sodium available)

1 tablespoon sugar

½ cup raspberries

> **COOK'S TIP:** Be sure to turn on your stovetop exhaust fan while cooking the sauce. The jalapeños will begin to "pop" slightly and can exude some potent fumes.

PER SERVING: Calories **206** • Total Fat **7.5 g** • Saturated Fat **2.0 g** • Trans Fat **0.0 g**
Polyunsaturated Fat **1.0 g** • Monounsaturated Fat **3.5 g** • Cholesterol **75 mg**
Sodium **396 mg** • Carbohydrates **9 g** • Fiber **2 g** • Sugars **7 g** • Protein **25 g**
DIETARY EXCHANGES: ½ other carbohydrate, 3 lean meat

Pork Tenderloin with Roasted Apple

SERVES 4
3 ounces pork and
½ cup apple mixture
per serving

PREP TIME
5 minutes

COOKING TIME
30 minutes

STANDING TIME
3 minutes

Cooking spray

1 teaspoon chopped fresh rosemary and ½ teaspoon chopped fresh rosemary, divided use

½ teaspoon garlic powder

½ teaspoon pepper and ⅛ teaspoon pepper, divided use

¼ teaspoon salt and ⅛ teaspoon salt, divided use

1 1-pound pork tenderloin, all visible fat discarded

1 teaspoon canola or corn oil and 2 teaspoons canola or corn oil, divided use

1 medium to large tart green apple (about 8 ounces), such as Granny Smith, cut into 8 wedges

1 medium onion, cut into 8 wedges

2 teaspoons sugar

Using the tenderloin rather than the loin reduces the roasting time without losing any slow-cooked flavor. Make room in the oven for Sweet Orange-Roasted Root Vegetables (page 247), which roast at the same temperature.

1. Preheat the oven to 425°F. Line a rimmed baking sheet with aluminum foil. Lightly spray the foil with cooking spray.

2. In a small bowl, stir together 1 teaspoon rosemary, the garlic powder, ½ teaspoon pepper, and ¼ teaspoon salt. Sprinkle all over the pork. Using your fingertips, gently press the mixture so it adheres to the pork.

3. In a large nonstick skillet, heat the oil over medium-high heat, swirling to coat the bottom. Cook the pork for 4 minutes, or until richly browned on the bottom. Turn over. Cook for 2 minutes, or until golden brown. Transfer to the baking sheet.

4. Roast for 15 minutes. Arrange the apple and onion around the pork. Lightly spray the apple and onion with cooking spray. Sprinkle the sugar over the apple and onion.

5. Roast for 5 minutes, or until the pork registers 145°F on an instant-read thermometer and is slightly pink in the center, and the apple and onion are tender-crisp.

6. Transfer the pork to a cutting board. Let stand for 3 minutes, or until the desired doneness. Cut crosswise into slices.

7. Keeping the apple mixture on the foil, stir in the remaining 2 teaspoons oil, ½ teaspoon rosemary, ⅛ teaspoon pepper, and ⅛ teaspoon salt. Serve the apple mixture with the pork.

PER SERVING: Calories 232 • Total Fat 8.5 g • Saturated Fat 2.0 g • Trans Fat 0.0 g
Polyunsaturated Fat 1.5 g • Monounsaturated Fat 4.5 g • Cholesterol 75 mg
Sodium 269 mg • Carbohydrates 14 g • Fiber 2 g • Sugars 10 g • Protein 25 g
DIETARY EXCHANGES: 1 fruit, 3 lean meat

Balsamic Pork with Pan-Popping Tomatoes

The pork, sauce, and topping are all cooked in just one pan, making cleanup a breeze. The acidity of the tomatoes balances the sweetness of the honey and the tanginess of the balsamic vinegar. *(See photo insert.)*

1. In a large skillet, heat 1 teaspoon oil over medium-high heat, swirling to coat the bottom. Cook the tomatoes and honey for 3 minutes, or until the tomatoes begin to pop and are lightly browned, stirring frequently. Transfer to a bowl. Cover to keep warm.

2. Sprinkle both sides of the pork with ¼ teaspoon salt and the pepper.

3. In the same skillet, still over medium-high heat, heat the remaining 1 teaspoon oil, swirling to coat the bottom. Cook the pork for 3 to 4 minutes on each side, or until it registers 145°F on an instant-read thermometer and is slightly pink in the center. Transfer to a platter. Let stand for 3 minutes, or until the desired doneness.

4. Meanwhile, in the same skillet, bring the vinegar and the remaining ⅛ teaspoon salt to a boil. Boil for 30 seconds, or until the mixture is reduced by half (to about 2 tablespoons). Spoon over the pork. Top with the tomato mixture.

TIPS, TRICKS & TIMESAVERS: Lightly spray a measuring spoon with cooking spray to keep honey from sticking to the spoon.

SERVES 4
3 ounces pork and 3 tablespoons tomato mixture per serving

PREP TIME
5 minutes

COOKING TIME
15 minutes

STANDING TIME
3 minutes

1 teaspoon canola or corn oil and 1 teaspoon canola or corn oil, divided use

1 cup grape tomatoes

1 tablespoon honey

4 boneless center-cut pork chops (about 4 ounces each), all visible fat discarded

¼ teaspoon salt and ⅛ teaspoon salt, divided use

¼ teaspoon pepper

¼ cup balsamic vinegar

PER SERVING: Calories 211 • Total Fat 8.5 g • Saturated Fat 2.0 g • Trans Fat 0.0 g
Polyunsaturated Fat 1.5 g • Monounsaturated Fat 4.0 g • Cholesterol 60 mg
Sodium 286 mg • Carbohydrates 10 g • Fiber 1 g • Sugars 9 g • Protein 23 g
DIETARY EXCHANGES: ½ other carbohydrate, 3 lean meat

4 boneless center-cut
pork chops (about
4 ounces each), all
visible fat discarded

½ teaspoon pepper

⅛ teaspoon salt and
⅛ teaspoon salt,
divided use

1 teaspoon olive oil and
1 tablespoon extra-
virgin olive oil, divided
use

½ cup water

2 medium green onions,
finely chopped

2 medium garlic cloves,
minced

1 packet (1 teaspoon) salt-
free instant chicken
bouillon

1 teaspoon Dijon mustard
(lowest sodium
available)

2 teaspoons chopped
fresh tarragon

Pork Chops with Tarragon Jus

Tarragon and Dijon mustard are a classic combo, giving pork chops a touch of sophisticated flavor. Spinach with Shallots and Thyme (page 242) and Orange-Soaked Apple Wedges (page 249) are simple-to-make, satisfying side dishes. Add a quick-cooking whole grain such as instant brown rice, quinoa, or barley to complete your meal.

1. Sprinkle both sides of the pork with the pepper and ⅛ teaspoon salt.

2. In a large skillet, heat 1 teaspoon oil over medium-high heat, swirling to coat the bottom. Cook the pork for 3 to 4 minutes on each side, or until it registers 145°F on an instant-read thermometer and is slightly pink in the center. Transfer to a plate. Let stand for 3 minutes, or until the desired doneness.

3. Meanwhile, in the same skillet, bring the water, green onions, garlic, bouillon, and mustard to a boil over medium-high heat. Boil for 3 minutes, or until the liquid is reduced by half (to about ¼ cup), scraping to dislodge any browned bits and stirring occasionally. Remove from the heat.

4. Stir in the tarragon and the remaining ⅛ teaspoon salt and 1 tablespoon oil. Spoon over the pork.

PER SERVING: Calories 195 • Total Fat **10.5 g** • Saturated Fat **2.5 g** • Trans Fat **0.0 g**
Polyunsaturated Fat **1.0 g** • Monounsaturated Fat **5.5 g** • Cholesterol **66 mg**
Sodium **219 mg** • Carbohydrates **2 g** • Fiber **1 g** • Sugars **1 g** • Protein **21 g**
DIETARY EXCHANGES: 3 lean meat

Mustard-Crusted Pork Medallions with Celery Root Purée

SERVES 4
2 pork medallions
and ¾ cup purée
per serving

PREP TIME
15 minutes

COOKING TIME
30 to 35 minutes

STANDING TIME
3 minutes

A smooth mixture of fat-free Greek yogurt and baked celery root makes for a healthy alternative to mashed potatoes and a cool accompaniment for this zesty pork. The taste of celery root (also called celeriac) is, of course, like celery but mellower, with flavors reminiscent of parsley and mild nuts, such as hazelnuts.

1. Preheat the oven to 375°F.

2. In a 13 × 9 × 2-inch baking pan or on a baking sheet, stir together the celery root, garlic, and oil. Arrange the mixture in a single layer. Bake for 27 to 30 minutes, or until the celery root and garlic are tender.

3. Meanwhile, in a small bowl, whisk together the thyme, mustard, paprika, and pepper. Spread on the top of the pork.

4. Lightly spray a large skillet with cooking spray. Heat the skillet over medium heat. Cook the pork with the mustard side down for 4 minutes. Turn over. Cook for 4 minutes, or until the internal temperature registers 145°F on an instant-read thermometer. Transfer the pork to a large plate. Cover loosely to keep warm. Let stand for 3 minutes.

5. In a food processor or blender, process the celery root mixture, yogurt, milk, and salt until smooth, scraping the side of the bowl once or twice. Add the green onions. Pulse to combine. Serve the purée with the pork.

1 pound peeled celery root, cut into 1-inch chunks

4 medium garlic cloves

1 tablespoon olive oil

2 tablespoons chopped fresh thyme

2 tablespoons stone-ground or coarse-grain mustard (lowest sodium available)

1 teaspoon paprika (smoked preferred)

½ teaspoon freshly ground pepper

1 1-pound pork tenderloin, all visible fat discarded, cut into 8 slices, pounded to ½-inch thickness

Olive oil cooking spray

½ cup fat-free Greek yogurt

½ cup fat-free milk

⅛ teaspoon salt

¼ cup chopped green onions (green part only)

PER SERVING: Calories 274 • Total Fat 9.5 g • Saturated Fat 2.5 g • Trans Fat 0.0 g
Polyunsaturated Fat 1.0 g • Monounsaturated Fat 4.5 g • Cholesterol 76 mg
Sodium 419 mg • Carbohydrates 17 g • Fiber 3 g • Sugars 5 g • Protein 30 g
DIETARY EXCHANGES: 3 vegetable, 3½ lean meat

Pork, Black Bean, and Broccoli Stir-Fry

With broccoli, red bell pepper, onion, and black beans, this dish is packed with fiber and provides a rainbow of colors. Serve it with instant brown rice or Green Rice (page 240) and Mango and Butter Lettuce Salad with Curry-Dijon Vinaigrette (page 80) for a fast and easy weeknight meal.

½ cup water and ½ cup water, divided use

¼ cup plain rice vinegar

2 tablespoons tamari sauce (lowest sodium available)

1 tablespoon brown sugar

1 tablespoon cornstarch

1 tablespoon toasted sesame oil

1 teaspoon canola or corn oil

12 ounces pork tenderloin, all visible fat discarded, cut into thin strips

1 medium red bell pepper, chopped into 1-inch squares

1 medium onion, chopped into 1-inch squares

2 teaspoons minced peeled gingerroot

10 ounces broccoli florets (1-inch pieces)

1 cup no-salt-added canned black beans, rinsed and drained

1. In a medium bowl, whisk together ½ cup water, the vinegar, tamari sauce, brown sugar, cornstarch, and sesame oil. Set aside.

2. In a large skillet, heat the canola oil over high heat, swirling to coat the bottom (the oil should be sizzling). Cook the pork for 3 minutes, or until no longer pink in the center, stirring constantly. Working quickly, transfer the pork to a plate. Set aside.

3. Stir in the bell pepper, onion, and gingerroot. Cook for 2 minutes, or until the vegetables are slightly softened, stirring constantly.

4. Quickly stir in the broccoli, beans, and the remaining ½ cup water. Cook for 2 minutes, or until the broccoli is tender-crisp, stirring frequently and scraping to dislodge any browned bits.

5. Stir the vinegar mixture. Pour into the skillet. Add the pork. Cook for 2 to 3 minutes, or until the sauce begins to bubble and thicken, stirring frequently. Remove from the heat. Serve immediately.

PER SERVING: Calories 281 • Total Fat 8.5 g • Saturated Fat 2.0 g • Trans Fat 0.0 g
Polyunsaturated Fat 2.0 g • Monounsaturated Fat 3.5 g • Cholesterol 56 mg
Sodium 371 mg • Carbohydrates 26 g • Fiber 6 g • Sugars 10 g • Protein 25 g
DIETARY EXCHANGES: 1 starch, 2 vegetable, 3 lean meat

Rosemary-Crusted Lamb Chops with Minted Pesto Chickpeas

Push aside the sugary mint jelly often served with lamb to make room for this minty chickpea condiment. It's so easy to make and uses fresh mint for a bolder, more natural flavor.

SERVES 4
1 lamb chop and scant ½ cup chickpeas per serving

PREP TIME
10 minutes

COOKING TIME
10 to 15 minutes

1. In a medium bowl, stir together the mint, 2 teaspoons oil, 1 garlic clove, ¼ teaspoon pepper, and ¼ teaspoon salt. Stir in the chickpeas. Cover and refrigerate until serving time.

2. In a small bowl, stir together the rosemary and the remaining 1 teaspoon oil, 3 garlic cloves, ¼ teaspoon pepper, and ¼ teaspoon salt. Sprinkle over both sides of the lamb. Using your fingertips, gently press the mixture so it adheres to the lamb.

3. Heat a large nonstick skillet or grill pan over medium heat. Cook the lamb for 5 to 6 minutes on each side, or until the desired doneness. Serve with the chickpea mixture.

¼ cup minced fresh mint

2 teaspoons extra-virgin olive oil and 1 teaspoon olive oil, divided use

1 medium garlic clove, minced, and 3 medium garlic cloves, minced, divided use

¼ teaspoon freshly ground pepper and ¼ teaspoon pepper, divided use

¼ teaspoon salt and ¼ teaspoon salt, divided use

1 15.5-ounce can no-salt-added chickpeas, rinsed and drained

1 tablespoon minced fresh rosemary

4 loin lamb chops with bone (about 6 ounces each), all visible fat discarded

TIPS, TRICKS & TIMESAVERS: To mince fresh rosemary, hold a thick, woody stem upright over a plate, at a slight angle so the leaves are pointing upward. Run your index finger and thumb down the length of the stem, starting at the top. The leaves will fall onto the plate. Transfer the leaves to a cup. Using kitchen scissors, snip the leaves into very small pieces.

PER SERVING: Calories 303 • Total Fat 11.0 g • Saturated Fat 3.0 g • Trans Fat 0.0 g
Polyunsaturated Fat 1.0 g • Monounsaturated Fat 5.5 g • Cholesterol 68 mg
Sodium 380 mg • Carbohydrates 21 g • Fiber 5 g • Sugars 1 g • Protein 28 g
DIETARY EXCHANGES: 1½ starch, 3 lean meat

VEGETARIAN ENTRÉES

Margherita Portobello Pizzas

SERVES 4
2 pizzas per serving

PREP TIME
5 minutes

COOKING TIME
25 minutes

These tri-colored pizzas, based on the colors of the Italian flag, start with a portobello mushroom "crust." Serve with a spinach salad dressed with Italian Vinaigrette (page 114).

1. Preheat the oven to 425°F.

2. Arrange the mushrooms with the gill side up on a rimmed baking sheet.

3. In a small bowl, stir together the oil, garlic, salt, and pepper. Brush the mixture over the mushrooms. Roast for 15 minutes. Remove from the oven, leaving the oven turned on.

4. Sprinkle with the basil. Top with the tomato and mozzarella. Bake for 5 minutes, or until the mozzarella is melted.

8 large portobello mushrooms, stems discarded

2 tablespoons plus 2 teaspoons olive oil

4 medium garlic cloves, minced

½ teaspoon salt

½ teaspoon cracked pepper

½ cup chopped fresh basil

1 cup seeded and chopped tomato

¾ cup shredded low-fat mozzarella cheese

PER SERVING: Calories **164** • Total Fat **11.5 g** • Saturated Fat **2.0 g** • Trans Fat **0.0 g** Polyunsaturated Fat **1.0 g** • Monounsaturated Fat **7.5 g** • Cholesterol **8 mg** Sodium **304 mg** • Carbohydrates **9 g** • Fiber **3 g** • Sugars **3 g** • Protein **9 g** DIETARY EXCHANGES: 2 vegetable, 2 lean meat, 2 fat

8 ounces dried whole-
grain spaghetti

3 cups cubed butternut
squash (¼-inch cubes)

1 cup fat-free, low-sodium
vegetable broth

½ cup chopped onion

2 medium garlic cloves,
minced

¼ teaspoon salt

¼ teaspoon pepper

2 cups trimmed, halved
sugar snap peas

2 tablespoons chopped
fresh sage

¼ cup shredded or grated
Parmesan cheese

Butternut Squash Pasta

The flavor of sage marries perfectly with any type of winter squash. In this hearty dish, the green sugar snap peas provide a striking visual contrast to the bright orange butternut squash.

1. Prepare the pasta using the package directions, omitting the salt. Drain well in a colander. Set aside.

2. In a large skillet, stir together the squash, broth, onion, garlic, salt, and pepper. Bring to a boil over medium-high heat. Reduce the heat and simmer for 5 minutes.

3. Stir in the peas. Return to a simmer and simmer for 7 to 10 minutes, or until the squash is tender and most of the liquid has evaporated.

4. Stir in the sage. Serve the squash mixture over the pasta. Sprinkle with the Parmesan.

SHOP & STORE: When choosing a butternut squash for this recipe, look for one that has a longer neck. The neck is easier to peel and chop since it doesn't have any seeds.

TIPS, TRICKS & TIMESAVERS: Some winter squash, such as butternut, are difficult to cut when raw. To make the job easy, pierce the squash several times with a fork and place the squash on a microwaveable plate. Microwave on 100 percent power (high) for 1 to 2 minutes. Let the squash stand for 5 minutes before cutting. Using a large, sturdy knife, cut off the stem end, then cut lengthwise from the stem end through the root end. Using a spoon, scoop out and discard the seeds and strings.

PER SERVING: Calories **298** • Total Fat **3.0 g** • Saturated Fat **1.0 g** • Trans Fat **0.0 g**
Polyunsaturated Fat **0.5 g** • Monounsaturated Fat **1.0 g** • Cholesterol **4 mg**
Sodium **243 mg** • Carbohydrates **59 g** • Fiber **9 g** • Sugars **7 g** • Protein **12 g**
DIETARY EXCHANGES: 3½ starch, 1 vegetable

Edamame Pasta

Marjoram tastes like a sweeter version of oregano, but it's actually a member of the mint family. Known for being distinctly aromatic, marjoram creates an enticing fragrance for this flavorful vegetable-and-rotini dish.

1. Prepare the pasta using the package directions, omitting the salt. Drain well in a colander. Set aside.

2. Meanwhile, in a large nonstick skillet, stir together the chard, edamame, broth, shallots, and garlic. Bring to a boil over medium-high heat. Boil gently for 6 to 8 minutes, or until the chard is tender.

3. Stir in the tomatoes, marjoram, thyme, salt, and pepper. Cook for 1 to 2 minutes, or until heated through, stirring frequently.

4. Transfer the chard mixture to a serving bowl. Add the pasta, tossing to combine. Sprinkle with the Parmesan.

SHOP & STORE: Edamame, or green soybeans, are available fresh for only a limited season (late spring to early fall), and you're most likely to find them at Asian markets and local farmers' markets. If you can't find them fresh or they are out of season, substitute frozen edamame, available year-round from most major supermarkets.

PER SERVING: Calories 331 • Total Fat **6.0 g** • Saturated Fat **1.0 g** • Trans Fat **0.0 g** • Polyunsaturated Fat **1.5 g** • Monounsaturated Fat **2.0 g** • Cholesterol **4 mg** • Sodium **324 mg** • Carbohydrates **56 g** • Fiber **11 g** • Sugars **8 g** • Protein **17 g**
DIETARY EXCHANGES: 3 starch, 2 vegetable, 1 lean meat

SERVES 4
1½ cups per serving

PREP TIME
10 minutes

COOKING TIME
15 to 20 minutes

8 ounces dried whole-grain rotini

4 cups coarsely chopped Swiss chard, tough stems discarded

2 cups edamame

⅓ cup fat-free, low-sodium vegetable broth

¼ cup thinly sliced shallots

2 medium garlic cloves, minced

2 cups quartered cherry or grape tomatoes

1 tablespoon chopped fresh marjoram

2 teaspoons chopped fresh thyme

¼ teaspoon salt

¼ teaspoon pepper

¼ cup shredded or grated Parmesan cheese

SERVES 5
1½ cups per serving

PREP TIME
10 minutes

COOKING TIME
15 to 20 minutes

7 ounces dried whole-grain penne

1 tablespoon olive oil

½ medium onion, thinly sliced

2 medium zucchini, halved lengthwise and cut crosswise into ¼-inch slices

1 tablespoon plus 2 teaspoons pine nuts

2 medium tomatoes, chopped (½-inch pieces)

½ cup tightly packed shredded fresh basil

½ cup water

10 kalamata olives, each cut into quarters

1 tablespoon capers, drained and chopped

½ teaspoon salt

¼ teaspoon freshly ground pepper

1 tablespoon plus 2 teaspoons shredded or grated Parmesan cheese

Pasta Provençal

Serve this dish during the summer months when fresh zucchini, basil, and tomatoes are at their peak. Add a mixed-greens salad with Raspberry-Blackberry Dressing (page 115) and you've got a summertime meal that incorporates some of the best from the season's bounty.

1. Prepare the pasta using the package directions, omitting the salt. Drain well in a colander. Set aside.

2. Meanwhile, in a large skillet, heat the oil over medium-high heat, swirling to coat the bottom. Cook the onion for 3 minutes, or until soft, stirring frequently.

3. Stir in the zucchini and pine nuts. Cook for 2 minutes, or until the zucchini is slightly soft, stirring frequently.

4. Stir in the tomatoes. Cook, covered, for 2 minutes, stirring occasionally.

5. Reduce the heat to medium. Stir in the basil, water, olives, capers, salt, pepper, and pasta. Cook for 2 minutes, stirring to combine.

6. Sprinkle with the Parmesan. Serve immediately.

COOK'S TIP ON WHOLE-GRAIN PASTA: Whole-grain pasta, which contains the bran and germ from the grain, takes longer to cook than pasta made from refined white flour, but it's worth the extra few minutes of cooking time because it provides a better blend of nutrients than white-flour pasta and has a chewier texture and nuttier taste.

PER SERVING: Calories 235 • Total Fat 8.0 g • Saturated Fat 1.0 g • Trans Fat 0.0 g
Polyunsaturated Fat 1.5 g • Monounsaturated Fat 4.5 g • Cholesterol 1 mg
Sodium 444 mg • Carbohydrates 36 g • Fiber 6 g • Sugars 6 g • Protein 8 g
DIETARY EXCHANGES: 2 starch, 1 vegetable, 1 fat

Tomato, Mushroom, and Arugula Fettuccine

SERVES 4
1 cup pasta and
½ cup mushroom
mixture per serving

PREP TIME
10 minutes

COOKING TIME
20 minutes

Arugula gives a peppery bite to this pasta dish. Using a variety of mushrooms provides an earthiness, and the bite-size tomatoes offer sweetness, a flavor combination not to be missed.

1. Prepare the pasta using the package directions, omitting the salt. Drain well in a colander. Set aside.

2. Meanwhile, in a large nonstick skillet, heat the oil over medium-high heat, swirling to coat the bottom. Cook the mushrooms, shallots, and garlic for 8 to 10 minutes, or until the mushrooms are tender and golden, stirring occasionally.

3. Stir in the tomatoes, broth, salt, and pepper. Cook for 7 to 9 minutes, or until most of the liquid has evaporated.

4. Add the arugula, stirring until wilted.

5. Serve the mushroom mixture over the pasta. Sprinkle with the Parmesan.

PER SERVING: Calories 300 • Total Fat 6.0 g • Saturated Fat 1.5 g • Trans Fat 0.0 g
Polyunsaturated Fat 1.0 g • Monounsaturated Fat 3.0 g • Cholesterol 4 mg
Sodium 253 mg • Carbohydrates 53 g • Fiber 9 g • Sugars 8 g • Protein 13 g
DIETARY EXCHANGES: 3 starch, 2 vegetable, ½ fat

8 ounces dried whole-grain fettuccine

2 teaspoons olive oil

4 cups sliced assorted mushrooms, such as button, brown (cremini), shiitake (stems discarded), or portobello

⅓ cup sliced shallots

2 medium garlic cloves, minced

2 cups quartered cherry or grape tomatoes

¼ cup fat-free, low-sodium vegetable broth

¼ teaspoon salt

¼ teaspoon pepper

4 cups baby arugula

¼ cup shredded or grated Parmesan cheese

SERVE 4

1½ cups per serving

PREP TIME

10 minutes

COOKING TIME

20 minutes

Barley, Beans, and Greens

The bright purple-red and green of the Swiss chard and the orange of the carrot against the creamy white barley and beans make this meal as enjoyable to look at as it is to eat.

1 cup uncooked quick-cooking barley

¾ cup fat-free, low-sodium vegetable broth

½ cup chopped onion

½ cup chopped carrot

4 large Swiss chard leaves, tough stems discarded, tender stems sliced and greens chopped, divided use

1 medium garlic clove, minced

1 15.5-ounce can no-salt-added cannellini beans or other no-salt-added white beans (such as Great Northern or navy beans), rinsed and drained

¼ teaspoon salt

¼ teaspoon pepper

⅓ cup chopped fresh parsley

¼ cup sliced almonds, dry-roasted

1. Prepare the barley using the package directions, omitting the salt. Drain well in a colander. Set aside.

2. Meanwhile, in a large skillet, stir together the broth, onion, carrot, chard stems, and garlic. Bring to a boil over medium-high heat. Boil gently for 6 to 8 minutes, or until the vegetables are tender, stirring occasionally.

3. Stir in the chard greens. Cook, covered, for 5 to 7 minutes, or until the greens are tender, stirring occasionally.

4. Stir in the beans, salt, and pepper. Cook for 1 to 2 minutes, or until heated through.

5. Stir in the barley. Just before serving, sprinkle with the parsley and almonds.

PER SERVING: Calories 266 • Total Fat 4.5 g • Saturated Fat 0.5 g • Trans Fat 0.0 g
Polyunsaturated Fat 1.0 g • Monounsaturated Fat 2.0 g • Cholesterol 0 mg
Sodium 231 mg • Carbohydrates 48 g • Fiber 10 g • Sugars 3 g • Protein 11 g
DIETARY EXCHANGES: 3 starch, 1 vegetable, ½ lean meat

Shiitake Barley

Hearty mushrooms, chewy barley, and earthy kale combine to make this a satisfying, filling dish, while the seasonings add a distinctly Asian flair. Cooking the shiitakes until they're slightly golden intensifies their flavor.

SERVES 4
1¼ cups per serving

PREP TIME
10 minutes

COOKING TIME
20 minutes

1. Prepare the barley using the package directions, omitting the salt. If you prefer more moisture in the finished dish, stop the cooking process before the barley has absorbed all the water. Set aside.

2. Meanwhile, in a large skillet, heat the oil over medium heat, swirling to coat the bottom. Cook the mushrooms, gingerroot, and garlic for 6 to 8 minutes, or until the mushrooms are slightly golden, stirring occasionally.

3. Stir in the kale and soy sauce. Cook, covered, for 6 to 8 minutes, or until the kale is tender, stirring occasionally. Stir in the barley, green onions, and pepper.

1½ cups uncooked quick-cooking barley

1 tablespoon olive oil

2 cups sliced shiitake mushrooms, stems discarded

1 tablespoon minced peeled gingerroot

2 medium garlic cloves, minced

4 cups chopped kale, any large stems discarded

1 tablespoon soy sauce (lowest sodium available)

½ cup thinly sliced green onions

¼ teaspoon pepper

PER SERVING: Calories **272** • Total Fat **5.0 g** • Saturated Fat **1.0 g** • Trans Fat **0.0 g** Polyunsaturated Fat **1.0 g** • Monounsaturated Fat **2.5 g** • Cholesterol **0 mg** Sodium **137 mg** • Carbohydrates **52 g** • Fiber **8 g** • Sugars **2 g** • Protein **9 g** DIETARY EXCHANGES: 3 starch, 2 vegetable, ½ fat

Bulgur with Chard and Feta

Swiss chard is a fresh change from spinach, which is more commonly used with the Mediterranean flavors of this dish. The relative mildness of potassium-rich chard is a natural complement to more assertive flavors such as the bite from red onion and the tanginess of feta.

¾ cup uncooked instant, or fine-grain, bulgur

2 cups coarsely chopped Swiss chard, tough stems discarded

¼ cup raw unsalted shelled pumpkin seeds, dry-roasted

¼ cup finely chopped red onion

1½ to 2 tablespoons chopped fresh dillweed

1 tablespoon grated lemon zest

1 tablespoon extra-virgin olive oil

2 medium garlic cloves, minced

1 teaspoon chopped fresh rosemary

4 ounces fat-free feta cheese, crumbled

1 medium lemon, cut into 4 wedges

1. Prepare the bulgur using the package directions, omitting the salt. Fluff with a fork.

2. Transfer the bulgur to a large bowl. Add the chard, pumpkin seeds, onion, dillweed, lemon zest, oil, garlic, and rosemary, gently stirring until the chard is slightly wilted. Gently stir in the feta. Serve with the lemon wedges.

PER SERVING: Calories **199** • Total Fat **7.5 g** • Saturated Fat **1.0 g** • Trans Fat **0.0 g**
Polyunsaturated Fat **2.0 g** • Monounsaturated Fat **3.5 g** • Cholesterol **0 mg**
Sodium **484 mg** • Carbohydrates **25 g** • Fiber **6 g** • Sugars **2 g** • Protein **12 g**
DIETARY EXCHANGES: 1½ starch, 1 lean meat, ½ fat

Poached Eggs with Pesto Bulgur

SERVES 4
1 egg and ½ cup bulgur mixture per serving

PREP TIME
10 minutes

COOKING TIME
15 minutes

This pesto replaces traditional olive oil with vegetable broth and trades the usual pine nuts for walnuts. It combines with a whole grain to create a hearty bed on which delicate poached eggs lie. *(See photo insert.)*

1. In a medium saucepan, prepare the bulgur using the package directions, omitting the salt and substituting 1⅓ cups broth for the water. Fluff with a fork.

2. Meanwhile, in a food processor or blender, process the basil, walnuts, garlic, salt, cayenne, and the remaining 2 tablespoons broth until smooth. Stir the basil mixture, bell pepper, and green onions into the bulgur.

3. In a large skillet, bring the water and vinegar to a boil over high heat. Reduce the heat and simmer. Break an egg into a cup and then carefully slip the egg into the simmering water. Repeat with the remaining eggs, placing them in the water so they don't touch. Simmer for 3 to 5 minutes, or until the whites are completely set and the yolks are beginning to set, but aren't hard. Using a slotted spoon, drain the eggs well and place on the bulgur mixture. Serve with the lemon wedges.

TIPS, TRICKS & TIMESAVERS: The vinegar helps the egg whites firm up faster and prevents them from spreading too much.

⅔ cup uncooked instant, or fine-grain, bulgur

1⅓ cups fat-free, low-sodium vegetable broth and 2 tablespoons fat-free, low-sodium vegetable broth, divided use

1 cup tightly packed fresh basil

2 tablespoons chopped walnuts, dry-roasted

1 small garlic clove, minced

⅛ teaspoon salt

Dash of cayenne

½ cup finely chopped yellow or red bell pepper

¼ cup thinly sliced green onions

4 cups water

1 tablespoon white vinegar

4 large eggs

1 medium lemon, cut into 4 wedges

PER SERVING: Calories 190 • Total Fat **7.5 g** • Saturated Fat **2.0 g** • Trans Fat **0.0 g** Polyunsaturated Fat **3.0 g** • Monounsaturated Fat **2.0 g** • Cholesterol **186 mg** Sodium **160 mg** • Carbohydrates **21 g** • Fiber **5 g** • Sugars **1 g** • Protein **11 g** DIETARY EXCHANGES: 1½ starch, 1 lean meat, ½ fat

SERVES 4
1¼ cups per serving

PREP TIME
10 minutes

COOKING TIME
20 to 30 minutes

3 cups water

¾ cup dried French green lentils or brown lentils, sorted for stones and shriveled lentils, rinsed, and drained

1 tablespoon olive oil

1 cup chopped onion

2 medium garlic cloves, minced

½ teaspoon salt

1½ cups fat-free, low-sodium vegetable broth or water

½ cup uncooked instant, or fine-grain, bulgur

1¼ cups chopped seeded tomatoes

½ cup chopped fresh parsley

¼ cup chopped fresh mint

¼ teaspoon pepper

¼ cup fat-free plain Greek yogurt

1 medium lemon, cut into 4 wedges

Lentils and Bulgur

This dish is like a hot tabbouleh salad. The addition of lentils makes it an excellent option for dinner. Use French green lentils, also called Puy lentils, which have a peppery flavor and hold their shape well during cooking. If you can't find them, you can always use brown lentils instead.

1. In a large microwaveable glass bowl, stir together the water and lentils. Cover with a glass lid. Microwave on 100 percent power (high) for 5 minutes, then microwave on 50 percent power (medium) for 15 to 20 minutes, or until the lentils are tender. Drain well in a fine-mesh sieve.

2. Meanwhile, in a large skillet, heat the oil over medium heat, swirling to coat the bottom. Cook the onion, garlic, and salt for 8 to 10 minutes, or until the onion is golden, stirring occasionally.

3. Stir in the broth and bulgur. Increase the heat to medium high and bring to a boil. Reduce the heat and simmer for 10 to 12 minutes, or until the liquid is absorbed.

4. Stir in the lentils, tomatoes, parsley, mint, and pepper. Cook for 1 to 2 minutes, or until heated through. Serve topped with the yogurt. Garnish with the lemon wedges.

COOK'S TIP: Be sure to use a microwaveable glass bowl when cooking the lentils. Plastic can melt and non-microwaveable glass can shatter.

PER SERVING: Calories 267 • Total Fat **4.0 g** • Saturated Fat **0.5 g** • Trans Fat **0.0 g**
Polyunsaturated Fat **0.5 g** • Monounsaturated Fat **2.5 g** • Cholesterol **0 mg**
Sodium **320 mg** • Carbohydrates **46 g** • Fiber **10 g** • Sugars **6 g** • Protein **16 g**
DIETARY EXCHANGES: 2½ starch, 1 vegetable, 1 lean meat

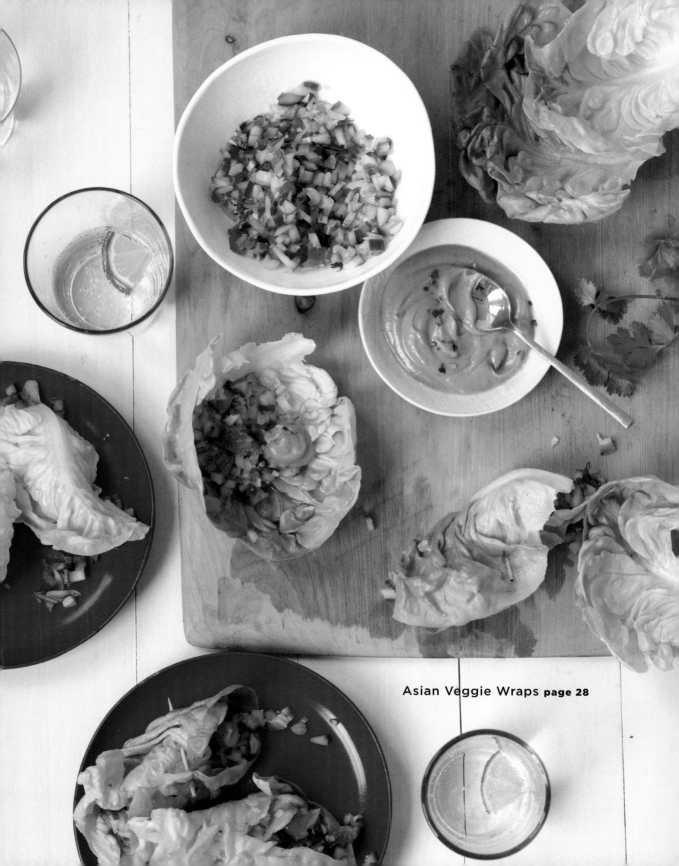

Asian Veggie Wraps **page 28**

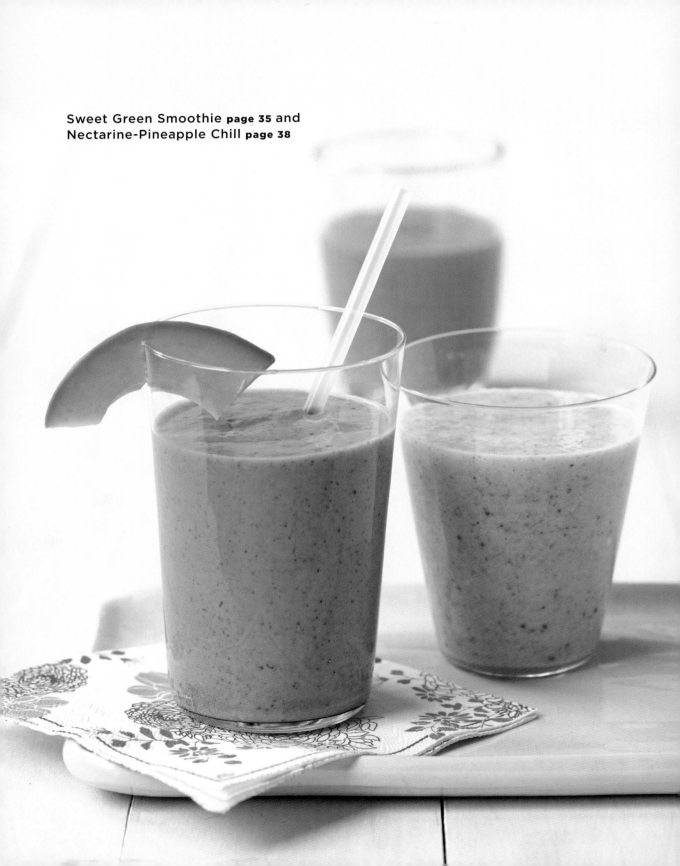

Sweet Green Smoothie **page 35** and
Nectarine-Pineapple Chill **page 38**

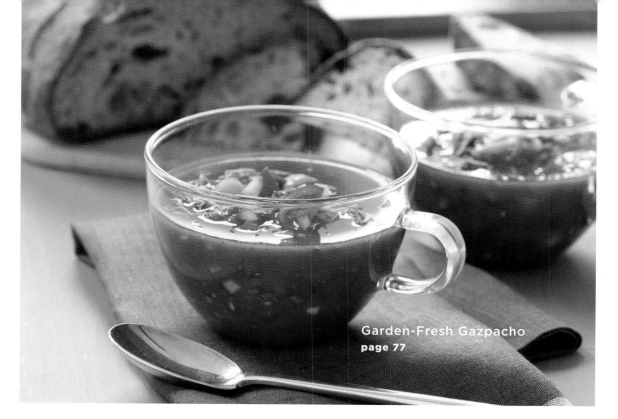

Garden-Fresh Gazpacho
page 77

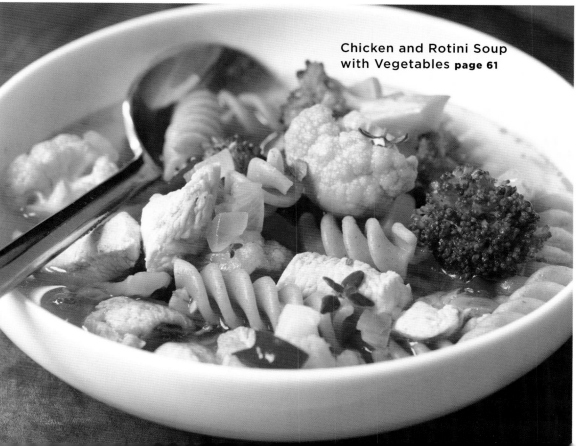

Chicken and Rotini Soup
with Vegetables **page 61**

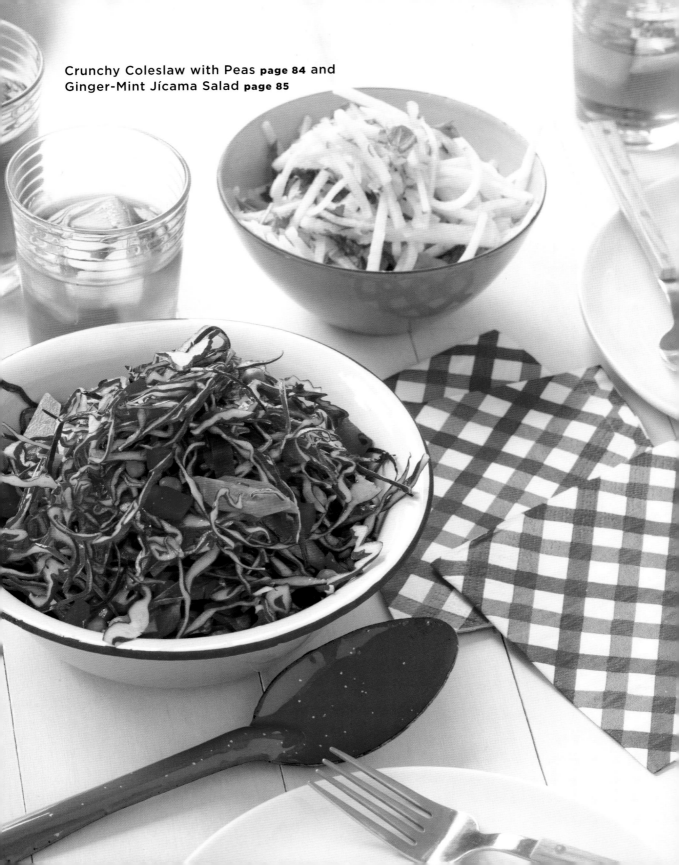

Crunchy Coleslaw with Peas **page 84** and
Ginger-Mint Jícama Salad **page 85**

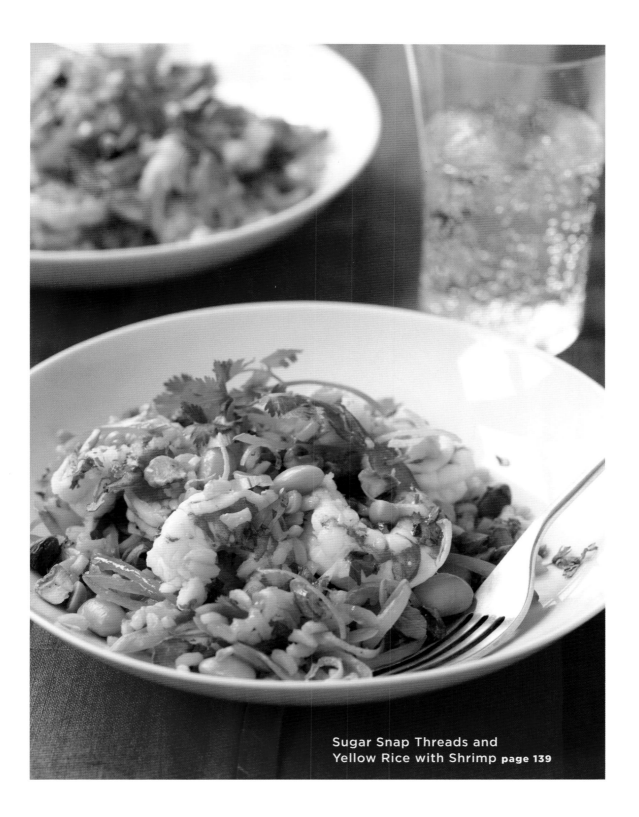

Sugar Snap Threads and
Yellow Rice with Shrimp **page 139**

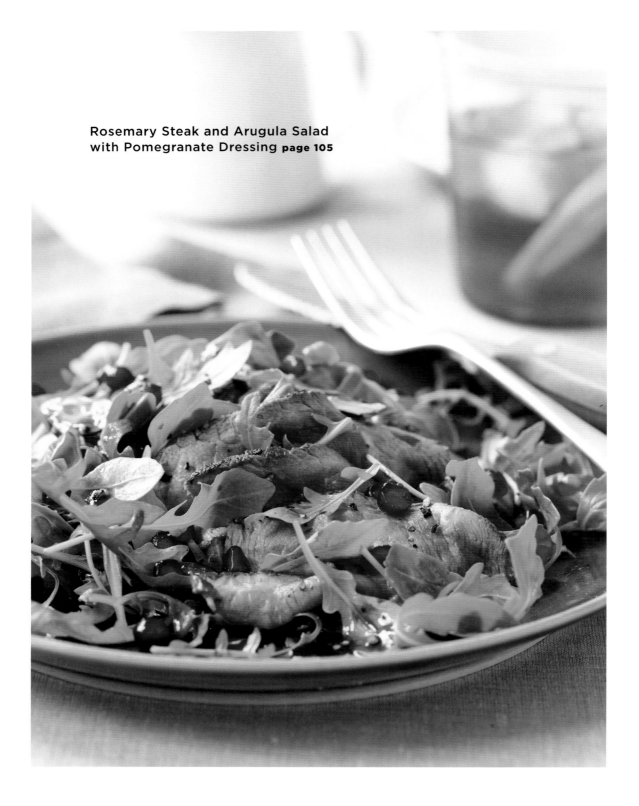

Rosemary Steak and Arugula Salad
with Pomegranate Dressing **page 105**

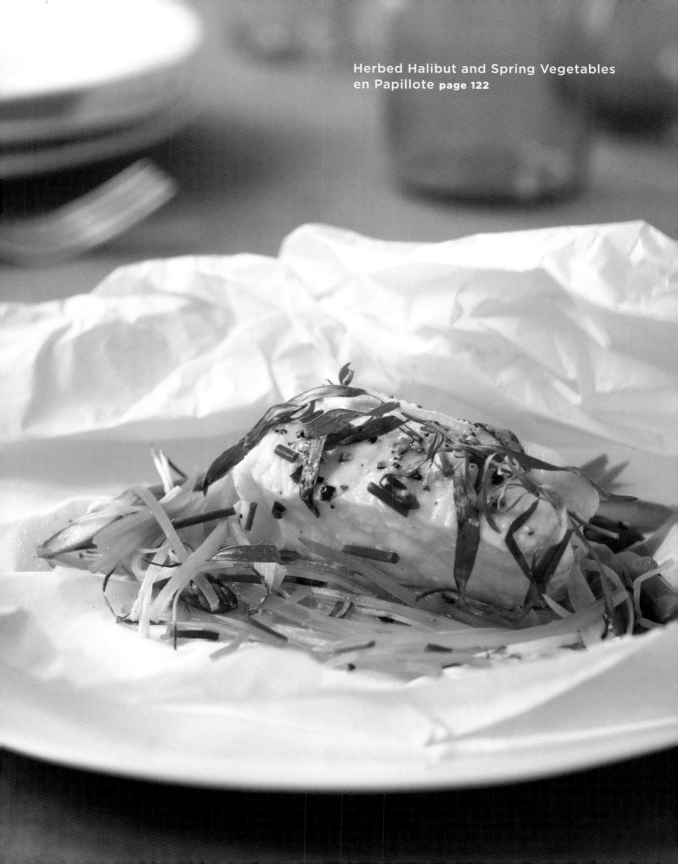

Herbed Halibut and Spring Vegetables
en Papillote **page 122**

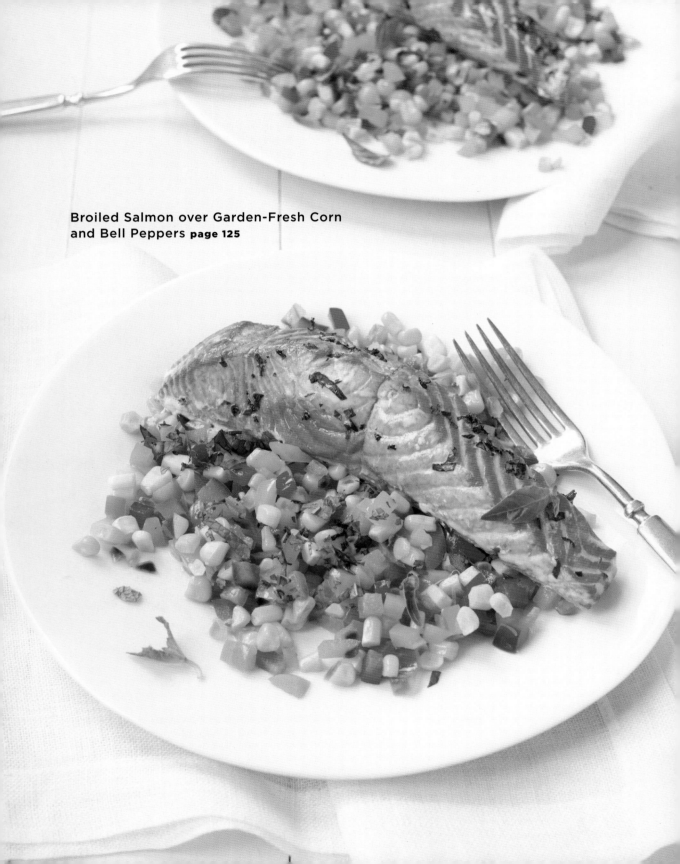

Broiled Salmon over Garden-Fresh Corn
and Bell Peppers **page 125**

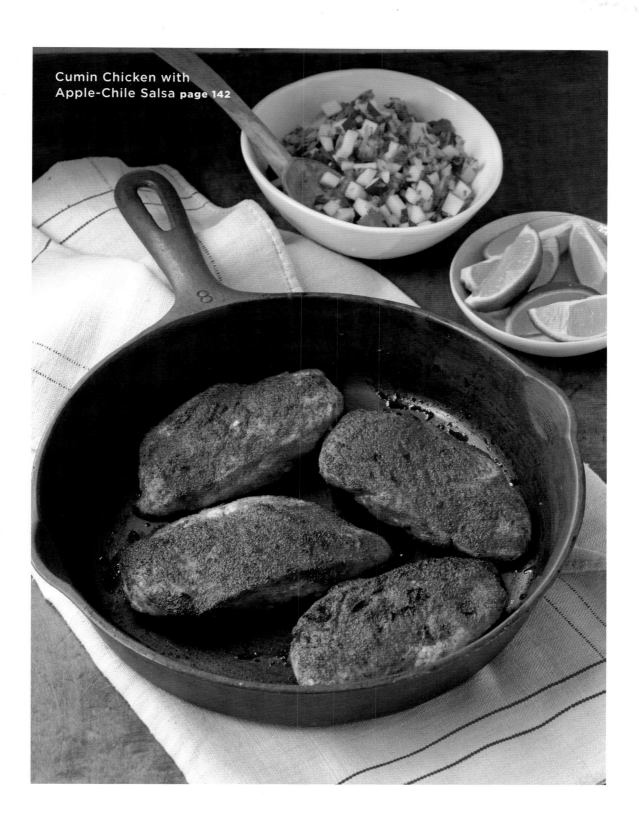

Cumin Chicken with
Apple-Chile Salsa **page 142**

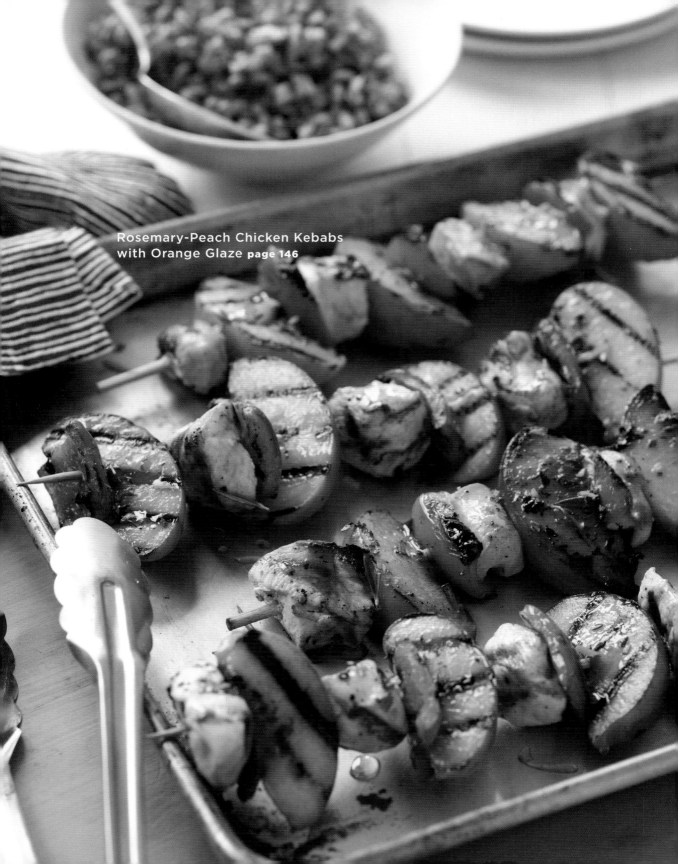

Rosemary-Peach Chicken Kebabs
with Orange Glaze **page 146**

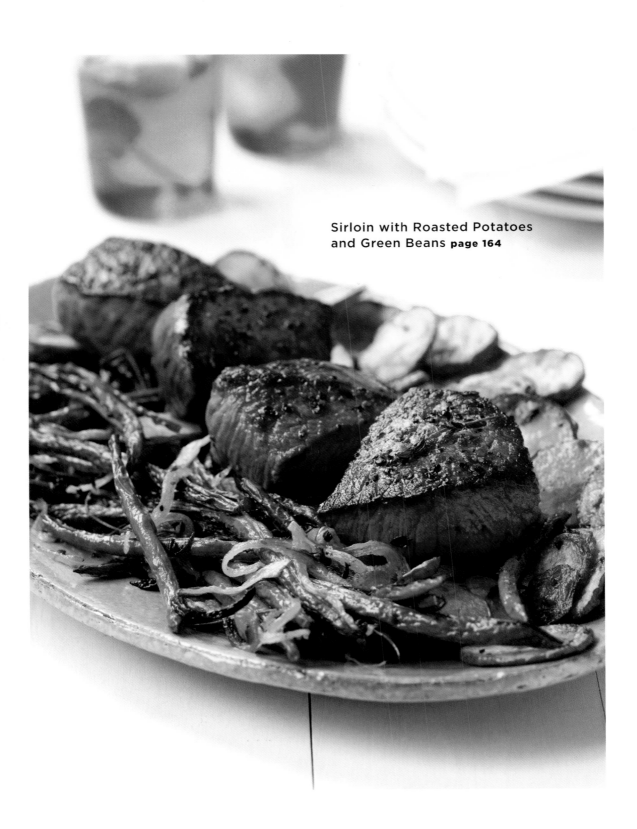

Sirloin with Roasted Potatoes
and Green Beans **page 164**

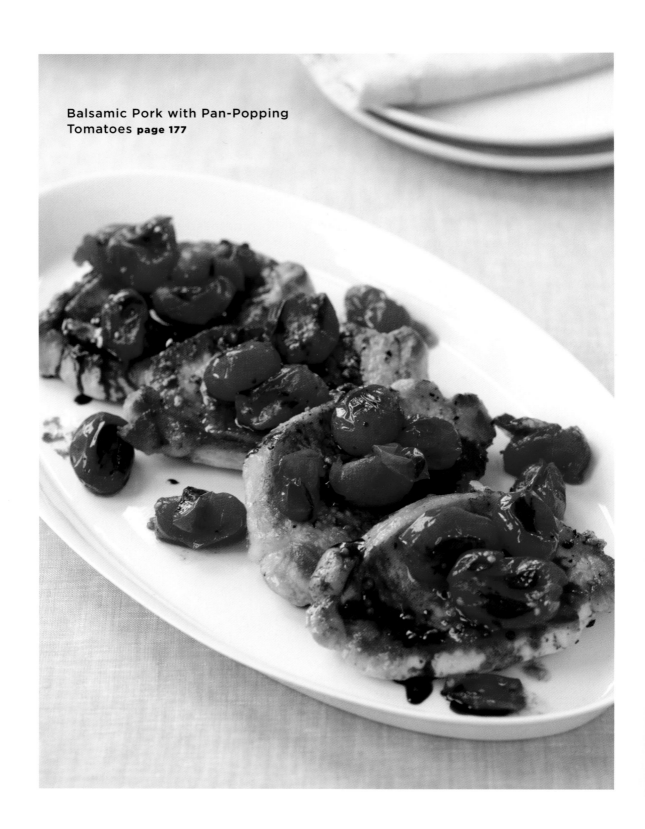

Balsamic Pork with Pan-Popping
Tomatoes **page 177**

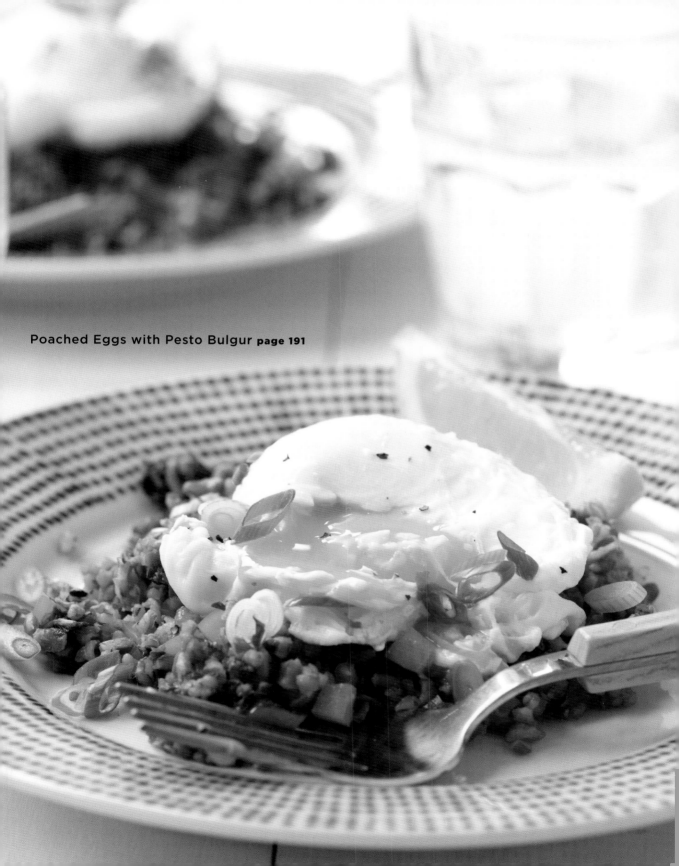

Poached Eggs with Pesto Bulgur **page 191**

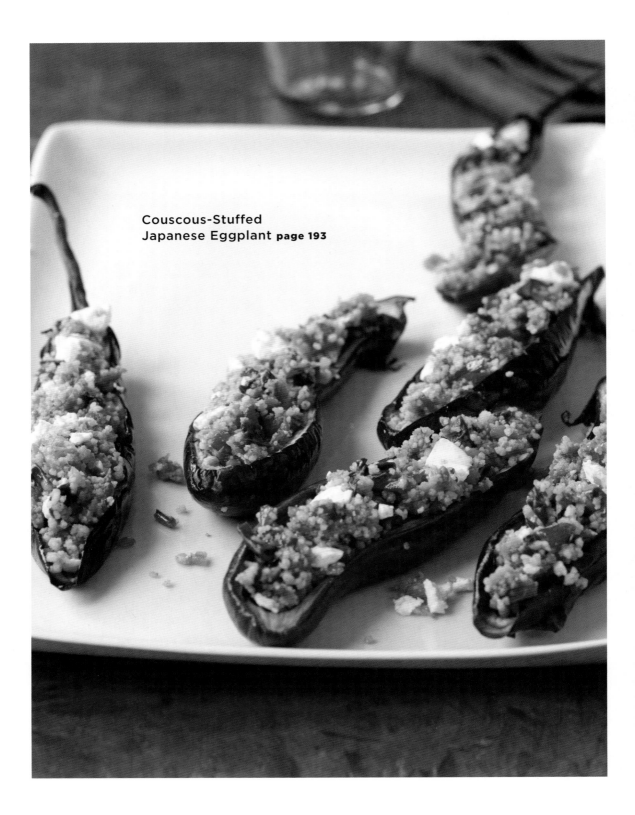

Couscous-Stuffed Japanese Eggplant page 193

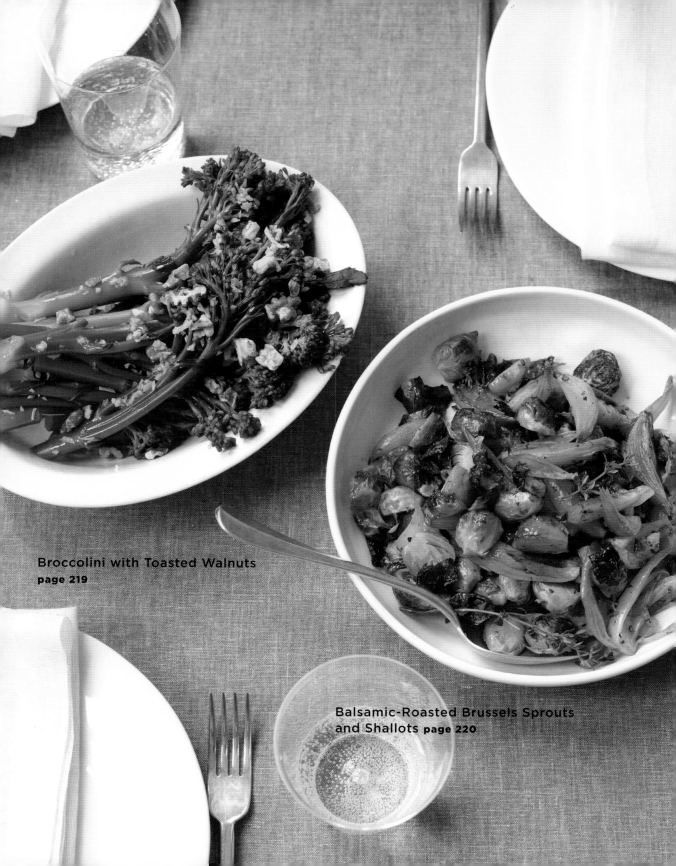

Broccolini with Toasted Walnuts
page 219

Balsamic-Roasted Brussels Sprouts
and Shallots **page 220**

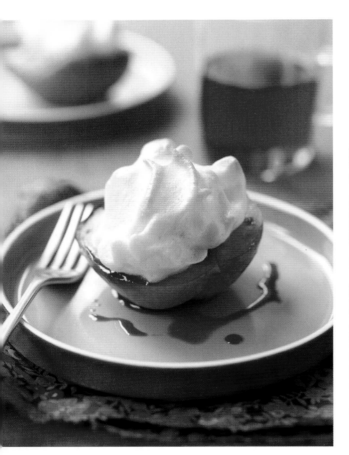

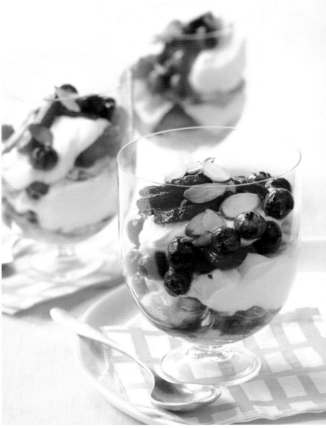

Broiled Vanilla Peaches Topped with Meringue page 298

Fruity Oatmeal Yogurt Parfaits page 286

Couscous-Stuffed Japanese Eggplant

Although this dish uses Japanese eggplant, its flavors from the olive oil, lemon, and feta are distinctively Greek. *(See photo insert.)*

1. Preheat the broiler.

2. Prepare the couscous using the package directions, omitting the salt. Fluff with a fork. Set aside.

3. Halve the eggplants lengthwise. Scoop out the pulp, leaving a ¼-inch border of the shell all the way around. Transfer the pulp to a cutting board.

4. Lightly spray the inside and outside of the shells with cooking spray. Arrange with the cut sides down on a baking sheet. Broil the shells about 4 inches from the heat for 8 to 10 minutes, or until tender, turning them over halfway through.

5. Meanwhile, chop the eggplant pulp.

6. In a large nonstick skillet, heat the oil over medium heat, swirling to coat the bottom. Cook the eggplant pulp, shallot, garlic, salt, and pepper for 5 to 7 minutes, or until the pulp is tender, stirring occasionally.

7. Stir in the spinach, tomatoes, and lemon zest. Cook for 1 to 2 minutes, or until the spinach is wilted, stirring frequently. Stir in the couscous and feta.

8. Put the shells on plates. Spoon the stuffing into the shells.

SHOP & STORE: Japanese eggplant is slender and has a thinner skin and sweeter flavor than the more familiar globe eggplant.

SERVES 4
2 stuffed eggplant halves per serving

PREP TIME
15 minutes

COOKING TIME
20 to 25 minutes

½ cup uncooked whole-wheat couscous

4 medium unpeeled Japanese eggplants

Cooking spray

2 teaspoons olive oil

2 tablespoons finely chopped shallot

1 medium garlic clove, minced

¼ teaspoon salt

¼ teaspoon pepper

2 cups shredded spinach

1¼ cups chopped seeded tomatoes

2 teaspoons grated lemon zest

1 ounce crumbled fat-free feta cheese

PER SERVING: Calories 208 • Total Fat 3.5 g • Saturated Fat 0.5 g • Trans Fat 0.0 g
Polyunsaturated Fat 0.5 g • Monounsaturated Fat 2.0 g • Cholesterol 0 mg
Sodium 315 mg • Carbohydrates 40 g • Fiber 13 g • Sugars 8 g • Protein 9 g
DIETARY EXCHANGES: 1½ starch, 3 vegetable, ½ fat

Roasted Winter Vegetables and Quinoa with Spinach Pesto

In this all-in-one entrée, winter vegetables are roasted until crisp, and then tossed with a whole grain and a tofu-based pesto, which adds creaminess and protein. Don't be put off by the number of ingredients. Once the vegetables are in the oven, the rest comes together quickly.

8 ounces peeled acorn squash, cut into 1-inch cubes

6 ounces brussels sprouts, each one quartered

6 ounces cauliflower florets, cut into 1-inch pieces

2 or 3 medium carrots, cut into ½-inch pieces

1 small onion, cut into ½-inch pieces

1 tablespoon olive oil

¼ teaspoon freshly ground pepper

¾ cup uncooked quinoa, rinsed and drained

PESTO

6½ ounces light firm tofu, drained and patted dry

6 ounces spinach

½ cup tightly packed fresh basil

¼ cup water

2 tablespoons olive oil

1 tablespoon chopped walnuts

1 tablespoon fresh lemon juice

2 medium garlic cloves, coarsely chopped

½ teaspoon salt

1. Preheat the oven to 425°F.

2. In a 14 × 10-inch roasting pan, toss together the squash, brussels sprouts, cauliflower, carrots, onion, oil, and pepper. Cover the pan with aluminum foil. Roast for 15 minutes. Uncover. Roast for 10 minutes.

3. Meanwhile, prepare the quinoa using the package directions, omitting the salt. Fluff with a fork.

4. In a food processor or blender, process the pesto ingredients for 2 minutes, or until smooth.

5. In a large serving bowl, gently stir together the vegetables, quinoa, and pesto. Serve immediately.

TIPS, TRICKS & TIMESAVERS: To save time, you can make the pesto a day or two in advance. Store in an airtight container and refrigerate until needed. Bring the pesto to room temperature or, in a microwaveable dish, microwave on 100 percent power (high) for 30 seconds, stirring once halfway through, before stirring it together with the vegetables and quinoa.

PER SERVING: Calories **224** • Total Fat **10.0 g** • Saturated Fat **1.5 g** • Trans Fat **0.0 g**
Polyunsaturated Fat **2.5 g** • Monounsaturated Fat **5.5 g** • Cholesterol **0 mg**
Sodium **263 mg** • Carbohydrates **28 g** • Fiber **6 g** • Sugars **6 g** • Protein **9 g**
DIETARY EXCHANGES: 1 starch, 2 vegetable, ½ lean meat, 1 fat

Grilled Veggies on Black Bean Quinoa

SERVES 4
1½ cups per serving

PREP TIME
10 minutes

COOKING TIME
20 minutes

A variety of tender-crisp vegetables blankets a coarse mixture of black beans, quinoa, and pine nuts. Blue cheese adds a pungent finishing touch.

1. Prepare the quinoa using the package directions, omitting the salt. Remove from the heat. Fluff with a fork.

2. Stir in the beans, pine nuts, pepper, and salt. Cover to keep warm. Set aside.

3. Meanwhile, lightly spray a grill pan with cooking spray. Heat over medium-high heat.

4. Lightly spray the mushrooms and both sides of the bell pepper halves, onion slices, and summer squash halves with cooking spray. Cook for 5 to 6 minutes on each side, or until the vegetables are tender-crisp, brushing occasionally with the vinegar. Transfer the vegetables to a cutting board. Coarsely chop them.

5. Transfer the quinoa mixture to a serving platter. Top with the vegetables. Sprinkle with the blue cheese.

> **TIPS, TRICKS & TIMESAVERS:** If you flatten each bell pepper half with the palm of your hand, it will cook more evenly.

½ cup uncooked quinoa, rinsed and drained

½ 15.5-ounce can no-salt-added black beans, rinsed and drained

¼ cup pine nuts, dry-roasted

½ teaspoon pepper

¼ teaspoon salt

Cooking spray

4 ounces whole button mushrooms

1 medium red bell pepper, halved lengthwise

1 medium onion, cut into 4 round slices

1 medium yellow summer squash, halved lengthwise

2 tablespoons balsamic vinegar

4 ounces low-fat blue cheese or low-fat feta cheese, crumbled

PER SERVING: Calories **284** • Total Fat **10.0 g** • Saturated Fat **4.5 g** • Trans Fat **0.0 g**
Polyunsaturated Fat **2.5 g** • Monounsaturated Fat **3.0 g** • Cholesterol **15 mg**
Sodium **538 mg** • Carbohydrates **33 g** • Fiber **7 g** • Sugars **10 g** • Protein **17 g**
DIETARY EXCHANGES: 1½ starch, 2 vegetable, 1½ lean meat, 1 fat

SERVES 4
1 stuffed pita half
and 2 tablespoons
yogurt per serving

PREP TIME
15 minutes

COOKING TIME
30 minutes

FILLING

1½ cups water

¼ cup dried lentils, sorted for stones and shriveled lentils, rinsed, and drained

¼ cup uncooked quinoa, rinsed and drained

1 cup spinach, coarsely chopped

½ cup finely chopped celery

½ cup diced red onion

¼ cup pine nuts, dry-roasted

1 tablespoon extra-virgin olive oil

1½ teaspoons fresh lime juice

1½ teaspoons cider vinegar

2 medium garlic cloves, minced

³⁄₈ teaspoon salt

* * *

2 6-inch whole-grain pita pockets, halved

½ cup fat-free plain Greek yogurt

2 tablespoons chopped fresh dillweed

Pita Pockets Stuffed with Lentils and Quinoa

You'll load up on wholesomeness with this garlicky, nutty legume and grain mixture stuffed into pita pockets. For variety, try serving the fiber-filled filling as a salad with baked whole-grain pita wedges on the side.

1. In a large saucepan, bring the water and lentils to a boil over high heat. Reduce the heat and simmer, covered, for 15 minutes. Stir in the quinoa. Return to a simmer and simmer, covered, for 12 minutes, or until the lentils are just tender. Transfer the mixture to a fine-mesh sieve. Rinse with cold water to cool quickly. Drain well. Transfer to a large bowl.

2. Stir in the remaining filling ingredients. Spoon into the pita pockets. Top with the yogurt and dillweed.

COOK'S TIP ON PITA: To make the pitas a little softer and more pliable, microwave them on 100 percent power (high) for 15 seconds.

PER SERVING: Calories 261 • Total Fat 8.5 g • Saturated Fat 1.5 g • Trans Fat 0.0 g
Polyunsaturated Fat 2.5 g • Monounsaturated Fat 4.0 g • Cholesterol 0 mg
Sodium 404 mg • Carbohydrates 37 g • Fiber 6 g • Sugars 5 g • Protein 13 g
DIETARY EXCHANGES: 2½ starch, 1 lean meat, ½ fat

Quinoa, Rice, and Red Beans

SERVES 4
1¼ cups per serving

PREP TIME
5 minutes

COOKING TIME
15 minutes

If you're not familiar with quinoa (KEEN-wah), then this dish is a perfect way to make its acquaintance. Quinoa is a rich source of protein, too, making it a complementary component of any vegetarian entrée.

1. In a medium saucepan, bring the water to a boil over high heat. Stir in the quinoa and rice. Reduce the heat and simmer, covered, for 10 to 12 minutes, or until the quinoa and rice are tender and the water is absorbed. Fluff with a fork. Set aside.

2. Meanwhile, in a large nonstick skillet, heat 1 teaspoon oil over medium-high heat, swirling to coat the bottom. Cook the onion and poblano for 3 minutes, or until the onion is soft, stirring frequently. Stir in the beans, tomatoes, and garlic. Cook for 2 minutes to heat through. Remove from the heat.

3. Stir in the quinoa mixture, adobo sauce, salt, and the remaining 2 tablespoons oil. Just before serving, top with the sour cream. Sprinkle with the green onions.

SHOP & STORE: Look in the Mexican food section of grocery stores for chipotle peppers (dried jalapeños that have a smoky flavor) canned in adobo sauce, a moderately spicy mixture of chiles, vinegar, garlic, and herbs. The leftovers freeze nicely. Spread the peppers with sauce in a thin layer on a medium plate covered with cooking parchment or wax paper, then freeze them, uncovered, for about 2 hours, or just until firm. (This step will keep the peppers from sticking together later.) Transfer the peppers to an airtight freezer bag and freeze.

2 cups water

⅓ cup uncooked quinoa, rinsed and drained

⅓ cup uncooked instant brown rice

1 teaspoon olive oil and 2 tablespoons extra-virgin olive oil, divided use

½ cup diced onion

1 medium poblano pepper, seeds and ribs discarded, diced (see Cook's Tip, page 261)

1 15.5-ounce can no-salt-added red or kidney beans, rinsed and drained

1 cup grape tomatoes, halved

2 medium garlic cloves, minced

1 to 2 teaspoons adobo sauce (from canned chipotle peppers in adobo sauce)

½ teaspoon salt

½ cup fat-free sour cream

1 to 2 medium green onions, chopped

PER SERVING: Calories 300 • Total Fat 10.0 g • Saturated Fat 1.0 g • Trans Fat 0.0 g Polyunsaturated Fat 1.5 g • Monounsaturated Fat 6.0 g • Cholesterol 5 mg Sodium 411 mg • Carbohydrates 42 g • Fiber 7 g • Sugars 7 g • Protein 11 g DIETARY EXCHANGES: 2 starch, 2 vegetable, ½ lean meat, 1 fat

SERVES 4
1½ cups per serving

PREP TIME
10 minutes

COOKING TIME
10 to 15 minutes

Cheesy Vegetable and Rice Skillet

This dish is a perfect choice for a Meatless Monday and an easy way to start off the workweek. You can have this one-dish meal on the table in less than half an hour from start to finish. Cleanup is quick, too, since it all cooks in one skillet.

1 teaspoon canola or corn oil

1 medium red bell pepper, chopped

½ cup chopped onion

8 ounces whole button mushrooms, halved or quartered if large

1 cup small broccoli florets

1 cup small cauliflower florets

¼ cup water and ¼ cup water, divided use

10 ounces frozen cooked brown rice

1 teaspoon fresh thyme

1 medium garlic clove, minced

¼ teaspoon pepper

½ teaspoon salt

1 cup shredded low-fat sharp Cheddar cheese

1. In a large skillet, heat the oil over medium-high heat, swirling to coat the bottom. Cook the bell pepper and onion for 2 minutes, stirring occasionally.

2. Stir in the mushrooms. Cook for 3 to 4 minutes, or until the mushrooms begin to release some of their juices, stirring frequently.

3. Stir in the broccoli, cauliflower, and ¼ cup water. Reduce the heat and simmer for 3 minutes, or until the vegetables are tender-crisp.

4. Stir in the rice, thyme, garlic, pepper, and the remaining ¼ cup water. Bring to a simmer over medium-high heat. Reduce the heat and simmer, covered, for 2 minutes, or until the rice is heated through.

5. Just before serving, stir in the salt. Sprinkle with the Cheddar.

PER SERVING: Calories 183 • Total Fat 4.0 g • Saturated Fat 1.5 g • Trans Fat 0.0 g Polyunsaturated Fat 0.5 g • Monounsaturated Fat 1.5 g • Cholesterol 6 mg Sodium 488 mg • Carbohydrates 25 g • Fiber 4 g • Sugars 4 g • Protein 13 g
DIETARY EXCHANGES: 1 starch, 2 vegetable, 1 lean meat

Garden Vegetable Fried Rice

SERVE 4
1½ cups per serving

PREP TIME
5 minutes

COOKING TIME
15 minutes

This Chinese food favorite is a great way to load up on veggies. Feel free to substitute any of the vegetables in your refrigerator for those in the recipe. Broccoli, mushrooms, eggplant, and zucchini would be good choices.

1. Prepare the rice using the package directions, omitting the salt and margarine. Set aside.

2. Meanwhile, in a large nonstick skillet, heat the oil over medium heat, swirling to coat the bottom. Cook the asparagus, snow peas, carrots, bell pepper, cauliflower, and garlic for 10 to 12 minutes, or until the vegetables are tender-crisp, stirring occasionally.

3. Meanwhile, in a small bowl, using a fork, beat together the eggs and soy sauce.

4. Stir the rice into the asparagus mixture. Push the mixture to the sides of the skillet. Pour the egg mixture into the center of the skillet. Using a heatproof rubber scraper, stir for 1 to 2 minutes, or until partially set.

5. Stir the asparagus mixture into the partially cooked egg mixture. Cook for 1 minute, or until the eggs are cooked through, stirring constantly.

6. Stir in the vinegar. Just before serving, sprinkle with the green onions and walnuts.

1 cup uncooked instant brown rice

2 teaspoons toasted sesame oil

1 cup chopped trimmed asparagus

1 cup trimmed, halved snow peas

1 cup shredded carrots

1 cup chopped red bell pepper

½ cup chopped cauliflower

2 medium garlic cloves, minced

2 large eggs

2 teaspoons soy sauce (lowest sodium available)

1 tablespoon plain rice vinegar

⅓ cup diagonally sliced green onions

2 tablespoons chopped walnuts, dry-roasted

PER SERVING: Calories **220** • Total Fat **8.0 g** • Saturated Fat **1.5 g** • Trans Fat **0.0 g**
Polyunsaturated Fat **3.5 g** • Monounsaturated Fat **2.5 g** • Cholesterol **93 mg**
Sodium **195 mg** • Carbohydrates **29 g** • Fiber **5 g** • Sugars **7 g** • Protein **8 g**
DIETARY EXCHANGES: 1½ starch, 2 vegetable, ½ lean meat, 1 fat

SERVES 4
½ cup vegetables
and ½ cup bean
purée per serving

PREP TIME
10 minutes

COOKING TIME
20 to 25 minutes

2 cups halved cherry or grape tomatoes

8 ounces asparagus spears, trimmed and cut into 1-inch pieces

¾ cup coarsely chopped onion

1 tablespoon olive oil

¼ teaspoon salt

¼ teaspoon pepper and ¼ teaspoon pepper, divided use

2 15.5-ounce cans no-salt-added cannellini beans, rinsed and drained

¼ cup fat-free, low-sodium vegetable broth

2 tablespoons chopped fresh parsley

1 tablespoon chopped fresh chives

1 teaspoon grated lemon zest

1 medium lemon, cut into 4 wedges

Roasted Tomato and Asparagus on White Bean Purée

This simple main dish works best with no-salt-added cannellini beans because of their creamy consistency, though you can use any no-salt-added canned beans. The white mashed beans provide a pillow on which colorful veggies seasoned with fresh parsley, chives, and citrus zest rest.

1. Preheat the oven to 450°F.

2. In a shallow roasting pan, arrange the tomatoes, asparagus, and onion in a single layer. Drizzle with the oil, tossing to coat. Sprinkle with the salt and ¼ teaspoon pepper. Roast for 15 to 20 minutes, or until the vegetables are just tender and slightly browned. Set aside.

3. Meanwhile, in a medium bowl, stir together the beans, broth, parsley, chives, lemon zest, and the remaining ¼ teaspoon pepper. Using a potato masher or the back of a spoon, mash the mixture until the desired texture. Transfer to a small saucepan.

4. Cook the bean mixture over medium heat for 5 to 7 minutes, or until heated through, stirring frequently. Transfer to plates. Top with the vegetables. Serve with the lemon wedges.

PER SERVING: Calories 249 • Total Fat **5.5 g** • Saturated Fat **0.5 g** • Trans Fat **0.0 g** Polyunsaturated Fat **1.0 g** • Monounsaturated Fat **3.0 g** • Cholesterol **0 mg** Sodium **228 mg** • Carbohydrates **40 g** • Fiber **12 g** • Sugars **7 g** • Protein **13 g** DIETARY EXCHANGES: 2 starch, 2 vegetable, 1 lean meat

Panini with Hummus and Basil

SERVES 4
¼ panini per serving

PREP TIME
10 minutes

COOKING TIME
10 minutes

Our panini is made of a hollowed-out loaf of whole-grain Italian bread and layered inside with homemade hummus, veggies, and basil, and then cooked to create a crusty, warm sandwich.

1. In a food processor or blender, process the beans, water, vinegar, and garlic until smooth. Transfer to a bowl.

2. Place the halves of the loaf on a flat work surface. Hollow out the inside of each half, leaving a ½-inch border of the shell all the way around. (You can freeze the bread from the hollowed-out center for later use.) Spread the bean mixture inside the bottom half. Top with, in order, the tomato, basil, and onion, slightly overlapping the ingredients in each layer. Place the top half of the loaf on the bottom, pressing down lightly.

3. In a large nonstick skillet, heat the oil over medium heat, swirling to coat the bottom. Place the panini in the skillet. Top with three dinner plates to weigh down the bread. Cook for 3 minutes. Remove the plates. Turn over the panini. Replace the plates and cook for 3 minutes, or until the panini is golden brown and heated through. Transfer to a cutting board. Cut crosswise into four pieces.

½ 15.5-ounce can no-salt-added navy beans, rinsed and drained

2 tablespoons water

2 teaspoons red wine vinegar

3 medium garlic cloves

1 12-ounce loaf whole-grain Italian bread (lowest sodium available), halved lengthwise

1 large tomato (about 6 ounces), cut into 8 slices

12 medium basil leaves

½ cup thinly sliced red onion

2 teaspoons canola or corn oil

PER SERVING: Calories 315 • Total Fat 5.5 g • Saturated Fat 1.0 g • Trans Fat 0.0 g
Polyunsaturated Fat 2.0 g • Monounsaturated Fat 2.0 g • Cholesterol 0 mg
Sodium 507 mg • Carbohydrates 55 g • Fiber 6 g • Sugars 3 g • Protein 11 g
DIETARY EXCHANGES: 3½ starch, 1 vegetable, ½ lean meat

Grilled Portobello Burgers with Spicy Avocado Sauce

SERVES 4
1 burger and
3 tablespoons sauce
per serving

PREP TIME
10 minutes

COOKING TIME
10 minutes

STANDING TIME
3 minutes

1 tablespoon fresh lemon
   juice

1 tablespoon balsamic
   vinegar

1 tablespoon canola or
   corn oil

Cooking spray

4 portobello mushroom
   caps

SAUCE

1 medium avocado,
   coarsely mashed

2 tablespoons chopped
   cilantro

2 tablespoons water

1 medium jalapeño with
   seeds and ribs, finely
   chopped (see Cook's
   Tip, page 261)

1 tablespoon fresh lemon
   juice

1 medium garlic clove,
   minced

¼ teaspoon salt

(continued)

You won't miss the beef with these mouthwatering "burgers." Meaty mushrooms with all the fixings are stuffed into pita pockets and dressed with a kickin' guacamolelike sauce.

1. Heat a grill pan over medium-high heat or preheat the grill on medium high.

2. In a medium bowl, whisk together the lemon juice, vinegar, and oil. Set aside.

3. Lightly spray both sides of the mushrooms with cooking spray. Grill the mushrooms for 5 minutes on each side, or until tender when pierced with a fork.

4. Meanwhile, in a small bowl, stir together the sauce ingredients.

5. Transfer the mushrooms to a cutting board. Cut into ½-inch slices. Stir into the lemon juice mixture, tossing to coat. Let stand for 3 minutes so the flavors blend.

6. Warm each pita individually using the package directions (or microwave on 100 percent power [high] for 12 to 15 seconds per pita). Put a tomato slice, an onion slice, and a cheese slice in each of the pita halves. Press to one side and spoon the mushroom mixture into each pita half. Top with the sauce.

TIPS, TRICKS & TIMESAVERS: To pit an avocado, halve the fruit lengthwise, cutting around the pit, and twist the two halves apart. Place the half with the pit on a cutting board and firmly strike the pit with the blade of a sharp knife, slightly embedding the blade in the pit. Gently twist the knife while lifting out the pit. Or insert a corkscrew into the pit and twist it to skewer the pit and remove it.

* * *

2 6-inch whole-grain pita pockets, halved

1 medium tomato, cut into 4 slices

4 thin onion slices (rounds)

4 very thin slices low-fat Swiss cheese

PER SERVING: Calories **297** • Total Fat **13.5 g** • Saturated Fat **2.0 g** • Trans Fat **0.0 g**
Polyunsaturated Fat **2.5 g** • Monounsaturated Fat **7.5 g** • Cholesterol **7 mg**
Sodium **377 mg** • Carbohydrates **37 g** • Fiber **10 g** • Sugars **11 g** • Protein **13 g**
DIETARY EXCHANGES: 1½ starch, 3 vegetable, 1 lean meat, 2 fat

SERVES 4
2 wraps per serving

PREP TIME
15 minutes

2 medium avocados,
coarsely mashed

2 tablespoons fresh lime
juice, or to taste

¼ to ½ teaspoon ground
cumin

¼ teaspoon salt

8 medium romaine leaves

4 ounces shredded
fat-free sharp Cheddar
cheese

1 15.5-ounce can no-salt-
added black beans,
rinsed and drained

1 cup fat-free sour cream

½ cup diced tomatoes

2 medium jalapeños,
seeds and ribs
discarded, diced (see
Cook's Tip, page 261)

½ cup chopped fresh
cilantro

1 medium lime, cut into
4 wedges

Avocado–Black Bean Lettuce Wraps

Crisp romaine leaves embrace guacamole, Cheddar cheese, black beans, sour cream, and tomato for a veggie wrap that's full of traditional Mexican flavors.

1. In a small bowl, stir together the avocados, lime juice, cumin, and salt. Spoon the mixture down the center of each romaine leaf.

2. In the order listed, layer the remaining ingredients except the lime wedges on the avocado mixture. For each wrap, fold the left and right sides of the romaine leaf toward the center (it will resemble a long burrito). Serve with the lime wedges.

PER SERVING: Calories **378** • Total Fat **15.0 g** • Saturated Fat **2.0 g** • Trans Fat **0.0 g** • Polyunsaturated Fat **2.0 g** • Monounsaturated Fat **10.0 g** • Cholesterol **15 mg** • Sodium **493 mg** • Carbohydrates **41 g** • Fiber **13 g** • Sugars **10 g** • Protein **22 g**
DIETARY EXCHANGES: 2½ starch, 2 lean meat, 1 fat

Roasted Vegetable Wraps

A fresh herb yogurt sauce—with just a hint of heat—provides a cooling spread on whole-grain tortillas that envelop raw greens and roasted veggies.

SERVES 6
1 wrap per serving

PREP TIME
15 minutes

COOKING TIME
25 to 30 minutes

1. Preheat the oven to 450°F.

2. On a baking sheet or in a shallow roasting pan, arrange the vegetables and asparagus in a single layer. Drizzle with the oil, tossing to coat. Roast for 15 to 20 minutes, or until the vegetables are just tender and slightly browned.

3. Meanwhile, in a small bowl, whisk together the yogurt, chives, parsley, garlic, lemon zest, and cayenne. Spread the mixture on the tortillas. Top with the arugula. Arrange the roasted vegetables and asparagus on the arugula, keeping them toward the center. Roll up the tortillas. Secure each wrap with a wooden toothpick. Serve immediately.

HEALTHY SWAP: Roast any combination of your favorite vegetables for these wraps. It's a quick and tasty way to use your garden's bounty.

5 cups assorted vegetables, such as red bell pepper cut into ½-inch wedges, zucchini cut into 3 × ½-inch strips, and onion cut into ½-inch wedges, or a combination

8 ounces thin asparagus spears, trimmed

1 tablespoon olive oil

½ cup fat-free plain Greek yogurt

1 tablespoon chopped fresh chives

1 tablespoon chopped fresh parsley

1 small garlic clove, minced

½ teaspoon grated lemon zest

⅛ teaspoon cayenne

6 8-inch whole-grain tortillas

1½ cups tightly packed baby arugula

PER SERVING: Calories 202 • Total Fat 4.5 g • Saturated Fat 0.5 g • Trans Fat 0.0 g
Polyunsaturated Fat 1.0 g • Monounsaturated Fat 2.5 g • Cholesterol 0 mg
Sodium 354 mg • Carbohydrates 35 g • Fiber 6 g • Sugars 8 g • Protein 8 g
DIETARY EXCHANGES: 1½ starch, 2 vegetable, ½ fat

SERVES 4
1 tortilla and ⅔ cup
topping per serving

PREP TIME
10 minutes

COOKING TIME
15 minutes

4 6-inch corn tortillas

1 teaspoon ground cumin

3 ounces soft goat cheese

¼ cup finely chopped
fresh mint

2 tablespoons finely
chopped fresh parsley

½ 15.5-ounce can no-salt-
added chickpeas,
rinsed and drained

½ cup diced red onion

2 medium tomatoes,
diced

¼ teaspoon salt and
⅛ teaspoon salt,
divided use

Corn Tortillas with Chickpeas, Goat Cheese, and Mint

Skip the usual Cheddar or Monterey Jack and try goat cheese for a soft cheesy layer that is a perfect textural contrast to the crunchy baked tortillas. Chickpeas, veggies, and fresh herbs top the tortillas and then they're quickly baked again.

1. Preheat the oven to 350°F.

2. Arrange the tortillas on a baking sheet. Sprinkle the cumin over the top of the tortillas. Using your fingertips, gently spread the cumin over the tortillas.

3. Bake for 3 minutes, or until the tortillas are heated but still soft. Remove from the oven.

4. Spread the goat cheese over the tortillas. Top with, in order, the mint, parsley, chickpeas, onion, and tomatoes. Sprinkle ¼ teaspoon salt over the tomatoes.

5. Bake for 5 minutes to heat slightly. Sprinkle with the remaining ⅛ teaspoon salt. Serve with a knife and fork.

PER SERVING: Calories **167** • Total Fat **5.5 g** • Saturated Fat **3.0 g** • Trans Fat **0.0 g**
Polyunsaturated Fat **0.5 g** • Monounsaturated Fat **1.0 g** • Cholesterol **10 mg**
Sodium **337 mg** • Carbohydrates **22 g** • Fiber **4 g** • Sugars **3 g** • Protein **9 g**
DIETARY EXCHANGES: 1 starch, 1 vegetable, 1 lean meat

Vegetable Curry

Cooks in India create their own curry seasonings based on the spices they prefer, rather than use a pre-made blend. Adding the spices individually, as in this recipe, increases the preparation time by only a few seconds but gives this entrée a more genuine curry flavor.

1. In a large nonstick skillet, heat the oil over medium-high heat, swirling to coat the bottom. Cook the cumin seeds for 30 seconds, stirring constantly.

2. Stir in the garam masala, gingerroot, turmeric, garlic, salt, and cayenne. Cook for 30 seconds, stirring constantly.

3. Stir in the water, tomatoes, potatoes, green beans, carrot, and raisins. Bring to a boil.

4. Stir in the rice and yogurt. Reduce the heat and simmer, covered, for 20 to 24 minutes, or until the rice is tender and the liquid is absorbed.

5. Just before serving, sprinkle the curry with the cilantro.

TIPS, TRICKS & TIMESAVERS: Prepare all the ingredients before you begin cooking because this dish goes together very quickly.

TIPS, TRICKS & TIMESAVERS: If you don't have a mortar and pestle to crush the cumin seeds, put them on a cutting board. Using the flat side of a chef's knife, press down on the seeds, and slide the knife over them to crush them. You can also use a metal measuring cup instead of the knife.

SERVES 4
1½ cups per serving

PREP TIME
15 minutes

COOKING TIME
25 to 30 minutes

1 tablespoon canola or corn oil

1 teaspoon cumin seeds, crushed

1 teaspoon garam masala

1 teaspoon minced peeled gingerroot

½ teaspoon ground turmeric

1 medium garlic clove, minced

¼ teaspoon salt

⅛ to ¼ teaspoon cayenne

3 cups water

2 cups seeded and chopped tomatoes

1½ cups diced peeled yellow potatoes, such as Yukon gold (¼-inch pieces)

1 cup cut green beans (1-inch pieces)

½ cup chopped carrot

¼ cup raisins

1 cup uncooked instant brown rice

1 cup fat-free plain Greek yogurt

¼ cup chopped fresh cilantro

PER SERVING: Calories 255 • Total Fat 5.0 g • Saturated Fat 0.5 g • Trans Fat 0.0 g
Polyunsaturated Fat 1.5 g • Monounsaturated Fat 2.5 g • Cholesterol 0 mg
Sodium 200 mg • Carbohydrates 45 g • Fiber 5 g • Sugars 13 g • Protein 10 g
DIETARY EXCHANGES: 2 starch, 1 vegetable, ½ fruit, ½ fat

Eggplant Parmesan

In our version of this classic, the eggplant is broiled, not breaded and fried, and then it's baked in a simple fresh tomato sauce with tofu for added creaminess and protein. The casserole is topped with a thin layer of mozzarella and Parmesan to add cheesiness without heaviness.

Cooking spray

1 unpeeled large eggplant, cut crosswise into ½-inch slices (about 12 slices)

14 ounces light firm tofu, drained, patted dry, and cut into ½-inch slices (about 8 slices)

1 teaspoon olive oil

1 small sweet onion, such as Vidalia, Maui, or Oso Sweet, halved crosswise and sliced

1 pound Italian plum (Roma) tomatoes, coarsely chopped

3 large garlic cloves, minced

⅓ cup chopped fresh basil

⅛ teaspoon salt and ⅛ teaspoon salt, divided use

(continued)

1. Preheat the broiler. Line a large rimmed baking sheet with aluminum foil. Lightly spray the foil with cooking spray. Lightly spray a 9-inch square glass baking dish with cooking spray.

2. Arrange the eggplant and tofu slices on the baking sheet. Broil about 4 to 6 inches from the heat for 3 minutes, or until the eggplant is browned. Turn over the eggplant (do not turn the tofu). Broil for 2 minutes, or until the eggplant is browned (the tofu will be dry on top but not browned). Turn off the broiler.

3. Preheat the oven to 400°F.

4. Meanwhile, in a large nonstick skillet, heat the oil over medium-high heat, swirling to coat the bottom. Cook the onion for 1 minute.

5. Stir in the tomatoes. Cook for 4 minutes, or until the tomatoes are slightly softened, gently mashing them with a spoon and stirring occasionally. Stir in the garlic during the last 30 seconds of cooking.

6. Stir in the basil, ⅛ teaspoon salt, and ⅛ teaspoon pepper.

7. Spread one-third of the sauce in the baking dish. Arrange half the eggplant on the sauce. Top with the tofu. Sprinkle half the Parmesan and the remaining ⅛ teaspoon salt and ⅛ teaspoon pepper over the tofu. Spoon half the remaining sauce over all. Top with the remaining eggplant. Spread the remaining sauce over the eggplant. Sprinkle with the remaining Parmesan and the mozzarella.

8. Bake for 20 minutes, or until golden brown and bubbling. Let stand for 3 to 5 minutes before serving.

⅛ teaspoon pepper and ⅛ teaspoon pepper, divided use

3 tablespoons shredded or grated Parmesan cheese

½ cup shredded low-fat mozzarella cheese

PER SERVING: Calories **170** • Total Fat **5.5 g** • Saturated Fat **1.5 g** • Trans Fat **0.0 g** Polyunsaturated Fat **1.5 g** • Monounsaturated Fat **2.0 g** • Cholesterol **8 mg** Sodium **353 mg** • Carbohydrates **16 g** • Fiber **7 g** • Sugars **8 g** • Protein **16 g** DIETARY EXCHANGES: 3 vegetable, 2 lean meat

VEGETABLES AND SIDE DISHES

SERVES 4
½ artichoke and
1 tablespoon sauce
per serving

PREP TIME
5 minutes

COOKING TIME
30 minutes

10 cups water

1 tablespoon cider
vinegar

2 medium whole
artichokes, 1 inch
trimmed from the tip,
½ inch trimmed from
the stem, small leaves
at the base discarded,
halved lengthwise

SAUCE

2 tablespoons extra-virgin
olive oil

2 teaspoons grated lemon
zest

1 tablespoon fresh lemon
juice

2 teaspoons finely
chopped fresh parsley

½ teaspoon
Worcestershire
sauce (lowest sodium
available)

⅛ teaspoon salt

Lemon Artichokes

Ordinarily, artichokes can take a long time to cook, but the secret is cutting them in half with a serrated knife to shorten the cooking time.

1. In a stockpot, bring the water and vinegar to a boil over high heat. Carefully add the artichokes. Return to a boil. Reduce the heat to medium and cook, covered, for 25 minutes, or until the leaves can be pulled off easily. Using tongs, remove the artichoke halves from the water, holding them over the pot so the excess water drains off. Place with the cut side down on a double layer of paper towels to absorb any additional water.

2. Meanwhile, in a small bowl, whisk together the sauce ingredients except the salt. Arrange the artichokes with the cut side up on a large plate. Gently scrape out and discard the inedible fuzzy center (the choke). Brush or spoon the sauce over the artichokes. Sprinkle with the salt.

COOK'S TIP ON ARTICHOKES: To eat an artichoke, pull off the outer leaves one at a time. Grip the top of each leaf and place the fleshy part into your mouth, using your teeth to scrape off the soft pulp. Eat the pulp and discard the rest of the leaf. When the leaves are finished, eat the bottom of the artichoke that was covered by the choke (known as the heart).

PER SERVING: Calories 93 • Total Fat 7.0 g • Saturated Fat 1.0 g • Trans Fat 0.0 g
Polyunsaturated Fat 1.0 g • Monounsaturated Fat 5.0 g • Cholesterol 0 mg
Sodium 150 mg • Carbohydrates 7 g • Fiber 4 g • Sugars 1 g • Protein 2 g
DIETARY EXCHANGES: 1 vegetable, 1½ fat

Asparagus Grill

A fresh herb vinaigrette enhances the smoky flavor of grilled asparagus in this double-duty recipe. Serve it hot as a delicious pairing to Grilled Salmon on Pasta and Greens (page 90) or Grilled Portobello Burgers with Spicy Avocado Sauce (page 202), or serve it at room temperature for a sophisticated side salad.

1. Lightly spray the grill rack with cooking spray. Preheat the grill on medium high.

2. Lightly spray both sides of the asparagus with cooking spray. Grill the asparagus for 3 to 4 minutes on each side, or until just tender-crisp. Transfer to a platter.

3. In a small bowl, whisk together the oil and vinegar. Spoon over the asparagus. Let stand for 10 minutes so the flavors blend.

4. Sprinkle the asparagus with the salt, then sprinkle with the cilantro and basil.

> **TIPS, TRICKS & TIMESAVERS:** To trim an asparagus spear, hold it at the top and the bottom, bend it, and snap off the woody end at the bending point.

SERVES 4
6 spears per serving

PREP TIME
5 minutes

COOKING TIME
10 to 15 minutes

STANDING TIME
10 minutes

Cooking spray

24 medium asparagus spears, trimmed

2 teaspoons toasted sesame oil

2 teaspoons balsamic vinegar

⅛ teaspoon salt

1 tablespoon chopped fresh cilantro

1 tablespoon chopped fresh basil

PER SERVING: Calories **42** • Total Fat **2.5 g** • Saturated Fat **0.5 g** • Trans Fat **0.0 g**
Polyunsaturated Fat **1.0 g** • Monounsaturated Fat **1.0 g** • Cholesterol **0 mg**
Sodium **86 mg** • Carbohydrates **4 g** • Fiber **2 g** • Sugars **2 g** • Protein **2 g**
DIETARY EXCHANGES: 1 vegetable, ½ fat

SERVES 8
½ cup per serving

PREP TIME
10 minutes

COOKING TIME
25 minutes

Barley "Risotto" with Sautéed Mushrooms and Garlic

Barley is a toothsome alternative to traditional Arborio rice because of its creamy texture, nutty taste, and extra-filling fiber. Mushrooms, thyme, and garlic add earthy overtones to this "risotto," which just needs minimal stirring while it cooks.

1½ teaspoons olive oil and 1½ teaspoons olive oil, divided use

¼ cup chopped onion

¼ cup chopped celery

¼ cup chopped carrot

2¼ cups fat-free, low-sodium beef broth

1 cup uncooked quick-cooking barley

8 ounces mixed exotic mushrooms, such as brown (cremini), oyster, and shiitake (stems discarded), sliced

1 tablespoon chopped fresh thyme and 1 tablespoon chopped fresh thyme, divided use

3 medium garlic cloves, minced

¼ teaspoon freshly ground pepper

1. In a medium saucepan, heat 1½ teaspoons oil over medium heat, swirling to coat the bottom. Cook the onion, celery, and carrot for 3 minutes, or until the onion is just beginning to soften, stirring occasionally.

2. Stir in the broth and barley. Increase the heat to high and bring to a boil. Reduce the heat and simmer for 12 minutes.

3. Meanwhile, in a medium skillet, heat the remaining 1½ teaspoons oil over medium heat, swirling to coat the bottom. Cook the mushrooms, 1 tablespoon thyme, the garlic, and pepper for 6 to 8 minutes, or until the mushrooms are soft, stirring occasionally.

4. Stir the mushroom mixture into the barley mixture. Bring to a simmer and simmer for 3 minutes, or until most of the liquid is absorbed. Sprinkle with the remaining 1 tablespoon thyme. Just before serving, sprinkle with additional pepper if desired.

PER SERVING: Calories 94 • Total Fat 2.0 g • Saturated Fat 0.5 g • Trans Fat 0.0 g
Polyunsaturated Fat 0.5 g • Monounsaturated Fat 1.5 g • Cholesterol 0 mg
Sodium 42 mg • Carbohydrates 16 g • Fiber 3 g • Sugars 1 g • Protein 4 g
DIETARY EXCHANGES: 1 starch

Barley with Strawberries and Avocado

The creaminess of the avocado contrasts with the juiciness of the strawberries and the crunch of the walnuts for a unique fruit and whole-grain side dish.

1. Prepare the barley using the package directions, omitting the salt. Drain well in a colander.

2. Meanwhile, in a large bowl, whisk together the orange zest, orange juice, oregano, oil, salt, and pepper.

3. Add the barley to the orange juice mixture, stirring to coat. Gently stir in the strawberries, avocado, and green onions. Sprinkle with the walnuts.

PER SERVING: Calories **159** • Total Fat **8.0 g** • Saturated Fat **1.0 g** • Trans Fat **0.0 g**
Polyunsaturated Fat **3.0 g** • Monounsaturated Fat **3.0 g** • Cholesterol **0 mg**
Sodium **79 mg** • Carbohydrates **22 g** • Fiber **5 g** • Sugars **4 g** • Protein **3 g**
DIETARY EXCHANGES: 1 starch, ½ fruit, 1½ fat

SERVES 8
½ cup per serving

PREP TIME
15 minutes

COOKING TIME
15 minutes

1 cup uncooked quick-cooking barley

1 teaspoon grated orange zest

⅓ cup fresh orange juice

1 tablespoon chopped fresh oregano

2 teaspoons walnut oil or extra-virgin olive oil

¼ teaspoon salt

¼ teaspoon pepper

2 cups chopped hulled strawberries

1 medium avocado, chopped

½ cup sliced green onions

¼ cup chopped walnuts, dry-roasted

SERVES 4
½ cup per serving

PREP TIME
5 minutes

COOKING TIME
35 minutes

1 teaspoon olive oil and
   1 tablespoon extra-
   virgin olive oil, divided
   use

2 ounces smoked turkey
   sausage, casings
   discarded, diced

⅓ cup diced celery

1 small poblano pepper,
   seeds and ribs
   discarded, diced (see
   Cook's Tip, page 261)

½ medium tomato, diced

1 teaspoon fresh thyme or
   chopped fresh sage

2 cups water

6 ounces frozen black-
   eyed peas

Black-Eyed Peas with Smoked Turkey Sausage

A Southern favorite, black-eyed peas are traditionally cooked for a very long time. In this recipe, though, they're cooked to the just-tender stage, which leaves these legumes with a firmer beanlike texture. Poblano pepper and tomato add color to the dish while turkey sausage adds a bit of smokiness.

1. In a large nonstick skillet, heat 1 teaspoon oil over medium heat, swirling to coat the bottom. Cook the sausage for 4 minutes, or until browned, stirring occasionally.

2. Stir in the celery and poblano. Cook for 4 minutes, or until tender-crisp, stirring frequently. Transfer the sausage mixture to a small bowl. Stir in the tomato and thyme. Cover to keep warm and retain moisture.

3. Increase the heat to medium high. In the same skillet, bring the water and peas to a simmer. Reduce the heat and simmer, covered, for 20 to 22 minutes, or until the peas are just tender. Remove from the heat.

4. Drain the peas, reserving 3 tablespoons of the cooking liquid. Return the peas and reserved liquid to the skillet. Stir in the sausage mixture. Drizzle with the remaining 1 tablespoon oil.

PER SERVING: Calories **214** • Total Fat **7.0 g** • Saturated Fat **1.5 g** • Trans Fat **0.0 g**
Polyunsaturated Fat **1.5 g** • Monounsaturated Fat **4.0 g** • Cholesterol **14 mg**
Sodium **113 mg** • Carbohydrates **27 g** • Fiber **9 g** • Sugars **5 g** • Protein **12 g**
DIETARY EXCHANGES: 2 starch, 1 lean meat, ½ fat

Bok Choy with Serranos and Ginger

Serrano pepper and ginger add heat and spiciness to bok choy, which is a mild Chinese cabbage. Pair this with Orange-Honey Salmon (page 124) or Tuna Kebabs with Asian Dipping Sauce (page 132).

SERVES 4
½ cup per serving

PREP TIME
10 minutes

COOKING TIME
10 minutes

1. In a large nonstick skillet, heat the oil over medium-high heat, swirling to coat the bottom. Cook the serrano, gingerroot, and garlic for 1 minute, stirring frequently.

2. Stir in the bok choy. Cook for 5 to 6 minutes, or until tender-crisp, stirring frequently.

3. Stir in the soy sauce.

2 teaspoons toasted sesame oil

1 medium serrano pepper or other hot red pepper, seeds and ribs discarded, finely chopped (see Cook's Tip, page 261)

1 tablespoon minced peeled gingerroot

2 medium garlic cloves, minced

8 cups bok choy, leaves chopped and stems thinly sliced

1½ teaspoons soy sauce (lowest sodium available)

PER SERVING: Calories 43 • Total Fat 2.5 g • Saturated Fat 0.5 g • Trans Fat 0.0 g Polyunsaturated Fat 1.0 g • Monounsaturated Fat 1.0 g • Cholesterol 0 mg Sodium 140 mg • Carbohydrates 4 g • Fiber 2 g • Sugars 2 g • Protein 2 g DIETARY EXCHANGES: 1 vegetable, ½ fat

SERVES 4
1 cup vegetables and
3 tablespoons sauce
per serving

PREP TIME
5 minutes

COOKING TIME
10 minutes

Broccoli and Red Bell Peppers with Parmesan Sauce

Dress up a simple white sauce with Parmesan cheese and fresh parsley, and drizzle it over brightly colored steamed broccoli and bell peppers to give any accompanying entrée a run for the starring role on the dinner plate.

5 cups broccoli florets

1 large red bell pepper, cut into 2 × ¼-inch strips

1 tablespoon all-purpose flour

⅛ teaspoon ground nutmeg

Dash of cayenne

⅔ cup fat-free milk

⅓ cup shredded or grated Parmesan cheese

2 tablespoons chopped fresh parsley or chives

1. In a medium saucepan, steam the broccoli and bell pepper, covered, for 5 to 7 minutes, or until tender, but still brightly colored. Drain well. Transfer the broccoli and bell pepper to a serving bowl.

2. Meanwhile, in a small saucepan, whisk together the flour, nutmeg, and cayenne. Gradually whisk in the milk until the mixture is smooth. Cook over medium heat for 5 to 6 minutes, or until thickened and bubbly, whisking constantly.

3. Whisk in the Parmesan until melted. Whisk in the parsley. Spoon the sauce over the vegetables.

PER SERVING: Calories **121** • Total Fat **3.5 g** • Saturated Fat **2.0 g** • Trans Fat **0.0 g**
Polyunsaturated Fat **0.0 g** • Monounsaturated Fat **1.0 g** • Cholesterol **8 mg**
Sodium **236 mg** • Carbohydrates **15 g** • Fiber **4 g** • Sugars **7 g** • Protein **10 g**
DIETARY EXCHANGES: 2 vegetable, ½ other carbohydrate, 1 lean meat

Broccolini with Toasted Walnuts

A simple topping of lemon zest, minced garlic, and crunchy walnuts is all you need to make steamed broccolini simply delicious. Try this side with Grilled Lemon-Tarragon Chicken (page 143). *(See photo insert.)*

1. In a large saucepan, steam the broccolini for 6 to 8 minutes, or until just tender. Drain well. Transfer to a serving bowl.

2. Meanwhile, in a small bowl, whisk together the remaining ingredients except the walnuts. Drizzle over the broccolini. Sprinkle with the walnuts.

PER SERVING: Calories **118** • Total Fat **8.5 g** • Saturated Fat **1.0 g** • Trans Fat **0.0 g** Polyunsaturated Fat **4.0 g** • Monounsaturated Fat **3.0 g** • Cholesterol **0 mg** Sodium **130 mg** • Carbohydrates **9 g** • Fiber **4 g** • Sugars **2 g** • Protein **4 g** DIETARY EXCHANGES: 2 vegetable, 2 fat

SERVES 4
4 ounces broccolini and 1 tablespoon walnuts per serving

PREP TIME
5 minutes

COOKING TIME
10 to 15 minutes

1 pound broccolini, trimmed

1 tablespoon olive oil

½ teaspoon grated lemon zest

1 small garlic clove, minced

¼ teaspoon pepper

⅛ teaspoon salt

¼ cup chopped walnuts, dry-roasted

SERVES 4
¾ cup per serving

PREP TIME
10 minutes

COOKING TIME
25 to 30 minutes

1 pound small brussels
sprouts, trimmed and
halved

4 large shallots, each cut
into 6 wedges

1 tablespoon olive oil

¼ teaspoon pepper

1 cup fat-free, low-sodium
chicken or vegetable
broth

1 tablespoon balsamic
vinegar

1 teaspoon sugar

1 teaspoon chopped fresh
thyme

Balsamic-Roasted Brussels Sprouts and Shallots

Concentrated flavors make this side dish stand out in front. Reducing the chicken broth intensifies its flavor and roasting the brussels sprouts and shallots brings out their natural sweetness. (See photo insert.)

1. Preheat the oven to 450°F.

2. In a large bowl, combine the brussels sprouts, shallots, and oil, stirring to coat. Arrange the brussels sprouts with the cut side down and the shallots in a single layer on a rimmed baking sheet. Sprinkle the pepper over the vegetables.

3. Roast for 15 to 20 minutes, or until the brussels sprouts are browned on the edges.

4. Meanwhile, in a large skillet, bring the broth to a boil over high heat. Boil for 8 to 10 minutes, or until reduced by three-fourths (to about ¼ cup). Remove from the heat.

5. Stir in the vinegar, sugar, and thyme. Add the vegetables to the broth mixture, stirring to coat.

PER SERVING: Calories 100 • Total Fat 3.5 g • Saturated Fat 0.5 g • Trans Fat 0.0 g Polyunsaturated Fat 0.5 g • Monounsaturated Fat 2.5 g • Cholesterol 0 mg Sodium 46 mg • Carbohydrates 15 g • Fiber 5 g • Sugars 5 g • Protein 5 g DIETARY EXCHANGES: 3 vegetable, 1 fat

Herbed Bulgur with Kalamatas

Fiber-rich bulgur studded with bits of red from onion and bell pepper teams up with classic Mediterranean ingredients—olives, oregano, and rosemary—in this whole-grain side dish. It goes well with Tomato-Basil Tilapia (page 129) or Turkey Lula Kebabs with Yogurt Sauce (page 157).

1. Prepare the bulgur using the package directions, omitting the salt. Remove from the heat. Fluff with a fork.

2. Stir in the remaining ingredients. Let stand for 10 minutes so the flavors blend.

PER SERVING: Calories 105 • Total Fat 4.0 g • Saturated Fat 0.5 g • Trans Fat 0.0 g
Polyunsaturated Fat 0.5 g • Monounsaturated Fat 3.0 g • Cholesterol 0 mg
Sodium 126 mg • Carbohydrates 16 g • Fiber 4 g • Sugars 1 g • Protein 3 g
DIETARY EXCHANGES: 1 starch, ½ fat

SERVES 4
½ cup per serving

PREP TIME
5 minutes

COOKING TIME
10 minutes

STANDING TIME
10 minutes

½ cup instant, or fine grain, bulgur

¼ cup finely chopped red onion

¼ cup finely chopped red bell pepper

8 kalamata olives, coarsely chopped

1½ teaspoons chopped fresh oregano

1½ teaspoons extra-virgin olive oil

1 medium garlic clove, minced

½ teaspoon chopped fresh rosemary

SERVES 4
2/3 cup per serving

PREP TIME
15 minutes

COOKING TIME
10 minutes

Sesame Carrots and Snow Peas

In this two-vegetable side dish, carrots and snow peas are seasoned with savory toasted sesame oil, sweet rice vinegar, and snappy orange zest. It's an ideal accompaniment for Citrus-Soy Tilapia (page 128).

2 teaspoons soy sauce (lowest sodium available)

1½ teaspoons toasted sesame oil

1½ teaspoons plain rice vinegar

1 teaspoon finely grated orange zest

1 teaspoon canola or corn oil

2 large or 4 medium carrots, thinly sliced

6 ounces snow peas, trimmed and halved diagonally

3 tablespoons chopped fresh cilantro

2 teaspoons sesame seeds, dry-roasted

1. In a small bowl, whisk together the soy sauce, sesame oil, vinegar, and orange zest. Set aside.

2. In a nonstick skillet, heat the canola oil over medium heat, swirling to coat the bottom. Cook the carrots for 4 minutes, or until tender, stirring occasionally.

3. Stir in the snow peas. Cook for 3 minutes, or until tender-crisp, stirring constantly. Remove from the heat.

4. Stir in the soy sauce mixture. Transfer the vegetable mixture to plates. Sprinkle with the cilantro and sesame seeds.

PER SERVING: Calories 70 • Total Fat **4.0 g** • Saturated Fat **0.5 g** • Trans Fat **0.0 g** Polyunsaturated Fat **1.5 g** • Monounsaturated Fat **2.0 g** • Cholesterol **0 mg** Sodium **93 mg** • Carbohydrates **7 g** • Fiber **2 g** • Sugars **4 g** • Protein **2 g** DIETARY EXCHANGES: 1 vegetable, 1 fat

Louisiana Chard

Swiss chard comes from the same family as beets and spinach. In this dish, a bit of vinegar balances the natural saline flavor of the chard and a hint of cayenne and a clove of garlic offset any bitterness from the greens.

SERVES 4
½ cup per serving

PREP TIME
5 minutes

COOKING TIME
5 minutes

1. In a small bowl, whisk together 2 teaspoons oil, the vinegar, and cayenne.

2. In a large nonstick skillet, heat the remaining 2 teaspoons oil over medium-high heat, swirling to coat the bottom. Cook the chard and garlic for 2 minutes, or until the chard begins to wilt, using two utensils to toss. Spoon the oil mixture over all. Cook for 30 seconds, stirring constantly.

2 teaspoons extra-virgin olive oil and
2 teaspoons olive oil, divided use

2 teaspoons white balsamic vinegar

⅛ teaspoon cayenne

7 ounces Swiss chard, tough stems discarded, coarsely chopped

1 medium garlic clove, minced

PER SERVING: Calories 53 • Total Fat 4.5 g • Saturated Fat 0.5 g • Trans Fat 0.0 g
Polyunsaturated Fat 0.0 g • Monounsaturated Fat 0.5 g • Cholesterol 0 mg
Sodium 107 mg • Carbohydrates 3 g • Fiber 1 g • Sugars 1 g • Protein 1 g
DIETARY EXCHANGES: 1 fat

SERVES 4
1 ear of corn
per serving

PREP TIME
5 minutes

COOKING TIME
25 to 30 minutes

4 medium ears of corn, husks and silk discarded

Cooking spray

1½ tablespoons light tub margarine

¼ teaspoon pepper

⅛ teaspoon paprika (smoked preferred)

⅛ teaspoon salt

Wrap-and-Grill Corn on the Cob

Spray it, wrap it, and toss it on the grill. This simply cooked and seasoned corn has maximum flavor with minimal work, and it tastes perfect every time!

1. Preheat the grill on medium high or heat a grill pan over medium-high heat.

2. Lightly spray the corn with cooking spray. Place each ear diagonally in the center of a 4½-inch square piece of aluminum foil. Roll the foil around the ear. Twist the ends to seal up the corn.

3. Grill the corn for 20 to 25 minutes, or until tender-crisp, turning occasionally.

4. Meanwhile, in a small bowl, stir together the margarine, pepper, paprika, and salt.

5. Remove the corn from the grill. Using the tines of a fork, carefully open the foil away from you (to prevent steam burns). Brush the margarine mixture all over the corn.

PER SERVING: Calories **103** • Total Fat **3.0 g** • Saturated Fat **0.5 g** • Trans Fat **0.0 g** Polyunsaturated Fat **1.0 g** • Monounsaturated Fat **1.5 g** • Cholesterol **0 mg** Sodium **122 mg** • Carbohydrates **19 g** • Fiber **2 g** • Sugars **6 g** • Protein **3 g** DIETARY EXCHANGES: 1½ starch, ½ fat

Israeli Couscous with Asparagus

Toasting the couscous deepens the flavor of the dish; lemon brightens it up.

1. In a large skillet, bring the broth and couscous to a boil over high heat. Reduce the heat and simmer for 2 minutes.

2. Stir in the asparagus and salt. Cook for 6 to 8 minutes, or until the broth is absorbed and the asparagus is tender-crisp. Stir in the lemon zest, lemon juice, and pepper.

> **TIPS, TRICKS & TIMESAVERS:** When using a rasp grater or four-sided (or "box") grater to zest lemons and oranges, turn the fruit often to avoid grating the white part of the peel, or pith, which has a bitter taste.
>
> ---
>
> **SHOP & STORE:** Look for Israeli couscous, which is larger than regular couscous, in the kosher foods section of the supermarket. To toast the couscous, heat a medium skillet over medium-high heat. Cook the couscous about 5 minutes, or until lightly golden, stirring frequently.

SERVES 8
½ cup per serving

PREP TIME
15 minutes

COOKING TIME
15 minutes

2¼ cups fat-free, low-sodium chicken or vegetable broth

1⅓ cups uncooked Israeli couscous, toasted

2 cups cut asparagus (¾-inch pieces)

⅛ teaspoon salt

2 teaspoons grated lemon zest

1½ tablespoons fresh lemon juice

½ teaspoon freshly ground pepper

PER SERVING: Calories **120** • Total Fat **0.0 g** • Saturated Fat **0.0 g** • Trans Fat **0.0 g**
Polyunsaturated Fat **0.0 g** • Monounsaturated Fat **0.0 g** • Cholesterol **0 mg**
Sodium **57 mg** • Carbohydrates **24 g** • Fiber **2 g** • Sugars **1 g** • Protein **5 g**
DIETARY EXCHANGES: 1½ starch

12 ounces unpeeled
eggplant, cut
crosswise into 8 slices

Cooking spray

2 teaspoons extra-virgin
olive oil

1 teaspoon red wine
vinegar

1 medium garlic clove,
minced

¼ cup chopped fresh
basil

4 kalamata olives,
chopped

¾ ounce crumbled
low-fat feta cheese

Grilled Eggplant with Feta

This Mediterranean-style eggplant dish is full of assertive flavors. When using kalamata olives and sharp feta, a little goes a long way.

1. Heat a grill pan over medium-high heat or preheat the grill on medium high.

2. Lightly spray both sides of the eggplant slices with cooking spray. Cook for 5 minutes. Turn over. Cook for 1 to 2 minutes, or until lightly browned and tender. Arrange the eggplant in a single layer on a large plate.

3. In a small bowl, whisk together the oil, vinegar, and garlic. Lightly brush over the top of each slice of eggplant. Sprinkle with the basil, olives, and feta. Let stand for 10 minutes so the flavors blend.

HEALTHY SWAP: If you prefer, you can broil the eggplant rather than grill it. To broil it, preheat the broiler. Lightly spray a baking sheet with cooking spray. Lightly spray both sides of the eggplant. Arrange the eggplant in a single layer on the baking sheet. Broil the eggplant about 5 to 6 inches from the heat for 5 minutes. Turn over. Broil for 1 to 2 minutes, or until lightly browned and tender.

PER SERVING: Calories **62** • Total Fat **4.0 g** • Saturated Fat **1.0 g** • Trans Fat **0.0 g** Polyunsaturated Fat **0.5 g** • Monounsaturated Fat **2.5 g** • Cholesterol **2 mg** Sodium **133 mg** • Carbohydrates **6 g** • Fiber **3 g** • Sugars **2 g** • Protein **2 g** DIETARY EXCHANGES: 1 vegetable, 1 fat

Asian Green Beans

Sesame and soy sauce coat these green beans with Asian flavor. Serve them with Garden Vegetable Fried Rice (page 199) or Pan-Seared Tuna Steaks on Bok Choy (page 134).

1. In a medium saucepan, steam the green beans for 6 to 8 minutes, or until tender. Drain well. Transfer to a serving plate.

2. In a small bowl, whisk together the sugar, soy sauce, and sesame oil. Spoon over the green beans. Sprinkle with the sesame seeds.

HEALTHY SWAP: For a variation, break asparagus spears into 2-inch pieces, steam as instructed for the green beans, and top with the sauce. Serve over a bed of brown rice.

SERVES 4
½ cup per serving

PREP TIME
5 minutes

COOKING TIME
10 minutes

12 ounces green beans, trimmed

1 tablespoon sugar

2½ teaspoons soy sauce (lowest sodium available)

2 teaspoons toasted sesame oil

1½ tablespoons sesame seeds, dry-roasted

PER SERVING: Calories 83 • Total Fat 4.5 g • Saturated Fat 0.5 g • Trans Fat 0.0 g
Polyunsaturated Fat 2.0 g • Monounsaturated Fat 1.5 g • Cholesterol 0 mg
Sodium 88 mg • Carbohydrates 10 g • Fiber 3 g • Sugars 6 g • Protein 3 g
DIETARY EXCHANGES: 1 vegetable, 1 fat

SERVES 8
½ cup per serving

PREP TIME
10 minutes

COOKING TIME
10 minutes

Country Greens

Try these southern-style greens quickly sautéed with jalapeño and garlic, with a bit of hot-pepper sauce splashed on just before serving to kick up the heat of these collards even more. Serve them with Turkey Patties with Mushroom Gravy (page 158).

2 tablespoons water

1 tablespoon Louisiana-style hot-pepper sauce

1 teaspoon sugar

1 teaspoon canola or corn oil and 1 teaspoon canola or corn oil, divided use

1 cup diced onion

1 medium jalapeño, seeds and ribs discarded, finely chopped (see Cook's Tip, page 261)

2 medium garlic cloves, minced

1 pound collard greens, any large stems discarded, coarsely chopped

1. In a small bowl, whisk together the water, hot sauce, and sugar. Set aside.

2. In a large heavy saucepan or Dutch oven, heat 1 teaspoon oil over medium-high heat, swirling to coat the bottom. Cook the onion for 5 to 6 minutes, or until golden brown, stirring occasionally.

3. Stir in the jalapeño and garlic. Cook for 30 seconds, stirring constantly.

4. Stir in the remaining 1 teaspoon oil and the collard greens. Cook for 3 to 4 minutes, or until the greens wilt, using two utensils to toss. Just before serving, sprinkle with the hot-sauce mixture.

PER SERVING: Calories 37 • Total Fat **1.5 g** • Saturated Fat **0.0 g** • Trans Fat **0.0 g** Polyunsaturated Fat **0.5 g** • Monounsaturated Fat **1.0 g** • Cholesterol **0 mg** Sodium **68 mg** • Carbohydrates **6 g** • Fiber **2 g** • Sugars **2 g** • Protein **1 g**
DIETARY EXCHANGES: 1 vegetable

Mexican Braised Kale with Cherry Tomatoes

Fresh, earthy kale—a rich source of calcium—is braised in a salsalike mixture and topped with cheese for a spicy, super sidekick to any Mexican entrée, such as Smoky Tostadas (page 172).

SERVES 6
½ cup per serving

PREP TIME
10 minutes

COOKING TIME
15 minutes

1. In a large skillet, bring the tomatoes, broth, and jalapeño to a boil over medium-high heat. Stir in the kale. Using tongs, turn it until slightly wilted. Reduce the heat and simmer, covered, for 8 to 10 minutes, or until the kale is tender.

2. Stir in the green onions and cilantro. Using a slotted spoon, transfer the mixture to a serving bowl. Sprinkle with the Monterey Jack.

PER SERVING: Calories 71 • Total Fat **2.0 g** • Saturated Fat **1.0 g** • Trans Fat **0.0 g**
Polyunsaturated Fat **0.5 g** • Monounsaturated Fat **0.5 g** • Cholesterol **5 mg**
Sodium **77 mg** • Carbohydrates **10 g** • Fiber **2 g** • Sugars **2 g** • Protein **5 g**
DIETARY EXCHANGES: 2 vegetable, ½ fat

1 cup quartered cherry or grape tomatoes

¼ cup fat-free, low-sodium chicken or vegetable broth

2 tablespoons finely chopped jalapeño, seeds and ribs discarded (see Cook's Tip, page 261)

8 ounces kale, any large stems discarded, coarsely chopped

¼ cup sliced green onions

¼ cup chopped fresh cilantro

¼ cup shredded low-fat Monterey Jack cheese or crumbled queso fresco

1⅓ cups water

⅓ cup dried brown lentils, sorted for stones and shriveled lentils, rinsed, and drained

1 teaspoon olive oil and 2 teaspoons olive oil, divided use

2 medium poblano peppers, seeds and ribs discarded, finely chopped (see Cook's Tip, page 261)

½ cup diced red onion

1 medium garlic clove, minced

2 tablespoons finely chopped fresh Italian (flat-leaf) parsley

1 teaspoon chopped fresh rosemary

1 teaspoon grated peeled gingerroot or grated lemon zest

⅛ teaspoon salt

Poblano-Lentil Pilaf

Lentils give this pilaf a chewier texture and a hefty helping of fiber. The poblano peppers and fresh ginger add a bit of bite.

1. In a large microwaveable glass bowl, stir together the water and lentils. Cover with a glass lid. Microwave on 100 percent power (high) for 5 minutes, then microwave on 50 percent power (medium) for 15 to 20 minutes, or until the lentils are tender. Drain well in a fine-mesh sieve.

2. Meanwhile, in a medium nonstick skillet, heat 1 teaspoon oil over medium-high heat, swirling to coat the bottom. Cook the poblanos and onion for 2 minutes, or until tender-crisp, stirring frequently.

3. Stir in the garlic. Cook for 15 seconds, stirring constantly. Remove from the heat.

4. Stir in the lentils, parsley, rosemary, gingerroot, and the remaining 2 teaspoons oil. Transfer the pilaf to a shallow serving dish. Sprinkle with the salt.

COOK'S TIP: Be sure to add the salt right at serving time, and not before then. The flavor will remain stronger. If you add it too early, the lentils will absorb and "hide" the salt.

PER SERVING: Calories 108 • Total Fat 3.5 g • Saturated Fat 0.5 g • Trans Fat 0.0 g
Polyunsaturated Fat 0.5 g • Monounsaturated Fat 2.5 g • Cholesterol 0 mg
Sodium 76 mg • Carbohydrates 15 g • Fiber 3 g • Sugars 3 g • Protein 6 g
DIETARY EXCHANGES: 1 starch, ½ lean meat

Lentils and Fennel

The fennel bulb has a slightly licorice taste—similar to anise, but milder and sweeter—that pairs well with earthy lentils and aromatic thyme. This rich and satisfying side dish would also make a great light entrée; just double the serving size.

1. In a large saucepan, heat the oil over medium heat, swirling to coat the bottom. Cook the fennel wedges, carrots, onion, and garlic for 8 to 10 minutes, or until the fennel and carrots are tender-crisp, stirring occasionally.

2. Stir in the broth. Bring to a boil over medium-high heat. Stir in the lentils, thyme, mustard, salt, and pepper. Reduce the heat and simmer, covered, for 15 to 20 minutes, or until the lentils are tender. Drain well in a fine-mesh sieve. Return the fennel mixture to the pan. Stir in the vinegar.

3. Arrange the tomato slices on serving plates. Spoon the fennel mixture over the tomatoes. Sprinkle with the fennel fronds.

PER SERVING: Calories 129 • Total Fat 1.5 g • Saturated Fat 0.0 g • Trans Fat 0.0 g
Polyunsaturated Fat 0.0 g • Monounsaturated Fat 1.0 g • Cholesterol 0 mg
Sodium 111 mg • Carbohydrates 23 g • Fiber 5 g • Sugars 4 g • Protein 9 g
DIETARY EXCHANGES: 1 starch, 1 vegetable, ½ lean meat

SERVES 8
½ cup lentils and
1 tomato slice
per serving

PREP TIME
15 minutes

COOKING TIME
30 to 35 minutes

2 teaspoons olive oil

1 small fennel bulb, cut into thin wedges or coarsely chopped (fronds reserved)

1 cup chopped carrots

½ cup finely chopped onion

1 medium garlic clove, minced

3 cups fat-free, low-sodium vegetable broth

1 cup uncooked brown or French green lentils, sorted for stones and shriveled lentils, rinsed, and drained

2 teaspoons chopped fresh thyme

½ teaspoon dry mustard

¼ teaspoon salt

¼ teaspoon pepper

1 tablespoon red wine vinegar

2 medium tomatoes, each cut into 4 slices

¼ cup chopped fennel fronds

Lima Beans with Mustard and Thyme

This recipe just might make lima beans a favorite in your home. The secret is to cook them until they are just tender, and then add mustard, onion, and a touch of thyme and cayenne to elevate their mild flavor.

2 cups water

8 ounces lima beans, shelled

½ cup diced onion

1 tablespoon yellow mustard (lowest sodium available)

1 tablespoon extra-virgin olive oil

1 teaspoon fresh thyme

Dash of cayenne (optional)

⅛ to ¼ teaspoon coarsely ground pepper

1. In a medium saucepan, bring the water to a boil over high heat. Stir in the beans and onion. Return to a boil. Reduce the heat and simmer, covered, for 10 minutes, or until the beans are tender. Drain well in a colander. Or, if using frozen beans, prepare them using the package directions, adding the onion.

2. Transfer the bean mixture to a medium serving bowl. Stir in the mustard, oil, thyme, and cayenne. Sprinkle with the pepper.

HEALTHY SWAP: For a slightly sweeter side dish, substitute diced shallots for the diced onion.

SHOP & STORE: Fresh lima beans can be difficult to find but are worth the search. However, if you can't find them, use frozen lima beans; just be sure to check the nutrition facts label and choose the brand with the lowest sodium. Either way, the beans pack plenty of potassium.

PER SERVING: Calories **101** • Total Fat **3.5 g** • Saturated Fat **0.5 g** • Trans Fat **0.0 g** Polyunsaturated Fat **0.5 g** • Monounsaturated Fat **2.5 g** • Cholesterol **0 mg** Sodium **141 mg** • Carbohydrates **13 g** • Fiber **4 g** • Sugars **2 g** • Protein **3 g** DIETARY EXCHANGES: 1 starch, ½ fat

Shallot-Garlic Mushrooms

A member of the onion family, shallots are formed like garlic into a head made of cloves. These large purple cloves taste a bit like sweet onion with just a hint of garlic. They add a unique, rich flavor to this side dish.

SERVES 4
½ cup per serving

PREP TIME
10 minutes

COOKING TIME
10 minutes

1. In a large nonstick skillet, heat the oil over medium-high heat, swirling to coat the bottom. Cook the shallots for 5 minutes, or until beginning to richly brown, stirring frequently.

2. Stir in the mushrooms. Cook for 3 minutes, or until beginning to brown, stirring occasionally. Remove from the heat.

3. Add the margarine, garlic, and salt, stirring until the margarine has melted.

1 teaspoon canola or corn oil

2 medium shallots, peeled and thinly sliced

12 ounces button mushrooms, quartered

2 tablespoons light tub margarine

1 medium garlic clove, minced

⅛ teaspoon salt

PER SERVING: Calories **56** • Total Fat **3.5 g** • Saturated Fat **0.0 g** • Trans Fat **0.0 g**
Polyunsaturated Fat **1.0 g** • Monounsaturated Fat **2.0 g** • Cholesterol **0 mg**
Sodium **123 mg** • Carbohydrates **4 g** • Fiber **1 g** • Sugars **2 g** • Protein **3 g**
DIETARY EXCHANGES: 1 vegetable, 1 fat

SERVES 4
½ cup okra and
2 tablespoons sauce
per serving

PREP TIME
10 minutes

COOKING TIME
20 minutes

Cornmeal-Crusted Okra with Cocktail Sauce

Give fried okra a healthy makeover with a paprika-spiked cornmeal coating that's roasted to a crisp golden brown. The spicy cocktail sauce gets its zing from horseradish, lemon juice, and hot sauce.

Cooking spray

2 teaspoons canola or corn oil and 1 table-spoon canola or corn oil, divided use

2 teaspoons cider vinegar

¾ cup yellow cornmeal

2 teaspoons paprika

10 ounces okra, trimmed and cut into ½-inch slices

SAUCE

½ cup no-salt-added ketchup

2 teaspoons grated peeled horseradish

2 teaspoons fresh lemon juice

1 teaspoon Worces-tershire sauce (lowest sodium available)

1 teaspoon Louisiana-style hot-pepper sauce

* * *

⅛ teaspoon salt

1 medium lemon, cut into 4 wedges

1. Preheat the oven to 475°F. Line a baking sheet with aluminum foil. Lightly spray the foil with cooking spray.

2. In a medium bowl, whisk together 2 teaspoons oil and the vinegar. In a pie pan, stir together the cornmeal and paprika. Set the bowl, pie pan, and baking sheet in a row, assembly-line fashion. Put the okra in the bowl, tossing to coat with the oil mixture. Working in small batches, dip the okra in the cornmeal mixture, turning to coat. Arrange in a single layer on the baking sheet, making sure the pieces don't touch. Drizzle the remaining 1 tablespoon oil over all.

3. Roast for 10 to 11 minutes, or until the okra is golden brown on the bottom.

4. Meanwhile, in a small bowl, whisk together the sauce ingredients.

5. Sprinkle the okra with the salt. Serve with the sauce and lemon wedges.

PER SERVING: Calories 139 • Total Fat **6.0 g** • Saturated Fat **0.5 g** • Trans Fat **0.0 g** Polyunsaturated Fat **2.0 g** • Monounsaturated Fat **4.0 g** • Cholesterol **0 mg** Sodium **99 mg** • Carbohydrates **21 g** • Fiber **3 g** • Sugars **8 g** • Protein **3 g** DIETARY EXCHANGES: ½ starch, 1 vegetable, ½ other carbohydrate, 1 fat

Roasted Parsnips and Carrots

Parsnips have a light licorice flavor and partner well with carrots, as you'll discover in this tasty side dish. Roasting these root vegetables brings out their natural sweetness.

1. Preheat the oven to 425°F. Line a baking sheet with aluminum foil. Lightly spray the foil with cooking spray.

2. Put the parsnips, carrots, onion, and garlic on the baking sheet. Drizzle the oil over the vegetables. Stir until well coated. Arrange in a single layer on the baking sheet.

3. Roast for 20 minutes, or until the vegetables begin to lightly brown, stirring once halfway through. Remove from the oven.

4. Sprinkle with the rosemary and salt. Pull together the edges of the foil and seal. Let stand for 10 minutes so the flavors blend.

PER SERVING: Calories **102** • Total Fat **4.0 g** • Saturated Fat **0.5 g** • Trans Fat **0.0 g**
Polyunsaturated Fat **1.0 g** • Monounsaturated Fat **2.5 g** • Cholesterol **0 mg**
Sodium **101 mg** • Carbohydrates **17 g** • Fiber **5 g** • Sugars **7 g** • Protein **1 g**
DIETARY EXCHANGES: 1 starch, 1 vegetable, ½ fat

SERVES 4
½ cup per serving

PREP TIME
10 minutes

COOKING TIME
30 minutes

STANDING TIME
10 minutes

Cooking spray

2 medium parsnips, peeled and cut crosswise into ½-inch slices

2 medium carrots, peeled and cut crosswise into ½-inch slices

1 medium onion, cut into 8 wedges

4 medium garlic cloves

1 tablespoon canola or corn oil

1 teaspoon chopped fresh rosemary

⅛ teaspoon salt

SERVES 4
½ cup per serving

PREP TIME
10 minutes

COOKING TIME
25 minutes

Potato-Veggie Bake

Potato casseroles often take at least an hour to bake, but in this recipe the potatoes are steamed first, then popped in the oven for a few minutes to give them that slow-baked flavor in less than half the time.

8 ounces Yukon gold potatoes, diced

2 ounces green beans, trimmed and broken into 1-inch pieces

½ medium poblano pepper, seeds and ribs discarded, diced (see Cook's Tip, page 261)

½ cup chopped green onions and 1 to 2 tablespoons chopped green onions, divided use

¼ cup fat-free sour cream

1 teaspoon grated peeled horseradish

½ ounce grated low-fat sharp Cheddar cheese

⅛ teaspoon salt

⅛ teaspoon pepper

1. Preheat the oven to 350°F.

2. In a large saucepan, steam the potatoes, green beans, and poblano for 8 minutes, or until the potatoes and green beans are just tender. Drain well.

3. In a 9-inch glass pie pan, stir together the potato mixture, ½ cup green onions, the sour cream, and horseradish. Bake for 10 minutes, or until heated through.

4. Sprinkle with the Cheddar and salt. Bake for 3 minutes, or until the Cheddar melts. Sprinkle with the pepper and the remaining 1 to 2 tablespoons green onions.

COOK'S TIP ON YUKON GOLD POTATOES: The skin and flesh of Yukon gold potatoes range from buttery yellow to golden. Their moist and almost succulent texture makes them perfect for healthy dishes because they don't need a lot of fat. Use them to make mashed potatoes, too.

PER SERVING: Calories **79** • Total Fat **0.5 g** • Saturated Fat **0.0 g** • Trans Fat **0.0 g**
Polyunsaturated Fat **0.0 g** • Monounsaturated Fat **0.0 g** • Cholesterol **3 mg**
Sodium **118 mg** • Carbohydrates **16 g** • Fiber **3 g** • Sugars **3 g** • Protein **3 g**
DIETARY EXCHANGES: 1 starch

Smoky Roasted Red Potatoes

Potatoes don't have to be loaded with fattening ingredients to taste delicious, but they do benefit from intense seasonings, such as smoked paprika and cayenne, because of their mild flavor.

1. Preheat the oven to 425°F. Line a baking sheet with aluminum foil. Lightly spray the foil with cooking spray.

2. Place the potatoes and onion on the baking sheet. Drizzle the oil over the vegetables. Sprinkle the vegetables with the paprika and cayenne. Stir until well coated. Arrange the vegetables in a single layer.

3. Roast for 20 minutes, stirring once halfway through. Remove from the oven.

4. Sprinkle the vegetables with the cilantro, lemon zest, lemon juice, and salt. Pull together the edges of the foil and seal. Let stand for 10 minutes so the flavors blend.

PER SERVING: Calories 130 • Total Fat 4.0 g • Saturated Fat 0.5 g • Trans Fat 0.0 g
Polyunsaturated Fat 1.0 g • Monounsaturated Fat 2.0 g • Cholesterol 0 mg
Sodium 96 mg • Carbohydrates 23 g • Fiber 3 g • Sugars 3 g • Protein 3 g
DIETARY EXCHANGES: 1½ starch, ½ fat

SERVES 4
¾ cup per serving

PREP TIME
5 minutes

COOKING TIME
30 minutes

STANDING TIME
10 minutes

Cooking spray

8 small red potatoes (about 2 ounces each)

1 cup diced onion

1 tablespoon canola or corn oil

1 teaspoon paprika (smoked preferred)

Dash of cayenne (optional)

¼ cup chopped fresh cilantro

2 teaspoons grated lemon zest

2 teaspoons to 1 tablespoon fresh lemon juice

⅛ teaspoon salt

SERVES 4
½ cup per serving

PREP TIME
5 minutes

COOKING TIME
15 minutes

½ **cup uncooked quinoa, rinsed and drained**

¼ **cup sliced almonds, dry-roasted and crushed**

1 **tablespoon sweetened flaked coconut, toasted**

½ **teaspoon grated orange zest (optional)**

¼ **to** ½ **teaspoon sugar**

⅛ **teaspoon salt**

Quinoa with Almonds and Toasted Coconut

This whole-grain side dish partners well with a beef roast or lean poultry. Add a green salad topped with some blueberries and some sliced hulled strawberries, and your dinner is ready.

1. Prepare the quinoa using the package directions, omitting the salt. Fluff with a fork.

2. Transfer to a bowl. Stir in the remaining ingredients.

TIPS, TRICKS & TIMESAVERS: To dry-roast the almonds and toast the coconut at the same time, heat a medium skillet over medium-high heat. Cook the almonds for 1 minute, stirring frequently. Stir in the coconut. Cook for 1 minute, or until the almonds and coconut begin to brown slightly, stirring constantly. Remove from the skillet immediately.

PER SERVING: Calories **127** • Total Fat **5.0 g** • Saturated Fat **1.0 g** • Trans Fat **0.0 g** Polyunsaturated Fat **1.5 g** • Monounsaturated Fat **2.5 g** • Cholesterol **0 mg** Sodium **78 mg** • Carbohydrates **16 g** • Fiber **3 g** • Sugars **2 g** • Protein **5 g** DIETARY EXCHANGES: 1 starch, 1 fat

Basil Brown Rice

Hot rice tossed with grape tomatoes, basil, garlic, and a hint of Parmesan perks up any simple entrée, such as baked chicken, broiled beef, or grilled fish, with Italian flavor.

SERVES 4
½ cup per serving

PREP TIME
5 minutes

COOKING TIME
15 minutes

1. Prepare the rice using the package directions, omitting the salt and margarine. Remove from the heat.

2. Stir in the remaining ingredients except the Parmesan. Stir in the Parmesan.

½ cup uncooked instant brown rice

½ cup grape tomatoes, quartered

⅓ cup chopped fresh basil

2 medium garlic cloves, minced

2 teaspoons extra-virgin olive oil

1 teaspoon cider vinegar

¼ teaspoon pepper

⅛ teaspoon salt

1 tablespoon shredded or grated Parmesan cheese

PER SERVING: Calories 77 • Total Fat 3.0 g • Saturated Fat 0.5 g • Trans Fat 0.0 g
Polyunsaturated Fat 0.5 g • Monounsaturated Fat 2.0 g • Cholesterol 1 mg
Sodium 100 mg • Carbohydrates 11 g • Fiber 1 g • Sugars 1 g • Protein 2 g
DIETARY EXCHANGES: ½ starch, ½ fat

SERVES 6
¾ cup per serving

PREP TIME
10 minutes

COOKING TIME
15 minutes

1 cup uncooked instant brown rice

1 cup cut asparagus (2-inch pieces)

¾ cup fat-free, low-sodium vegetable broth

¾ cup edamame

¾ cup snow peas, trimmed and cut into thirds

¼ cup finely chopped carrot

¼ cup finely chopped shallot

2 medium garlic cloves, minced

¼ cup chopped fresh parsley

¼ teaspoon salt

¼ teaspoon pepper

Green Rice

This dish is named for the three green main ingredients—asparagus, snow peas, and edamame—that are added to the rice. Diced carrot adds a flash of orange for visual contrast and a bit more crunch.

1. Prepare the rice using the package directions, omitting the salt and margarine.

2. Meanwhile, in a large skillet, stir together the asparagus, broth, edamame, snow peas, carrot, shallot, and garlic. Bring to a boil over medium-high heat. Boil gently for 6 to 8 minutes, or until the vegetables are tender and most of the liquid has evaporated. Stir in the rice, parsley, salt, and pepper.

PER SERVING: Calories 93 • Total Fat 1.5 g • Saturated Fat 0.0 g • Trans Fat 0.0 g Polyunsaturated Fat 0.0 g • Monounsaturated Fat 0.0 g • Cholesterol 0 mg Sodium 111 mg • Carbohydrates 17 g • Fiber 3 g • Sugars 2 g • Protein 4 g DIETARY EXCHANGES: 1 starch

Garlic-Ginger Snow Peas

Sometimes called Chinese pea pods, snow peas not only make a delicious side dish on their own but also can be used as a colorful, crunchy bed for a stir-fry as an unconventional alternative to rice.

SERVES 4
½ cup per serving

PREP TIME
5 minutes

COOKING TIME
5 to 10 minutes

1. In a large nonstick skillet, heat the oil over medium-high heat, swirling to coat the bottom. Cook the snow peas and bell pepper for 4 to 5 minutes, or until tender-crisp, stirring frequently.

2. Stir in the green onions, garlic, and gingerroot. Cook for 30 seconds, stirring constantly. Remove from the heat. Sprinkle with the sugar and salt.

1 teaspoon canola or corn oil

6 ounces snow peas, trimmed

½ medium yellow bell pepper, thinly sliced

2 medium green onions, chopped

2 medium garlic cloves, minced

1½ teaspoons grated peeled gingerroot

¼ teaspoon sugar

⅛ teaspoon salt

PER SERVING: Calories 40 • Total Fat 1.5 g • Saturated Fat 0.0 g • Trans Fat 0.0 g
Polyunsaturated Fat 0.5 g • Monounsaturated Fat 1.0 g • Cholesterol 0 mg
Sodium 78 mg • Carbohydrates 6 g • Fiber 2 g • Sugars 3 g • Protein 1 g
DIETARY EXCHANGES: 1 vegetable

SERVES 4
½ cup per serving

PREP TIME
5 minutes

COOKING TIME
5 minutes

1 teaspoon canola or corn
oil and 1 teaspoon
canola or corn oil,
divided use

½ cup thinly sliced
shallots

10 ounces spinach

1 to 1½ teaspoons fresh
thyme

1 teaspoon light tub
margarine

⅛ teaspoon salt

Spinach with Shallots and Thyme

Browned shallots top this super easy-to-make side to add a deep, rich flavor to wilted spinach. It's a perfect complement to Nutty Baked Flounder (page 120).

1. In a large nonstick skillet, heat 1 teaspoon oil over medium-high heat, swirling to coat the bottom. Cook the shallots for 3 minutes, or until they begin to brown, stirring frequently. Transfer to a small plate or bowl. Set aside.

2. In the same skillet, heat the remaining 1 teaspoon oil over medium-high heat, swirling to coat the bottom. Stir in the spinach, thyme, and margarine. Cook for 1 minute, or until the spinach is just beginning to wilt, using two utensils to toss. Remove from the heat. Sprinkle with the salt. Top with the shallots.

COOK'S TIP ON SHALLOTS: Use browned shallots as a topping for asparagus spears, brown rice, or your favorite veggie.

PER SERVING: Calories 55 • Total Fat **3.0 g** • Saturated Fat **0.0 g** • Trans Fat **0.0 g**
Polyunsaturated Fat **1.0 g** • Monounsaturated Fat **1.5 g** • Cholesterol **0 mg**
Sodium **139 mg** • Carbohydrates **6 g** • Fiber **2 g** • Sugars **2 g** • Protein **3 g**
DIETARY EXCHANGES: 1 vegetable, ½ fat

Split Peas with Canadian Bacon

SERVES 4
½ cup per serving

PREP TIME
10 minutes

COOKING TIME
30 minutes

Split peas aren't just for soup. In this entrée accompaniment, Canadian bacon and onion flavor this hearty legume. Try it with Spicy Turkey Cutlets and Olives (page 155).

1 teaspoon canola or corn oil and 1 teaspoon canola or corn oil, divided use

1 ounce Canadian bacon, finely chopped

1 cup diced onion

2 cups water

¾ cup dried green split peas, sorted for stones and shriveled peas, rinsed, and drained

1 or 2 tablespoons chopped fresh parsley

⅛ teaspoon coarsely ground pepper

1. In a medium saucepan, heat 1 teaspoon oil over medium heat, swirling to coat the bottom. Cook the Canadian bacon for 2 minutes, or until browned, stirring frequently. Transfer to a bowl.

2. Increase the heat to medium high. In the same pan, heat the remaining 1 teaspoon oil, swirling to coat the bottom. Cook the onion for 4 minutes, or until richly browned, stirring occasionally. Stir into the Canadian bacon. Set aside.

3. Increase the heat to high and bring the water and peas to a simmer. Reduce the heat and simmer, covered, for 22 minutes, or until the peas are tender and the liquid is almost absorbed. Remove from the heat. Transfer to a serving dish.

4. Stir in the parsley. Top with the Canadian bacon mixture. Sprinkle with the pepper.

PER SERVING: Calories 172 • Total Fat 3.0 g • Saturated Fat 0.5 g • Trans Fat 0.0 g
Polyunsaturated Fat 1.0 g • Monounsaturated Fat 2.0 g • Cholesterol 4 mg
Sodium 84 mg • Carbohydrates 26 g • Fiber 10 g • Sugars 5 g • Protein 11 g
DIETARY EXCHANGES: 1½ starch, 1 vegetable, 1 lean meat

SERVES 4
½ cup per serving

_____

PREP TIME
5 minutes

_____

COOKING TIME
5 minutes

1 teaspoon canola or corn oil

8 ounces sugar snap peas, trimmed

⅛ teaspoon crushed red pepper flakes

3 tablespoons chopped fresh mint

2 tablespoons chopped fresh cilantro

2 tablespoons finely chopped red onion

⅛ teaspoon salt

Crisp Sugar Snaps with Mint and Cilantro

This crisp dish snaps with crunch and adds brightness to any meal any night of the week. Serve it hot or at room temperature.

1. In a large nonstick skillet, heat the oil over medium heat, swirling to coat the bottom. Cook the peas and red pepper flakes for 4 to 5 minutes, or until the peas are just tender-crisp, stirring frequently. Remove from the heat.

2. Gently stir in the mint, cilantro, and onion. Just before serving, sprinkle with the salt.

TIPS, TRICKS & TIMESAVERS: To trim sugar snap peas, use a paring knife to cut off the ends of the peas and pull the string that runs along the inside curve of the peas and discard it.

PER SERVING: Calories 38 • Total Fat **1.5 g** • Saturated Fat **0.0 g** • Trans Fat **0.0 g** • Polyunsaturated Fat **0.5 g** • Monounsaturated Fat **1.0 g** • Cholesterol **0 mg** • Sodium **78 mg** • Carbohydrates **5 g** • Fiber **2 g** • Sugars **3 g** • Protein **2 g** • DIETARY EXCHANGES: 1 vegetable

Ginger-Honey Sweet Potatoes

Simply pop nutrient-rich sweet potatoes into the microwave to cook them in a fraction of the time it would take in a conventional oven. They're topped with a warm honey-ginger mixture that makes sweet potatoes that much sweeter.

1. Wrap each sweet potato in a paper towel to prevent splatters. Put the sweet potatoes in a microwaveable pie pan or on a large rimmed plate. Microwave on 100 percent power (high) for 10 to 11 minutes, or until tender when pierced with a fork. Remove from the microwave. Let stand for 2 minutes.

2. Meanwhile, in a small bowl, whisk together the remaining ingredients.

3. Halve the sweet potatoes lengthwise. Fluff the pulp with a fork. Top with the margarine mixture.

PER SERVING: Calories **134** • Total Fat **1.5 g** • Saturated Fat **0.0 g** • Trans Fat **0.0 g** Polyunsaturated Fat **0.5 g** • Monounsaturated Fat **1.0 g** • Cholesterol **0 mg** Sodium **93 mg** • Carbohydrates **29 g** • Fiber **3 g** • Sugars **11 g** • Protein **2 g** DIETARY EXCHANGES: 2 starch

SERVES 4
1 potato half and 2 teaspoons margarine mixture per serving

PREP TIME
5 minutes

COOKING TIME
10 minutes

STANDING TIME
2 minutes

2 8-ounce sweet potatoes, pierced with a fork in several places

1 tablespoon plus 1 teaspoon light tub margarine, melted

1 tablespoon plus 1 teaspoon honey

½ teaspoon grated peeled gingerroot

½ teaspoon vanilla extract

SERVES 4
½ cup per serving

PREP TIME
5 minutes

COOKING TIME
10 minutes

STANDING TIME
5 minutes

1 teaspoon canola or
corn oil

½ cup diced onion

2 medium zucchini,
quartered lengthwise
and cut crosswise into
2½- to 3-inch pieces

¼ teaspoon pepper

1 tablespoon chopped
fresh oregano

⅛ teaspoon salt

¾ ounce shredded or
grated Parmesan
cheese

Sautéed Zucchini with Parmesan

Zucchini spears are lightly browned and then sprinkled with fresh oregano to heighten the flavor of mild summer squash.

1. In a large nonstick skillet, heat the oil over medium-high heat, swirling to coat the bottom. Cook the onion for 2 minutes, or until beginning to soften, stirring frequently.

2. Stir in the zucchini. Cook for 6 minutes, or until tender-crisp, stirring frequently. Transfer to a serving platter.

3. Sprinkle with the remaining ingredients in the order listed. Let stand for 5 minutes.

PER SERVING: Calories 59 • Total Fat 3.0 g • Saturated Fat 1.0 g • Trans Fat 0.0 g
Polyunsaturated Fat 0.5 g • Monounsaturated Fat 1.0 g • Cholesterol 5 mg
Sodium 163 mg • Carbohydrates 5 g • Fiber 1 g • Sugars 3 g • Protein 4 g
DIETARY EXCHANGES: 1 vegetable, ½ fat

Sweet Orange-Roasted Root Vegetables

When beets, carrots, and onions are richly roasted to deepen their natural flavors, and then seasoned with a bit of brown sugar and orange zest, the result is sweet perfection.

SERVES 4
½ cup per serving

PREP TIME
10 minutes

COOKING TIME
30 minutes

1. Preheat the oven to 425°F. Line a baking sheet with aluminum foil. Lightly spray the foil with cooking spray.

2. Put the beets, carrots, and onion on the baking sheet. Drizzle the oil over the vegetables. Stir until well coated. Arrange in a single layer on the baking sheet. Roast for 22 minutes, or until the onion is richly browned on the edges and the beets and carrots are tender-crisp when pierced with a fork, stirring once halfway through. Remove from the oven.

3. Sprinkle the vegetables with the brown sugar, orange zest, and salt.

Cooking spray

3 medium beets (about 3 ounces each), peeled and quartered

2 medium carrots, peeled and cut crosswise into 2-inch slices

1 small onion, cut into 8 wedges

1 tablespoon canola or corn oil

2 teaspoons firmly packed dark brown sugar

1 teaspoon grated orange zest

⅛ teaspoon salt

TIPS, TRICKS & TIMESAVERS: Peel fresh beets under running water to prevent the beet juice from staining your hands. The water rinses the juice away from your fingers before the color has time to stain your skin.

PER SERVING: Calories 87 • Total Fat **3.5 g** • Saturated Fat **0.5 g** • Trans Fat **0.0 g**
Polyunsaturated Fat **1.0 g** • Monounsaturated Fat **2.0 g** • Cholesterol **0 mg**
Sodium **144 mg** • Carbohydrates **13 g** • Fiber **3 g** • Sugars **9 g** • Protein **2 g**
DIETARY EXCHANGES: 2 vegetable, 1 fat

PREP TIME
15 minutes

COOKING TIME
15 minutes

12 medium button mushroom caps

1 medium zucchini, cut crosswise into 12 1/2-inch slices

12 medium green onions, trimmed to 6 inches

12 grape tomatoes

Cooking spray

SAUCE

2 tablespoons finely chopped fresh cilantro

1 teaspoon grated lime zest

1 1/2 tablespoons fresh lime juice

1 tablespoon canola or corn oil

2 teaspoons soy sauce (lowest sodium available)

2 teaspoons Worcestershire sauce (lowest sodium available)

Soy-Lime Veggie Kebabs

It's easy to get your kids to stick around for dinner and eat their veggies with these tangy kebabs. Serve them with burgers or grilled steak or chicken at your next family barbecue.

1. Soak four 12-inch bamboo skewers for at least 10 minutes in cold water to keep them from charring, or use metal skewers. Using 3 each of the mushrooms, zucchini, green onions, and tomatoes per skewer, alternate the vegetables as you thread them onto the skewers, folding the green onions in half. Lightly spray the kebabs with cooking spray.

2. Lightly spray the grill rack. Preheat the grill on medium high. Or lightly spray a grill pan and heat over medium-high heat. Grill the kebabs for 10 to 12 minutes, or until the vegetables are tender-crisp, turning occasionally. Transfer the kebabs to serving plates.

3. Meanwhile, in a small bowl, whisk together the sauce ingredients. Brush the kebabs with the sauce.

HEALTHY SWAP: If you prefer to broil the kebabs, preheat the broiler. Lightly spray a broiler rack and pan with cooking spray. Place the kebabs on the broiler rack. Broil about 2 to 3 inches from the heat for 5 minutes on each side, or until the vegetables are tender-crisp, turning occasionally.

PER SERVING: Calories 96 • Total Fat 4.0 g • Saturated Fat 0.5 g • Trans Fat 0.0 g
Polyunsaturated Fat 1.0 g • Monounsaturated Fat 2.0 g • Cholesterol 0 mg
Sodium 102 mg • Carbohydrates 13 g • Fiber 5 g • Sugars 7 g • Protein 3 g
DIETARY EXCHANGES: 2 vegetable, 1 fat

Orange-Soaked Apple Wedges

Citrus and cinnamon complement the sweet tartness of apples in this autumnal side dish that you're sure to fall in love with.

SERVES 4
¾ cup per serving

PREP TIME
5 minutes

COOKING TIME
10 minutes

STANDING TIME
10 minutes

1. In a large skillet, bring all the ingredients to a boil over medium-high heat. Boil for 4 minutes, or until the apples are just tender-crisp and the liquid is slightly thickened, stirring frequently. Remove from the heat.

2. Let stand, covered, for 10 minutes so the flavors blend.

2 medium unpeeled red apples, such as Gala or Jonathan (about 8 ounces each), cut into 8 wedges each

½ cup fresh orange juice

1 tablespoon sugar

1 teaspoon ground cinnamon

> **COOK'S TIP:** Don't skip the standing step. It not only gives the apples time to absorb the other flavors, but it also allows them to continue gently cooking without drying out or browning as they might over direct heat.

PER SERVING: Calories **82** • Total Fat **0.0 g** • Saturated Fat **0.0 g** • Trans Fat **0.0 g**
Polyunsaturated Fat **0.0 g** • Monounsaturated Fat **0.0 g** • Cholesterol **0 mg**
Sodium **0 mg** • Carbohydrates **21 g** • Fiber **2 g** • Sugars **17 g** • Protein **1 g**
DIETARY EXCHANGES: 1½ fruit

SAUCES AND CONDIMENTS

Arugula Pesto with Basil

Basil takes a back seat in this pesto. Arugula, with its slightly assertive, peppery taste, drives the flavor in our version. Almonds are used rather than the more traditional pine nuts.

In a food processor or blender, process all the ingredients until smooth.

> **TIPS, TRICKS & TIMESAVERS:** Don't let citrus zest go to waste. When zesting a lemon, as in this recipe, zest the entire fruit. Separate the zest into ½-teaspoon piles on a plate and place the plate in the freezer. When the zest is frozen, transfer the piles to an airtight container or a resealable plastic freezer bag and return to the freezer.

4 cups arugula (about 2½ ounces)

½ cup fresh basil

¾ ounce Parmesan cheese

2 tablespoons water

1 tablespoon slivered or sliced almonds, dry-roasted

1 teaspoon grated lemon zest

1 tablespoon fresh lemon juice

2 medium garlic cloves

1½ teaspoons capers, drained

PER SERVING: Calories **42** • Total Fat **2.5 g** • Saturated Fat **1.0 g** • Trans Fat **0.0 g** Polyunsaturated Fat **0.5 g** • Monounsaturated Fat **1.0 g** • Cholesterol **5 mg** Sodium **119 mg** • Carbohydrates **2 g** • Fiber **1 g** • Sugars **1 g** • Protein **3 g** DIETARY EXCHANGES: ½ fat

⅔ cup fat-free plain
Greek yogurt

⅓ cup unpeeled zucchini,
shredded

⅓ cup unpeeled seedless
cucumber, finely diced

1 tablespoon chopped
fresh cilantro

1 teaspoon chopped fresh
mint

¼ teaspoon ground
cumin, toasted

⅛ teaspoon pepper

⅛ teaspoon salt

Cucumber-Zucchini Raita with Mint

Raita, a yogurt-based sauce, cools down spicy curries and grilled foods. In our version, cucumber and zucchini are bathed in thick and creamy Greek yogurt that's perked up with cilantro, mint, and cumin.

In a medium bowl, stir together all the ingredients until blended.

SHOP & STORE: Seedless cucumbers, also called English cucumbers, are long, slender cucumbers with thin skins and very few seeds. They are usually sold wrapped in plastic in the produce section of the supermarket. If seedless cucumbers are not available, use a regular cucumber, but remove the seeds by halving the cucumber lengthwise and running a spoon down the middle to scoop them out.

COOK'S TIP ON TOASTING CUMIN: Toast cumin in a small, dry skillet over medium heat for 30 seconds to 1 minute, or until the cumin darkens slightly and becomes fragrant, stirring constantly.

PER SERVING: Calories **24** • Total Fat **0.0 g** • Saturated Fat **0.0 g** • Trans Fat **0.0 g**
Polyunsaturated Fat **0.0 g** • Monounsaturated Fat **0.0 g** • Cholesterol **0 mg**
Sodium **86 mg** • Carbohydrates **2 g** • Fiber **0 g** • Sugars **2 g** • Protein **4 g**
DIETARY EXCHANGES: ½ lean meat

Tzatziki Sauce with Capers

Greek yogurt, which makes a great substitute for sour cream, brings rich and creamy texture and a punch of protein to this sauce.

In a small bowl, stir together all the ingredients.

> **COOK'S TIP:** A topping of tzatziki sauce adds a new dimension of flavor to grilled meat, poultry, or seafood, and even cooked vegetables. Use it to dress raw cucumber or tomato slices for an easy salad, or serve it as a dip with crudités.

PER SERVING: Calories **32** • Total Fat **2.5 g** • Saturated Fat **0.5 g** • Trans Fat **0.0 g**
Polyunsaturated Fat **0.0 g** • Monounsaturated Fat **1.5 g** • Cholesterol **0 mg**
Sodium **104 mg** • Carbohydrates **1 g** • Fiber **0 g** • Sugars **1 g** • Protein **2 g**
DIETARY EXCHANGES: ½ fat

SERVES 4
2 tablespoons per serving

PREP TIME
5 minutes

⅓ cup fat-free plain Greek yogurt

2 tablespoons diced peeled cucumber

1½ tablespoons capers, drained and finely chopped

1 tablespoon minced fresh Italian (flat-leaf) parsley

2 teaspoons extra-virgin olive oil

½ medium garlic clove, minced

½ teaspoon grated lemon zest

SERVES 4
2 tablespoons
per serving

PREP TIME
5 minutes

COOKING TIME
5 minutes

STANDING TIME
5 minutes

Orange and Red Pepper Sauce

This fiery-colored sauce makes a tangy topper for grilled pork, chicken, or shrimp. Up the heat by adding some crushed red pepper flakes.

⅓ cup fresh orange juice

¼ cup finely chopped red bell pepper

1 tablespoon sugar

2 teaspoons cider vinegar

½ teaspoon cornstarch

⅛ teaspoon crushed red pepper flakes (optional)

½ teaspoon grated orange zest

1. In a small saucepan, combine all the ingredients except the orange zest, whisking until the cornstarch is dissolved. Bring to a boil over high heat. Boil for 1 minute. Remove from the heat.

2. Stir in the zest. Pour into a shallow bowl to cool quickly. Let stand for 5 minutes.

PER SERVING: Calories 27 • Total Fat 0.0 g • Saturated Fat 0.0 g • Trans Fat 0.0 g
Polyunsaturated Fat 0.0 g • Monounsaturated Fat 0.0 g • Cholesterol 0 mg
Sodium 1 mg • Carbohydrates 6 g • Fiber 0 g • Sugars 5 g • Protein 0 g
DIETARY EXCHANGES: ½ other carbohydrate

Fresh Herb and Olive Oil Sauce

SERVES 4
1 tablespoon
per serving

PREP TIME
5 minutes

CHILLING TIME
Up to 8 hours
(optimal)

The fusion of basil, rosemary, and oregano in olive oil makes this sauce explode with Italian flavor. Drizzle it on steamed or roasted vegetables or brush it on thin slices of a crunchy, toasted whole-grain baguette.

In a small bowl, whisk together the vinegar, water, oil, salt, and pepper until well blended. Stir in the remaining ingredients. Serve immediately or cover and refrigerate for up to 8 hours for peak flavor and texture.

PER SERVING: Calories **42** • Total Fat **4.0 g** • Saturated Fat **0.5 g** • Trans Fat **0.0 g**
Polyunsaturated Fat **0.5 g** • Monounsaturated Fat **3.0 g** • Cholesterol **0 mg**
Sodium **120 mg** • Carbohydrates **1 g** • Fiber **0 g** • Sugars **1 g** • Protein **0 g**
DIETARY EXCHANGES: 1 fat

1 tablespoon balsamic vinegar

1 tablespoon water

1 tablespoon extra-virgin olive oil

⅛ teaspoon salt

⅛ teaspoon pepper

3 kalamata olives, finely chopped

1 tablespoon chopped fresh basil

1 teaspoon chopped fresh rosemary

½ teaspoon chopped fresh oregano

⅛ teaspoon crushed red pepper flakes

Cooking spray

4 cups cherry tomatoes, halved

1 medium onion, cut into ¼-inch slices

2 large garlic cloves, minced

2 tablespoons chopped fresh oregano

2 teaspoons olive oil

¼ teaspoon pepper

⅛ teaspoon salt

Oven-Roasted Cherry Tomato Sauce

Cherry tomatoes give you that fresh-from-the-vine flavor, even in the middle of winter. Their year-round availability makes them a staple in the kitchen, and roasting intensifies their natural sweetness. Use this chunky-style sauce to top whole-grain pasta or homemade pizza or to accompany juicy sirloin steaks, chicken breasts, or pork tenderloin.

1. Preheat the oven to 450°F. Lightly spray a large rimmed baking sheet with cooking spray.

2. In a large bowl, toss together all the ingredients until the vegetables are lightly coated with oil. Arrange in a single layer on the baking sheet.

3. Roast for 10 to 13 minutes, or until the tomatoes are wilted and tender and the onion is slightly charred. Just before serving, sprinkle with additional pepper if desired.

PER SERVING: Calories **84** • Total Fat **3.0 g** • Saturated Fat **0.5 g** • Trans Fat **0.0 g**
Polyunsaturated Fat **0.5 g** • Monounsaturated Fat **2.0 g** • Cholesterol **0 mg**
Sodium **95 mg** • Carbohydrates **15 g** • Fiber **3 g** • Sugars **9 g** • Protein **2 g**
DIETARY EXCHANGES: 3 vegetable, ½ fat

Spaghetti Sauce with Sausage and Eggplant

SERVES 4
½ cup per serving

PREP TIME
10 minutes

COOKING TIME
10 minutes

Turn your favorite whole-grain pasta into a complete meal with this hearty meat sauce made with turkey sausage—as a bonus, the vegetables are included, too!

1. In a large nonstick skillet, heat the oil over medium-high heat, swirling to coat the bottom. Cook the sausage for 4 minutes, or until browned on the outside and no longer pink in the center, stirring frequently to turn and break up the sausage.

2. Stir in the tomatoes, eggplant, bell pepper, water, onion, garlic, and tomato paste. Bring to a boil. Reduce the heat and simmer, covered, for 5 minutes, or until the eggplant is tender. Remove from the heat.

3. Stir in the basil and salt.

TIPS, TRICKS & TIMESAVERS: Double the batch and freeze half for later use. For added freshness, stir in 2 tablespoons of chopped fresh basil after reheating.

1 teaspoon canola or corn oil

4 ounces low-fat Italian turkey sausage, casings discarded

2 cups grape tomatoes, quartered

1½ cups diced eggplant

1 medium green bell pepper, diced

⅔ cup water

½ cup diced onion

4 medium garlic cloves, minced

2 tablespoons no-salt-added tomato paste

¼ cup chopped fresh basil, or to taste

⅛ teaspoon salt

PER SERVING: Calories **103** • Total Fat **4.0 g** • Saturated Fat **1.0 g** • Trans Fat **0.0 g**
Polyunsaturated Fat **1.0 g** • Monounsaturated Fat **2.0 g** • Cholesterol **24 mg**
Sodium **289 mg** • Carbohydrates **11 g** • Fiber **3 g** • Sugars **5 g** • Protein **6 g**
DIETARY EXCHANGES: 2 vegetable, 1 lean meat

SERVES 4
2 tablespoons
per serving

PREP TIME
5 minutes

¼ cup chopped fresh cilantro

3 tablespoons fresh lime juice

2 tablespoons diced red onion

2 tablespoons low-sodium smooth peanut butter

1 medium jalapeño with seeds and ribs (see Cook's Tip, page 261)

1 tablespoon sugar

¾ teaspoon soy sauce (lowest sodium available)

⅛ teaspoon salt

Spicy Peanut-Lime Stir-Fry Sauce

Toss this rich and zesty sauce with whole-grain vermicelli or steamed broccoli, serve it over pan-seared chicken or tofu, or use it to stir-fry shrimp and vegetables.

In a food processor or blender, process all the ingredients until smooth.

PER SERVING: Calories 66 • Total Fat 4.0 g • Saturated Fat 1.0 g • Trans Fat 0.0 g
Polyunsaturated Fat 1.0 g • Monounsaturated Fat 2.0 g • Cholesterol 0 mg
Sodium 99 mg • Carbohydrates 7 g • Fiber 1 g • Sugars 5 g • Protein 2 g
DIETARY EXCHANGES: ½ other carbohydrate, 1 fat

Orange-Hoisin Stir-Fry Sauce

SERVES 4
2 tablespoons
per serving

PREP TIME
5 minutes

Add Asian flair with a zing of citrus to shrimp, chicken, pork, or vegetables with this sauce that's infused with hoisin, a spicy-sweet mixture of soybeans, garlic, chiles, and spices.

In a small bowl, whisk together all the ingredients.

PER SERVING: Calories **42** • Total Fat **0.5 g** • Saturated Fat **0.0 g** • Trans Fat **0.0 g** Polyunsaturated Fat **0.0 g** • Monounsaturated Fat **0.0 g** • Cholesterol **0 mg** Sodium **103 mg** • Carbohydrates **9 g** • Fiber **0 g** • Sugars **9 g** • Protein **0 g** DIETARY EXCHANGES: ½ other carbohydrate

½ teaspoon grated orange zest

⅓ cup fresh orange juice

2 tablespoons hoisin sauce (lowest sodium available)

1½ tablespoons sugar

1 to 1½ tablespoons cider vinegar

1 teaspoon grated peeled gingerroot

Ancho-Tequila Marinade

MAKES ¾ CUP
enough for
1 to 1½ pounds of
poultry or meat

PREP TIME
10 minutes

Make any meal a fiesta with this south-of-the-border marinade. Use it to marinate flank or sirloin steak, pork chops, or chicken.

In a small bowl, whisk together all the ingredients.

COOK'S TIP ON MAKING ANCHO POWDER: In a food processor or blender, process extra ancho peppers, stems and some seeds discarded, for 1 to 2 minutes, or until finely ground. Use the powder to season meat, fish, vegetables, and dips, or in recipes such as Ancho Chicken and Black Bean Salad with Cilantro-Lime Dressing (page 96).

PER SERVING: Calories **44** • Total Fat **2.5 g** • Saturated Fat **0.5 g** • Trans Fat **0.0 g** Polyunsaturated Fat **0.5 g** • Monounsaturated Fat **1.5 g** • Cholesterol **0 mg** Sodium **1 mg** • Carbohydrates **2 g** • Fiber **0 g** • Sugars **1 g** • Protein **0 g** DIETARY EXCHANGES: ½ fat

¼ cup tequila

2 ancho peppers, minced

2 tablespoons minced fresh cilantro

2 tablespoons fresh lime juice

2 tablespoons fresh orange juice

1 tablespoon olive oil

3 medium garlic cloves, minced

¼ teaspoon cayenne

MAKES ¼ CUP
enough for 1 pound
of poultry or meat

PREP TIME
5 minutes

Italian Herb Marinade

Combine a few heady ingredients—including rosemary, oregano, garlic, and cider vinegar—in one little bowl and you'll have a mighty marinade.

3 tablespoons cider vinegar

1 tablespoon extra-virgin olive oil

⅛ teaspoon salt

2 tablespoons finely chopped fresh Italian (flat-leaf) parsley

1½ teaspoons chopped fresh rosemary

1 teaspoon chopped fresh oregano

1 medium garlic clove, minced

1. In a small bowl, whisk together the vinegar, oil, and salt.

2. Stir in the remaining ingredients.

PER SERVING: Calories 35 • Total Fat 3.5 g • Saturated Fat 0.5 g • Trans Fat 0.0 g
Polyunsaturated Fat 0.5 g • Monounsaturated Fat 2.5 g • Cholesterol 0 mg
Sodium 75 mg • Carbohydrates 1 g • Fiber 0 g • Sugars 0 g • Protein 0 g
DIETARY EXCHANGES: 1 fat

Basil-Jalapeño Rub

For a change from marinades, try a rub instead. It's just as flavorful, and it's faster because you eliminate the marinating time. Before grilling meat, poultry, or seafood, rub it with this spicy, fresh herb mixture.

In a small bowl, stir together all the ingredients.

> **COOK'S TIP ON HANDLING HOT CHILES:** Hot chiles, such as jalapeños, contain oils that can burn your skin, lips, and eyes. Wear disposable gloves or wash your hands thoroughly with warm, soapy water after handling the peppers.

PER SERVING: Calories **34** • Total Fat **3.5 g** • Saturated Fat **0.5 g** • Trans Fat **0.0 g** Polyunsaturated Fat **0.5 g** • Monounsaturated Fat **2.5 g** • Cholesterol **0 mg** Sodium **73 mg** • Carbohydrates **1 g** • Fiber **0 g** • Sugars **0 g** • Protein **0 g** DIETARY EXCHANGES: ½ fat

MAKES ABOUT ¼ CUP enough for 1 pound of poultry, meat, or seafood

PREP TIME 5 minutes

1 tablespoon minced fresh basil

1 tablespoon extra-virgin olive oil

1½ teaspoons minced fresh oregano

1½ teaspoons cider vinegar

2 medium garlic cloves, minced

1 medium jalapeño, seeds and ribs discarded, minced

⅛ teaspoon salt

MAKES ABOUT
¼ CUP
enough for 1 pound
of poultry or meat

PREP TIME
5 minutes

Country Garden Sage and Green Onion Rub

Parsley, sage, and green onions contribute country-fresh flavor to this rub that elevates savory roasted poultry or pork to a whole new level.

2 tablespoons very finely chopped fresh parsley

2 tablespoons minced green onions

1 tablespoon canola or corn oil

2 teaspoons minced fresh sage

3 medium garlic cloves, minced

⅛ teaspoon salt

In a small bowl, stir together all the ingredients.

SHOP & STORE: Many recipes use only part of the green onion. If you need only the dark part, cut off the green tops to about 3 inches above the white bulbs, and set the green onions in a glass, bulb end down. Add about 2 inches of water. Place the glass on a sunny windowsill and change the water daily. You'll have new green tops in about a week.

PER SERVING: Calories 37 • Total Fat 3.5 g • Saturated Fat 0.5 g • Trans Fat 0.0 g Polyunsaturated Fat 1.0 g • Monounsaturated Fat 2.0 g • Cholesterol 0 mg Sodium 75 mg • Carbohydrates 1 g • Fiber 0 g • Sugars 0 g • Protein 0 g DIETARY EXCHANGES: 1 fat

Avocado-Tomatillo Salsa

SERVES 8
¼ cup per serving

PREP TIME
10 minutes

The tangy tomatillo may look like a little green tomato, but it definitely doesn't taste like one. Tomatillos, which are commonly used in Mexican cuisine, have a slightly acidic taste with hints of lemon.

In a medium bowl, gently stir together all the ingredients.

1 medium avocado, diced

1 medium poblano pepper, seeds and ribs discarded, diced (see Cook's Tip, page 261)

1 medium tomatillo, papery husk discarded, diced

½ medium tomato, diced

¼ cup diced red onion

¼ cup chopped fresh cilantro

2 tablespoons fresh lime juice

1 medium garlic clove, minced

⅛ teaspoon salt

SHOP & STORE: Choose hard-fleshed tomatillos, discard the husks just before use, and wash the tomatillos well. To store them, leave the husks on and refrigerate the tomatillos in a paper bag for up to one month. Roasting or grilling them tames the tartness and gives them a sweeter taste.

PER SERVING: Calories 50 • Total Fat **4.0 g** • Saturated Fat **0.5 g** • Trans Fat **0.0 g**
Polyunsaturated Fat **0.5 g** • Monounsaturated Fat **2.5 g** • Cholesterol **0 mg**
Sodium **40 mg** • Carbohydrates **4 g** • Fiber **2 g** • Sugars **1 g** • Protein **1 g**
DIETARY EXCHANGES: 1 vegetable, 1 fat

SERVES 6
⅓ cup per serving

PREP TIME
10 minutes

STANDING TIME
5 minutes

1½ cups diced seeded
watermelon

¼ cup diced seeded
tomato

2 tablespoons chopped
fresh cilantro

1½ to 2 teaspoons grated
peeled gingerroot

1 medium jalapeño with
seeds and ribs, finely
chopped (see Cook's
Tip, page 261)

Spicy Watermelon Salsa

Pair this icy-hot salsa with grilled tuna steaks or pork. Team it with toasted pita chips that have been tossed with a hint of cinnamon and sugar for a lively and unusual snack.

In a small bowl, stir together all of the ingredients. Let stand for 5 minutes so the flavors blend. Serve within 2 hours for peak flavor and texture.

PER SERVING: Calories **14** • Total Fat **0.0 g** • Saturated Fat **0.0 g** • Trans Fat **0.0 g**
Polyunsaturated Fat **0.0 g** • Monounsaturated Fat **0.0 g** • Cholesterol **0 mg**
Sodium **1 mg** • Carbohydrates **3 g** • Fiber **0 g** • Sugars **3 g** • Protein **0 g**
DIETARY EXCHANGES: Free

Pomegranate-Citrus Salsa

Pomegranate seeds, or arils, add a tart snap to this citrusy fruit salsa while the onion and red pepper flakes add bite.

In a medium bowl, gently stir together all the ingredients.

> **SHOP & STORE:** Look for packages of fresh pomegranate seeds, or arils, in the produce section of large supermarkets. To remove the arils from a whole pomegranate, cut off the crown and then cut the fruit into sections. Put the sections in a bowl of water. Using your fingers, roll the arils out, discarding the membrane and rind. Strain the arils in a fine-mesh sieve. Pomegranates are a delicious source of fiber, vitamin C, and potassium.

PER SERVING: Calories **64** • Total Fat **0.5 g** • Saturated Fat **0.0 g** • Trans Fat **0.0 g**
Polyunsaturated Fat **0.0 g** • Monounsaturated Fat **0.0 g** • Cholesterol **0 mg**
Sodium **1 mg** • Carbohydrates **15 g** • Fiber **2 g** • Sugars **12 g** • Protein **1 g**
DIETARY EXCHANGES: 1 fruit

SERVES 4
½ cup per serving

PREP TIME
5 minutes

¾ cup pomegranate seeds, or arils

½ teaspoon grated orange zest

½ cup orange sections, diced

½ cup grapefruit sections, diced (see Cook's Tip, page 40)

2 tablespoons finely chopped red onion

1 tablespoon sugar

1 teaspoon vanilla extract

⅛ teaspoon crushed red pepper flakes

½ cup fat-free plain Greek yogurt

2 tablespoons sugar

1½ tablespoons fresh orange juice

½ teaspoon curry powder

½ teaspoon vanilla extract

1 medium apricot, diced

Apricot Curry Dipping Sauce

This sauce has a hint of curry and citrus to balance the sweetness from the apricot. Use it to dip chunks of fresh pineapple, whole strawberries, pear and apple slices, and even melon cubes.

In a small bowl, whisk together all the ingredients except the apricot. Stir in the apricot.

PER SERVING: Calories 49 • Total Fat 0.0 g • Saturated Fat 0.0 g • Trans Fat 0.0 g Polyunsaturated Fat 0.0 g • Monounsaturated Fat 0.0 g • Cholesterol 0 mg Sodium 11 mg • Carbohydrates 9 g • Fiber 0 g • Sugars 9 g • Protein 3 g DIETARY EXCHANGES: ½ other carbohydrate

2 cups blackberries

1 medium pear, diced

⅓ cup sugar

2 tablespoons water

2 teaspoons cornstarch

¼ teaspoon ground cardamom or allspice

1½ teaspoons vanilla extract

½ teaspoon almond extract

Blackberry-Pear Fruit Spread

The secret ingredient in this spread is cardamom, the high-powered "cousin" to allspice. Enjoy it on toast or in yogurt.

1. In a medium saucepan, combine the blackberries, pear, sugar, water, cornstarch, and cardamom, stirring until the cornstarch is dissolved. Bring to a boil over medium-high heat. Reduce the heat to medium and cook for 2 minutes, or until slightly thickened, stirring occasionally. Remove from the heat.

2. Whisk in the vanilla and almond extracts, breaking up larger pieces of the fruit. Serve immediately for a warm sauce or cool completely, cover, and refrigerate until needed.

PER SERVING: Calories 34 • Total Fat 0.0 g • Saturated Fat 0.0 g • Trans Fat 0.0 g Polyunsaturated Fat 0.0 g • Monounsaturated Fat 0.0 g • Cholesterol 0 mg Sodium 1 mg • Carbohydrates 8 g • Fiber 1 g • Sugars 6 g • Protein 0 g DIETARY EXCHANGES: ½ fruit

Cinnamon-Stick Cranberry Relish with Apples

SERVES 8
scant ½ cup
per serving

PREP TIME
5 minutes

COOKING TIME
5 minutes

CHILLING TIME
15 minutes

Diced apples add an unexpected flavor and crunch to this relish that you can use to liven up a pork, turkey, or chicken dish at any time of year. And once it's cooked and you're waiting for it to cool, put the cinnamon sticks in a saucepan with some water and simmer on your back burner to create a delicious aroma that will fill your whole house, enticing the family to dinner.

1. In a large saucepan, stir together the water and sugar. Bring to a boil over high heat.

2. Stir in the remaining ingredients. Return to a boil and boil for 2 minutes, or until the cranberries pop.

3. Pour into a 13 × 9 × 2-inch glass baking dish. Discard the cinnamon sticks. Transfer the dish to the freezer for 15 minutes to cool slightly. Serve the relish warm or cover and refrigerate to serve cold.

1 cup water

¾ cup sugar

2 large unpeeled red apples, such as Jonathan or Gala, diced

12 ounces fresh cranberries

4 whole cinnamon sticks (each about 3 inches long)

⅛ teaspoon ground cloves

SHOP & STORE: To freeze cranberry relish, spoon the cooled relish into an airtight freezer container and freeze for up to one year.

PER SERVING: Calories **122** • Total Fat **0.0 g** • Saturated Fat **0.0 g** • Trans Fat **0.0 g**
Polyunsaturated Fat **0.0 g** • Monounsaturated Fat **0.0 g** • Cholesterol **0 mg**
Sodium **3 mg** • Carbohydrates **32 g** • Fiber **3 g** • Sugars **26 g** • Protein **0 g**
DIETARY EXCHANGES: 1 fruit, 1 other carbohydrate

1 medium mango, peeled
and chopped

¼ cup diced red onion

¼ cup diced red bell
pepper

2 tablespoons sugar

2 tablespoons white
balsamic vinegar

2 tablespoons water

½ teaspoon grated
orange zest

Mango-Orange Chutney

Chutney is usually made with fruit, vinegar, sugar, and spices or other flavorings, such as citrus zest. Chutneys are in the same family as salsas and relishes—that is, they're all condiments. Try this as a sweet spread on sandwiches or as a topping for toasted whole-grain English muffins.

1. In a medium saucepan, stir together all the ingredients except the orange zest. Bring to a boil over medium-high heat. Reduce the heat and simmer, covered, for 5 minutes, or until the bell pepper is soft. Remove from the heat.

2. Stir in the zest. Let stand for 10 minutes. Serve warm or chilled.

HEALTHY SWAP: As a change from mango, substitute fresh plums when they come into season—they're an underused fruit that bursts with flavor.

PER SERVING: Calories 36 • Total Fat 0.0 g • Saturated Fat 0.0 g • Trans Fat 0.0 g Polyunsaturated Fat 0.0 g • Monounsaturated Fat 0.0 g • Cholesterol 0 mg Sodium 2 mg • Carbohydrates 9 g • Fiber 1 g • Sugars 8 g • Protein 0 g DIETARY EXCHANGES: ½ fruit

Sugar-and-Spice Tomato Chutney

SERVES 4
2 tablespoons
per serving

PREP TIME
5 minutes

COOKING TIME
10 minutes

STANDING TIME
10 minutes

The texture of a chutney can be chunky or smooth and its flavor hot or mild. This one is chunky, with a mild heat from the ginger and a bit of smokiness from the cumin. Serve it with meat or poultry, or use it as a unique sandwich spread.

1. In a medium nonstick skillet, heat the oil over medium heat, swirling to coat the bottom. Cook the onion for 2 minutes, or until just tender-crisp, stirring frequently.

2. Stir in the tomato and garlic. Increase the heat to medium high and bring to a boil. Boil for 2 minutes, or until the mixture is slightly thickened. Remove from the heat.

3. Stir in the remaining ingredients. Spoon the mixture into a shallow glass pan, such as a pie pan. Let stand for 10 minutes to cool.

PER SERVING: Calories **35** • Total Fat **1.5 g** • Saturated Fat **0.0 g** • Trans Fat **0.0 g**
Polyunsaturated Fat **0.5 g** • Monounsaturated Fat **1.0 g** • Cholesterol **0 mg**
Sodium **76 mg** • Carbohydrates **6 g** • Fiber **1 g** • Sugars **4 g** • Protein **1 g**
DIETARY EXCHANGES: 1 vegetable

1 teaspoon canola or corn oil

½ cup diced onion

1 medium tomato, diced

1 medium garlic clove, minced

2 teaspoons sugar

2 teaspoons white balsamic vinegar

1 teaspoon grated peeled gingerroot

⅛ to ¼ teaspoon ground cumin

⅛ teaspoon salt

BREADS AND BREAKFASTS

Lemon-Rosemary Oatmeal Mini Muffins

SERVES 12
2 mini muffins
per serving

PREP TIME
10 minutes

COOKING TIME
20 minutes

Lemon zest and rosemary infuse these muffins with a delicate savoriness, and because they're minis, they bake almost twice as fast as regular-size muffins. Try these with soup or salad; they're ideal for tucking into brown bag lunches.

1. Preheat the oven to 425°F. Lightly spray a 24-cup mini muffin pan with cooking spray.

2. In a large bowl, stir together the flour, oats, sugar, baking powder, baking soda, and salt.

3. In a small bowl, whisk together the remaining ingredients. Pour into the flour mixture, stirring just until moistened but no flour is visible. Don't overmix; the batter should be lumpy. Spoon the batter into the muffin cups.

4. Bake for 10 minutes, or until a wooden toothpick inserted in the center comes out clean. Turn the muffins out of the pan.

5. Serve warm or at room temperature. Store any leftover muffins in an airtight container in a cool, dry place for up to two days. Or freeze in an airtight freezer bag for up to one month.

Cooking spray

1⅓ cups all-purpose flour

¾ cup uncooked rolled oats

1½ tablespoons sugar

1¾ teaspoons baking powder

¼ teaspoon baking soda

⅛ teaspoon salt

1 cup low-fat buttermilk

2 large egg whites

3 tablespoons canola or corn oil

½ to 1 teaspoon finely chopped fresh rosemary

½ to 1 teaspoon grated lemon zest

PER SERVING: Calories **118** • Total Fat **4.0 g** • Saturated Fat **0.5 g** • Trans Fat **0.0 g**
Polyunsaturated Fat **1.0 g** • Monounsaturated Fat **2.5 g** • Cholesterol **1 mg**
Sodium **140 mg** • Carbohydrates **17 g** • Fiber **1 g** • Sugars **3 g** • Protein **4 g**
DIETARY EXCHANGES: 1 starch, ½ fat

Peach-Perfect Muffins

SERVES 12
1 muffin per serving

PREP TIME
10 minutes

COOKING TIME
25 minutes

STANDING TIME
5 minutes

Cooking spray

1½ cups uncooked quick-cooking oats

1 cup white whole-wheat flour

¼ cup wheat bran

1 teaspoon ground cinnamon and ¼ teaspoon ground cinnamon, divided use

½ teaspoon ground nutmeg

½ teaspoon baking soda

¼ teaspoon salt

1 cup low-fat buttermilk

½ cup sugar and 1½ tablespoons sugar, divided use

¼ cup canola or corn oil

2 large egg whites

2 teaspoons grated lemon zest

½ cup diced peaches and 1½ cups diced peaches, divided use (about 3 medium peaches total)

Filled with oats and fresh peaches, these muffins offer both fiber and fruit in this grab-and-go breakfast or snack. Try smearing Blackberry-Pear Fruit Spread (page 266) on them for a new fruit flavor sensation.

1. Preheat the oven to 350°F. Lightly spray a standard 12-cup muffin pan with cooking spray.

2. In a large bowl, stir together the oats, flour, wheat bran, 1 teaspoon cinnamon, the nutmeg, baking soda, and salt.

3. In a medium mixing bowl, whisk together the buttermilk, ½ cup sugar, the oil, egg whites, and lemon zest until well blended.

4. Stir the buttermilk mixture and ½ cup peaches into the oats mixture just until moistened but no flour is visible. Don't overmix; the batter should be lumpy. Spoon the batter into the muffin cups. Top the batter with the remaining 1½ cups peaches.

5. Bake for 20 minutes, or until a wooden toothpick inserted in the center comes out clean.

6. Meanwhile, in a small bowl, stir together the remaining 1½ tablespoons sugar and ¼ teaspoon cinnamon.

7. When the muffins are done, transfer the pan to a cooling rack. Sprinkle the muffins with the sugar mixture. Let stand in the pan for 5 minutes. Serve warm or at room temperature.

COOK'S TIP: Freeze any leftovers in an airtight freezer container for up to one month.

PER SERVING: Calories 177 • Total Fat 6.0 g • Saturated Fat 0.5 g • Trans Fat 0.0 g
Polyunsaturated Fat 1.5 g • Monounsaturated Fat 3.5 g • Cholesterol 1 mg
Sodium 132 mg • Carbohydrates 27 g • Fiber 3 g • Sugars 14 g • Protein 5 g
DIETARY EXCHANGES: 2 starch, 1 fat

Nutty Spiced Granola

Enjoy this as a breakfast cereal with fat-free milk or as a midmorning snack sprinkled over fat-free yogurt. Divide it into individual snack-size baggies ahead of time so it's easy to grab on your way to work or bring in the car for the kids to munch on the way to school or sports practice.

1. Preheat the oven to 300°F. Lightly spray a large baking sheet with cooking spray.

2. In a medium bowl, stir together the cereal clusters, oats, cereal twigs, pumpkin seeds, almonds, sugar, and oil.

3. Spread the cereal mixture in an even layer on the baking sheet. Bake for 25 minutes, or until lightly golden, stirring two or three times while baking. Transfer to a bowl.

4. Stir in the remaining ingredients. Let stand for 15 minutes, or until cool.

COOK'S TIP: This granola can be stored for up to two weeks in an airtight container. Keep it in a cool, dark place, such as a pantry.

PER SERVING: Calories 182 • Total Fat 7.5 g • Saturated Fat 1.5 g • Trans Fat 0.0 g
Polyunsaturated Fat 2.5 g • Monounsaturated Fat 3.0 g • Cholesterol 0 mg
Sodium 95 mg • Carbohydrates 26 g • Fiber 6 g • Sugars 8 g • Protein 7 g
DIETARY EXCHANGES: 2 starch, 1 fat

SERVES 14
½ cup per serving

PREP TIME
5 minutes

COOKING TIME
30 minutes

STANDING TIME
15 minutes (optional)

Cooking spray

3 cups high-fiber cereal clusters

2 cups uncooked rolled oats

1 cup bran cereal twigs

½ cup raw unsalted shelled pumpkin seeds

½ cup slivered almonds or shelled, dry-roasted, unsalted pistachios

3 tablespoons sugar

1 tablespoon toasted sesame oil

⅓ cup sweetened flaked coconut

1 tablespoon grated peeled gingerroot

1½ teaspoons grated orange zest

1 teaspoon ground cinnamon

¼ teaspoon salt

SERVES 4
¾ cup cereal and
⅓ cup pear mixture
per serving

PREP TIME
5 minutes

COOKING TIME
5 minutes

STANDING TIME
5 minutes

2 cups water

⅔ cup uncooked quinoa
flakes

⅓ cup cranberries, halved

¾ teaspoon ground
cinnamon

¼ teaspoon ground
allspice

⅛ teaspoon salt

2 tablespoons firmly
packed light brown
sugar

TOPPING

1 medium pear, diced

2 tablespoons firmly
packed light brown
sugar

¼ cup chopped walnuts

½ teaspoon vanilla
extract

¼ teaspoon almond
extract

Hot Cereal with Cranberries and Pear

This cereal will warm you up on a cold morning, and it's an interesting change from the more-familiar apple-cinnamon oatmeal or cream of wheat. Quinoa flakes cook in a matter of minutes, so you'll have breakfast on the table in a flash.

1. In a large saucepan, bring the water to a boil over high heat. Stir in the quinoa flakes, cranberries, cinnamon, allspice, and salt. Boil for 1½ minutes, stirring frequently. Remove from the heat.

2. Stir in 2 tablespoons brown sugar. Let stand for 5 minutes, or until the mixture is slightly thickened.

3. Meanwhile, in a small bowl, stir together the topping ingredients.

4. Spoon the cereal into bowls. Spoon the topping onto the cereal.

COOK'S TIP: Be sure to let the cereal stand for 5 minutes. The standing time allows it to become creamier and more tender.

COOK'S TIP ON QUINOA FLAKES: The quinoa seed is flattened into quinoa flakes, which resemble uncooked rolled oats. The flakes cook very quickly, make a great hot cereal, and can be used as a substitute for rolled oats in baking.

PER SERVING: Calories 237 • Total Fat 6.5 g • Saturated Fat 0.5 g • Trans Fat 0.0 g
Polyunsaturated Fat 4.5 g • Monounsaturated Fat 1.0 g • Cholesterol 0 mg
Sodium 83 mg • Carbohydrates 41 g • Fiber 5 g • Sugars 20 g • Protein 5 g
DIETARY EXCHANGES: 1½ starch, ½ fruit, 1 other carbohydrate, 1 fat

Maple-Pumpkin Oatmeal with Apple and Spiced Yogurt Topping

SERVES 6
1 cup per serving

PREP TIME
10 minutes

COOKING TIME
20 minutes

Celebrate the traditional autumnal flavors of maple, pumpkin, and apple with this oatmeal. It's so warm and creamy that you'll want to make it all through the fall season!

3 cups water

⅛ teaspoon salt

2 cups uncooked rolled oats

2 medium red apples, such as Jazz or Gala, diced

1 cup canned solid-pack pumpkin (not pie filling)

¼ cup pure maple syrup

1 teaspoon pumpkin pie spice and ½ teaspoon pumpkin pie spice, divided use

½ cup fat-free vanilla Greek yogurt

1. In a large saucepan, bring the water and salt to a boil, covered, over high heat. Stir in the oats and apples. Reduce the heat and simmer, covered, for 10 minutes, or until the liquid is absorbed, stirring occasionally.

2. Stir in the pumpkin, maple syrup, and 1 teaspoon pumpkin pie spice. Cook for 2 minutes, or until heated through, stirring occasionally.

3. In a small bowl, whisk together the yogurt and the remaining ½ teaspoon pumpkin pie spice. Spoon the oatmeal into bowls. Top with the yogurt mixture.

COOK'S TIP ON MAPLE SYRUP: Pure maple syrup is made from maple sap. The primary ingredient in maple-flavored, imitation maple, or pancake syrup is high fructose corn syrup. Such syrups also contain added sodium.

PER SERVING: Calories **198** • Total Fat **2.5 g** • Saturated Fat **0.5 g** • Trans Fat **0.0 g**
Polyunsaturated Fat **0.5 g** • Monounsaturated Fat **0.5 g** • Cholesterol **1 mg**
Sodium **70 mg** • Carbohydrates **41 g** • Fiber **6 g** • Sugars **19 g** • Protein **5 g**
DIETARY EXCHANGES: 2 starch, 1 fruit

SERVES 4
1 cup oatmeal and
¼ cup topping
per serving

PREP TIME
10 minutes

COOKING TIME
10 minutes

Peach-Pecan Oatmeal

Loaded with the goodness of chopped peaches and dry-roasted pecans, this oatmeal is a tasty way to get you going in the morning.

¼ cup chopped pecans, dry-roasted

2 tablespoons firmly packed dark brown sugar and 2 tablespoons firmly packed dark brown sugar, divided use

1 tablespoon plus 1 teaspoon wheat germ

3¾ cups water

2 cups uncooked quick-cooking oats

1 medium unpeeled peach, chopped, and 1 medium unpeeled peach, chopped, divided use

1 teaspoon vanilla, butter, and nut flavoring or vanilla extract

⅛ teaspoon salt

1. In a small bowl, stir together the pecans, 2 tablespoons brown sugar, and the wheat germ. Set aside.

2. In a medium saucepan, bring the water to a boil over high heat. Stir in the oats and 1 chopped peach. Reduce the heat and simmer for 3 minutes, stirring occasionally. Remove from the heat.

3. Stir in the remaining 2 tablespoons brown sugar, the flavoring, and salt.

4. Spoon the oatmeal into bowls. Sprinkle with the pecan mixture. Top with the remaining chopped peach.

PER SERVING: Calories 293 • Total Fat 7.5 g • Saturated Fat 1.0 g • Trans Fat 0.0 g
Polyunsaturated Fat 2.5 g • Monounsaturated Fat 3.5 g • Cholesterol 0 mg
Sodium 85 mg • Carbohydrates 50 g • Fiber 6 g • Sugars 21 g • Protein 8 g
DIETARY EXCHANGES: 2 starch, ½ fruit, 1 other carbohydrate, 1 fat

Strawberry-Almond Oatmeal with Ginger

Hot creamy oats are topped with ginger-kissed strawberries. Toasted almonds add a nutty crunch to wake up your palate.

SERVES 4
1 cup oatmeal and ½ cup topping per serving

PREP TIME
10 minutes

COOKING TIME
15 minutes

1. In a small bowl, gently stir together the strawberries, 1 tablespoon sugar, and the gingerroot. Set aside.

2. In a medium saucepan, bring the water to a boil over high heat. Stir in the oats. Reduce the heat and simmer for 3 minutes, stirring occasionally. Remove from the heat.

3. Stir in the almond extract, salt, and the remaining 3 tablespoons sugar.

4. Spoon the oatmeal into bowls. Spoon the strawberry mixture onto the oatmeal. Sprinkle with the almonds.

2 cups diced hulled strawberries

1 tablespoon sugar and 3 tablespoons sugar, divided use

1 teaspoon grated peeled gingerroot

3¾ cups water

2 cups uncooked quick-cooking oats

¼ teaspoon almond extract

⅛ teaspoon salt

¼ cup slivered almonds, dry-roasted

PER SERVING: Calories 273 • Total Fat 6.5 g • Saturated Fat 0.5 g • Trans Fat 0.0 g
Polyunsaturated Fat 2.0 g • Monounsaturated Fat 3.0 g • Cholesterol 0 mg
Sodium 82 mg • Carbohydrates 48 g • Fiber 7 g • Sugars 18 g • Protein 9 g
DIETARY EXCHANGES: 2 starch, ½ fruit, ½ other carbohydrate, 1 fat

SERVES 6
3 pancakes and
⅓ cup topping
per serving

PREP TIME
10 minutes

COOKING TIME
10 minutes

STANDING TIME
10 to 15 minutes
(optional)

1 cup white whole-wheat
flour

½ cup whole-wheat
pastry flour

½ cup uncooked quick-
cooking oats

1 tablespoon light or dark
brown sugar

1 teaspoon baking
powder

1 teaspoon baking soda

½ teaspoon cinnamon
and ¼ teaspoon
cinnamon, divided use

1 teaspoon grated orange
zest

1 cup unsweetened soy
milk or fat-free milk

2 large eggs

½ cup low-fat buttermilk

1 cup sliced hulled
strawberries

2 medium oranges,
sectioned

(continued)

Oatmeal Pancakes with Strawberry-Orange Topping

Whole-grain pancakes get your day off to a healthy start.
Strawberries and oranges mingle in maple syrup for the topping.

1. In a medium bowl, whisk together the flours, oats, brown
   sugar, baking powder, baking soda, ½ teaspoon cinnamon,
   and the orange zest.

2. In a small bowl, whisk together the soy milk, eggs, and
   buttermilk. Slowly pour into the flour mixture, stirring until
   well blended and no flour is visible. For a cakelike pancake,
   let the batter stand for 10 to 15 minutes (see Cook's Tip).
   For thinner, more eggy pancakes, skip the standing time and
   cook the batter immediately.

3. Meanwhile, in a medium bowl, gently stir together the
   strawberries, oranges, orange juice, maple syrup, and the
   remaining ¼ teaspoon cinnamon. Set aside.

4. Preheat the oven to 200°F.

5. Lightly spray an electric griddle with cooking spray. Preheat
   to 375°F. Or lightly spray a large skillet and heat over
   medium-high heat. Test the temperature by sprinkling a
   few drops of water on the griddle. If the water evaporates
   quickly, the griddle is ready.

6. Drop the batter by large spoonfuls onto the griddle,
   spreading it into 3½-inch circles. (You may need to make
   several batches, depending on the size of your griddle.)
   Cook for 2 minutes, or until the tops begin to bubble slightly
   and the edges are browned. Turn over. Cook for 2 minutes.
   Transfer the pancakes to a baking sheet and put in the oven
   to keep warm while you cook the remaining batter.

7. Just before serving, top the pancakes with the strawberry
   mixture. Serve immediately.

2 tablespoons fresh
 orange juice

1 tablespoon pure maple
 syrup

Cooking spray

COOK'S TIP: Pancakes made with whole grains often take longer to cook than those made with white flour, thus the heat needs to be a bit lower to cook them properly. Other differences to note are that the batter is thicker and fewer of the characteristic bubbles form as the pancakes cook. The best way to see if they're ready to flip is to lift the edges a bit to check if they're browned.

COOK'S TIP: Letting the pancake batter stand for 10 to 15 minutes allows the grains to absorb the liquid and gives the leaveners a head start, producing a lighter, fluffier pancake. The batter will thicken slightly.

PER SERVING: Calories **236** • Total Fat **3.5 g** • Saturated Fat **1.0 g** • Trans Fat **0.0 g**
Polyunsaturated Fat **1.0 g** • Monounsaturated Fat **1.0 g** • Cholesterol **63 mg**
Sodium **338 mg** • Carbohydrates **43 g** • Fiber **5 g** • Sugars **12 g** • Protein **9 g**
DIETARY EXCHANGES: 2 starch, 1 fruit, ½ lean meat

Sweet Potato Pancakes with Caramelized Cinnamon Apples

These pancakes are made with uncooked sweet potatoes, making them similar to potato pancakes or latkes, except that their batter is bright orange. A warm cinnamon apple mixture tops them for a sweet finishing touch.

Cooking spray

TOPPING

1 pound unpeeled sweet apples such as Golden Delicious, Fuji, Gala, or Cortland, cut into ¼-inch slices

2 tablespoons firmly packed dark brown sugar

½ cup 100% apple juice

½ teaspoon ground cinnamon

(continued)

1. Preheat the oven to 250°F.

2. Lightly spray a large skillet with cooking spray and heat over medium-high heat. Cook the apples for 5 to 7 minutes, or until they begin to soften and brown, stirring occasionally.

3. Reduce the heat to medium low. Stir in the brown sugar. Cook for 3 minutes, or until the apples begin to caramelize, stirring frequently.

4. Stir in the apple juice and cinnamon. Increase the heat to medium high. Cook for 1 to 2 minutes, or until the apples are tender and the liquid is reduced by half (to about ¼ cup). Remove from the heat. Cover to keep warm.

5. In a food processor or blender, process the pancake ingredients until the sweet potatoes are finely chopped and the mixture is almost smooth but some texture remains.

6. Preheat the oven to 200°F.

7. Preheat an electric griddle to 350°F or heat a large skillet over medium heat. Test the temperature by sprinkling a few drops of water on the griddle. If the water evaporates quickly, the griddle is ready. Brush with about ½ teaspoon of oil, or enough to lightly coat the griddle.

8. Using ¼ cup for each pancake, pour the batter onto the griddle, spreading it into 4-inch circles. (You may need to make two batches, depending on the size of your griddle.) Cook for 4 minutes, or until bubbles form and pop on the tops, and the bottoms are golden brown. Turn over. Cook for 3 minutes, or until the bottoms are golden brown. Transfer the pancakes to a baking sheet and put in the oven to keep warm while you cook the remaining batter, using the remaining oil.

9. Just before serving, top the pancakes with the apple mixture. Serve immediately.

PER SERVING: Calories 316 • Total Fat **4.5 g** • Saturated Fat **1.0 g** • Trans Fat **0.0 g**
Polyunsaturated Fat **1.0 g** • Monounsaturated Fat **2.0 g** • Cholesterol **94 mg**
Sodium **311 mg** • Carbohydrates **63 g** • Fiber **7 g** • Sugars **28 g** • Protein **8 g**
DIETARY EXCHANGES: 2½ starch, 1½ fruit, ½ lean meat

PANCAKES

1 pound sweet potatoes, peeled and coarsely chopped into ¾-inch pieces

½ cup all-purpose flour

½ cup fat-free milk

2 large eggs

½ teaspoon baking powder

¼ teaspoon salt

* * *

1½ teaspoons canola or corn oil

SERVES 4
3 sticks and
2 tablespoons sauce
per serving

PREP TIME
10 minutes

COOKING TIME
15 minutes

4 large egg whites

1 large egg

2 tablespoons fat-free milk

6 ounces multigrain Italian bread (lowest sodium available), cut into 4 slices, each slice cut lengthwise into 3 strips

2 teaspoons canola or corn oil and 2 teaspoons canola or corn oil, divided use

SAUCE

1 teaspoon grated orange zest

⅓ cup fresh orange juice

2 tablespoons sugar

½ teaspoon ground cinnamon

2 tablespoons light tub margarine

1 teaspoon vanilla extract

French Toast Sticks with Orange Dipping Sauce

French toast is a popular breakfast choice, but it's usually reserved for leisurely weekend mornings. These sticks are easy enough to make before heading out the door on weekdays, too.

1. Preheat the oven to 200°F.

2. In a shallow dish, whisk together the egg whites, egg, and milk. Working quickly with half the strips, lightly dip in the egg white mixture, turning to coat. Transfer to a large plate. Repeat with the remaining strips and egg white mixture.

3. In a large nonstick skillet, heat 2 teaspoons oil over medium heat, swirling to coat the bottom. Cook half the strips for 4 minutes, turning every minute, or until golden brown all over. Transfer to a baking sheet and put in the oven to keep warm while you cook the remaining strips, using the remaining 2 teaspoons oil.

4. In a small saucepan, whisk together the orange zest, orange juice, sugar, and cinnamon. Increase the heat to medium high and bring to a boil. Remove from the heat. Whisk in the margarine and vanilla until the margarine is melted.

5. Serve the dipping sauce with the French toast sticks.

TIPS, TRICKS & TIMESAVERS: Some of the bread strips might have slightly curved edges. To brown the strips evenly, use the back of a fork or spoon to gently press the bread down while it cooks.

PER SERVING: Calories 232 • Total Fat **7.5 g** • Saturated Fat **1.0 g** • Trans Fat **0.0 g**
Polyunsaturated Fat **2.0 g** • Monounsaturated Fat **3.5 g** • Cholesterol **47 mg**
Sodium **370 mg** • Carbohydrates **31 g** • Fiber **2 g** • Sugars **9 g** • Protein **9 g**
DIETARY EXCHANGES: 2 starch, 1 lean meat, ½ fat

Black Bean Chilaquiles

SERVES 4
¾ cup per serving

PREP TIME
15 minutes

COOKING TIME
10 minutes

Chilaquiles is a traditional Mexican breakfast dish in which crisp tortillas are simmered in salsa or mole sauce and then combined with eggs, queso fresco (fresh Mexican cheese), and beans. In this version, fresh tomato, cilantro, and jalapeño add more flavor. For a spicier dish, leave in the jalapeño seeds.

1. In a large bowl, using a fork, lightly beat the egg whites, eggs, and salt. Stir in the tortilla squares and ½ cup queso fresco.

2. In a small bowl, stir together the beans and chipotle powder. Fold into the egg white mixture. Set aside so the tortillas can soften.

3. In a large nonstick skillet, heat the oil over medium heat, swirling to coat the bottom. Cook the onion and jalapeño for 3 minutes, stirring occasionally.

4. Stir the tomatoes into the egg white mixture. Pour into the skillet. Cook for 4 to 5 minutes, or until the eggs are set, stirring occasionally. Just before serving, sprinkle with the cilantro and the remaining ¼ cup queso fresco.

PER SERVING: Calories 235 • Total Fat **9.0 g** • Saturated Fat **3.5 g** • Trans Fat **0.0 g**
Polyunsaturated Fat **1.5 g** • Monounsaturated Fat **3.5 g** • Cholesterol **108 mg**
Sodium **345 mg** • Carbohydrates **20 g** • Fiber **4 g** • Sugars **5 g** • Protein **18 g**
DIETARY EXCHANGES: 1 starch, 1 vegetable, 2½ lean meat

6 large egg whites

2 large eggs

¼ teaspoon salt

3 6-inch corn tortillas, stacked, cut into ¾-inch strips, then cut crosswise into 1-inch squares

½ cup crumbled queso fresco or farmer's cheese and ¼ cup crumbled queso fresco or farmer's cheese, divided use

¾ cup canned no-salt-added black beans, rinsed and drained

1 teaspoon chipotle powder

2 teaspoons canola or corn oil

½ cup chopped onion

1 medium jalapeño, seeds and ribs discarded if desired, chopped (see Cook's Tip, page 261)

1½ cups chopped seeded tomatoes

⅓ cup chopped fresh cilantro

SERVES 2
one-half omelet
per serving

PREP TIME
10 minutes

COOKING TIME
10 to 15 minutes

Garden Omelet

This omelet is overflowing with a mushroom sauté, so don't worry if some spills out onto the plate—it's just a sneak peek at the deliciousness waiting inside.

1 teaspoon olive oil and
 2 teaspoons olive oil,
 divided use

1 cup sliced button or
 cremini (brown)
 mushrooms

¼ cup chopped yellow
 bell pepper

¼ teaspoon salt

2 cups loosely packed
 baby spinach

½ cup quartered cherry
 or grape tomatoes

2 tablespoons chopped
 fresh basil

Dash of cayenne

3 large egg whites

1 large egg

1 tablespoon chopped
 fresh chives

1 tablespoon water

2 tablespoons goat
 cheese crumbles

1. In a large nonstick skillet, heat 1 teaspoon oil over medium-high heat, swirling to coat the bottom. Cook the mushrooms, bell pepper, and salt for 4 to 5 minutes, or until the vegetables are tender, stirring occasionally. Stir in the spinach, tomatoes, basil, and cayenne. Cook for 1 to 2 minutes, or until the spinach is wilted, stirring frequently. Transfer the mushroom mixture to a medium bowl. Set aside.

2. Wipe the skillet with paper towels.

3. In a medium bowl, whisk together the egg whites, egg, chives, and water.

4. In the same skillet, still over medium-high heat, heat the remaining 2 teaspoons oil, swirling to coat the bottom. Pour the egg white mixture into the skillet, swirling to coat the bottom. Cook for 30 seconds, or until beginning to set. Using a spatula, carefully lift the cooked edge of the omelet and tilt the skillet so the uncooked portion flows under the edge. Cook until no runniness remains, repeating the lift-and-tilt procedure once or twice at other places along the edge if needed. Spread the mushroom mixture over half of the omelet. Remove from the heat.

5. Sprinkle with the goat cheese. Using a spatula, carefully fold the half with no filling over the other half. Gently slide the omelet onto a large plate. Cut the omelet in half. Transfer half to another plate.

PER SERVING: Calories **186** • Total Fat **12.0 g** • Saturated Fat **3.5 g** • Trans Fat **0.0 g** Polyunsaturated Fat **1.5 g** • Monounsaturated Fat **6.5 g** • Cholesterol **100 mg** Sodium **464 mg** • Carbohydrates **7 g** • Fiber **2 g** • Sugars **4 g** • Protein **13 g** DIETARY EXCHANGES: 1 vegetable, 1½ lean meat, 1½ fat

Asparagus Omelet with Creamy Yogurt Sauce

This omelet is quick enough for a weekday breakfast. You can prepare the yogurt sauce the night before.

SERVES 2
one-half omelet and 2 tablespoons sauce per serving

PREP TIME
5 minutes

COOKING TIME
10 to 15 minutes

1. In a small bowl, whisk together the yogurt, olive oil, mustard, and ½ teaspoon tarragon. Set aside.

2. In a separate small bowl, whisk together the egg whites, egg, and milk. Set aside.

3. In a medium nonstick skillet, bring the water and asparagus to a boil over medium-high heat. Reduce the heat and simmer, covered, for 1½ to 2 minutes, or until the asparagus is just tender-crisp. Drain immediately in a colander.

4. In a medium bowl, stir together the asparagus, bell pepper, salt, and the remaining 1½ teaspoons tarragon. Cover to keep warm. Set aside.

5. Wipe the skillet with paper towels. Heat the canola oil over medium heat, swirling to coat the bottom. Pour the egg white mixture into the skillet, swirling to coat the bottom. Cook for 30 seconds, or until beginning to set. Using a spatula, carefully lift the cooked edge of the omelet and tilt the skillet so the uncooked portion flows under the edge. Cook until no runniness remains, repeating the lift-and-tilt procedure once or twice at other places along the edge if needed. Spread the asparagus mixture over half of the omelet. Remove from the heat.

6. Top with the yogurt mixture. Using a spatula, carefully fold the half with no filling over the other half. Gently slide the omelet onto a large plate. Cut the omelet in half. Transfer half to another plate. Garnish each half with a tarragon sprig.

¼ cup fat-free plain yogurt

1½ teaspoons extra-virgin olive oil

¼ teaspoon yellow mustard (lowest sodium available)

½ teaspoon chopped fresh tarragon and 1½ teaspoons chopped fresh tarragon, divided use

2 large egg whites

1 large egg

3 tablespoons fat-free milk

½ cup water

4 ounces asparagus spears, trimmed and cut into ½-inch pieces

¼ cup diced red bell pepper

¼ teaspoon salt

2 teaspoons canola or corn oil

2 sprigs of fresh tarragon (optional)

PER SERVING: Calories **168** • Total Fat **10.5 g** • Saturated Fat **1.5 g** • Trans Fat **0.0 g**
Polyunsaturated Fat **2.0 g** • Monounsaturated Fat **6.5 g** • Cholesterol **94 mg**
Sodium **423 mg** • Carbohydrates **7 g** • Fiber **2 g** • Sugars **6 g** • Protein **11 g**
DIETARY EXCHANGES: 1 vegetable, 1½ lean meat, 1 fat

SERVES 4
1 parfait per serving

PREP TIME
10 minutes

COOKING TIME
10 minutes

2 cups sliced hulled
  strawberries

2 cups blueberries or
  halved blackberries, or
  a combination

1 tablespoon plus
  1 teaspoon honey

2 teaspoons ground
  cinnamon

2 cups water

1 cup uncooked rolled
  oats

2 cups fat-free plain
  Greek yogurt

¼ cup sliced almonds
  or chopped shelled
  dry-roasted, unsalted
  pistachios

Fruity Oatmeal Yogurt Parfaits

Warm, chewy oatmeal, layers of cool, creamy yogurt, and sweet, cinnamon-laced berries add up to a high-powered breakfast. If you want to bump up the fiber in these quick-and-easy parfaits, try sprinkling some flax seed meal on top. You can also substitute any fruit for the berries—apples and pears make a great choice for a fall or wintertime breakfast parfait. *(See photo insert.)*

1. In a medium bowl, gently stir together the strawberries, blueberries, honey, and cinnamon. Set aside.

2. In a medium saucepan, bring the water and oats to a boil over medium-high heat. Boil for about 5 minutes, or until the oatmeal begins to thicken, stirring occasionally.

3. In each parfait glass, layer the ingredients as follows: ¼ cup oatmeal, ¼ cup strawberry mixture, ¼ cup yogurt, and ¼ cup strawberry mixture. Repeat the layers, ending with the strawberry mixture. Sprinkle with the almonds.

COOK'S TIP ON GREEK YOGURT: Greek yogurt is thicker, denser, and creamier than regular yogurt and it has almost twice the protein. Substitute fat-free Greek yogurt for full-fat sour cream, heavy cream, regular mayonnaise, or regular cream cheese to save on saturated fat and calories.

PER SERVING: Calories 264 • Total Fat 4.5 g • Saturated Fat 0.5 g • Trans Fat 0.0 g
Polyunsaturated Fat 1.5 g • Monounsaturated Fat 2.5 g • Cholesterol 0 mg
Sodium 49 mg • Carbohydrates 43 g • Fiber 7 g • Sugars 22 g • Protein 16 g
DIETARY EXCHANGES: 1½ starch, 1½ fruit, 1½ lean meat

Mango and Pineapple Tropical Parfaits

SERVES 4
1 parfait per serving

PREP TIME
10 minutes

Dig down deep so you'll capture the ripe fruit, silky yogurt, and crunchy granola in every spoonful of this paradisiacal parfait. Ruby-red pomegranate "jewels" and lacy coconut top off this island treasure.

1 medium mango, peeled and chopped

2 cups fat-free plain Greek yogurt

½ cup low-fat granola

½ cup diced pineapple

1 medium banana, sliced

¼ cup pomegranate seeds, or arils

2 tablespoons sweetened flaked coconut

1. In each parfait glass, layer the ingredients as follows: one-fourth of the mango, ¼ cup yogurt, 1 tablespoon granola, 2 tablespoons pineapple, one-fourth of the banana slices, and ¼ cup yogurt. Top with the remaining granola. Sprinkle with the pomegranate seeds and coconut.

2. Serve immediately for peak flavor and texture.

PER SERVING: Calories **216** • Total Fat **2.0 g** • Saturated Fat **1.0 g** • Trans Fat **0.0 g**
Polyunsaturated Fat **0.5 g** • Monounsaturated Fat **0.5 g** • Cholesterol **0 mg**
Sodium **79 mg** • Carbohydrates **40 g** • Fiber **4 g** • Sugars **27 g** • Protein **12 g**
DIETARY EXCHANGES: 1½ fruit, 1 fat-free milk, ½ starch

DESSERTS

Mini Fruited Phyllo Tarts

These dessert bites look colorfully impressive with deep indigo blueberries, golden-orange apricots, and bright green kiwifruit, but they're simple to make—even on a busy weekday. Use your favorite fresh fruits for some variations.

In a small bowl, gently stir together the blueberries, apricot, and kiwifruit. Spoon about 1 tablespoon of yogurt into each phyllo shell. Top each shell with about 1 tablespoon of the blueberry mixture. Serve immediately for peak flavor and texture.

> **TIPS, TRICKS & TIMESAVERS:** If you want to make these ahead, you may prepare, cover, and refrigerate the individual ingredients for up to 48 hours, but don't assemble the tarts until serving time. Once they are filled, these tarts will begin to lose their crispness.
>
> ---
>
> **TIPS, TRICKS & TIMESAVERS:** To peel a kiwifruit easily and with no mess, cut off the ends of the fruit. Gently press a thin teaspoon between the skin and the flesh of the fruit. Holding the fruit in the palm of your hand, gently rotate the spoon around the fruit, loosening the skin. Slide the skin off in one piece.

SERVES 5
3 mini tarts per serving

PREP TIME
10 minutes

½ cup blueberries

1 medium apricot, diced

1 medium kiwifruit, peeled and diced

1 cup fat-free vanilla yogurt

15 frozen mini phyllo tart shells, thawed

PER SERVING: Calories 117 • Total Fat 3.0 g • Saturated Fat 0.0 g • Trans Fat 0.0 g
Polyunsaturated Fat 1.5 g • Monounsaturated Fat 1.0 g • Cholesterol 1 mg
Sodium 72 mg • Carbohydrates 20 g • Fiber 1 g • Sugars 12 g • Protein 3 g
DIETARY EXCHANGES: 1 starch, ½ fruit, ½ fat

PREP TIME
10 minutes

COOKING TIME
25 minutes

CHILLING TIME
1 to 1½ hours
(optional)

½ cup uncooked instant
brown rice

2 cups fat-free
half-and-half

1 large egg

1 tablespoon sugar

¼ teaspoon ground
cardamom

Dash of ground allspice

2 cups raspberries

¼ cup slivered almonds,
dry-roasted

Nordic Raspberry-Almond Rice Pudding

This traditional Scandinavian holiday dessert is lightened up and made healthier with whole grains, fresh fruit, and fat-free dairy. Serve the pudding warm or at room temperature.

1. Prepare the rice using the package directions, omitting the salt and margarine.

2. Meanwhile, in a medium bowl, whisk together the half-and-half, egg, sugar, cardamom, and allspice until blended. Slowly stir the mixture into the cooked rice. Simmer for 8 to 10 minutes, or until the pudding is thick and creamy, stirring frequently.

3. If serving warm, spoon into ramekins, custard cups, or dessert bowls. Top with the raspberries. Sprinkle with the almonds. If serving at room temperature, refrigerate the pudding, uncovered, for 1 to 1½ hours, stirring occasionally. Just before serving, top with the raspberries and sprinkle with the almonds.

PER SERVING: Calories **149** • Total Fat **3.5 g** • Saturated Fat **0.5 g** • Trans Fat **0.0 g** Polyunsaturated Fat **1.0 g** • Monounsaturated Fat **2.0 g** • Cholesterol **31 mg** Sodium **94 mg** •.Carbohydrates **24 g** • Fiber **4 g** • Sugars **9 g** • Protein **9 g** DIETARY EXCHANGES: 1 fat-free milk, ½ starch, ½ fruit

Dark Chocolate Pudding with Banana Slices

SERVES 4
½ cup pudding and scant ¼ cup banana per serving

PREP TIME
5 minutes

COOKING TIME
10 minutes

CHILLING TIME
1 to 1½ hours (optional)

Dark cocoa powder intensifies the flavor of this chocolate pudding, which tops slices of fresh banana. Crunchy pecans provide a nice texture contrast to the creaminess of the homemade pudding, which can be served warm or chilled.

1. In a heavy medium saucepan, whisk together the milk, egg substitute, sugar, cornstarch, and cocoa. Cook over medium-high heat for 8 to 10 minutes, or until the mixture comes to a full boil and begins to thicken, whisking constantly. Remove from the heat. Stir in the vanilla.

2. Put the banana slices in custard cups or parfait glasses. Spoon the pudding over the banana slices.

3. Sprinkle the pecans over the pudding.

> **COOK'S TIP:** If you prefer to serve the pudding chilled, cover and refrigerate it for 1 hour before sprinkling it with the pecans.

2 cups fat-free milk

1 large egg

3 tablespoons sugar

2 tablespoons cornstarch

2 tablespoons unsweetened dark cocoa powder

2 teaspoons vanilla extract

1 medium banana, sliced

2 tablespoons plus 2 teaspoons chopped pecans, dry-roasted if desired

PER SERVING: Calories 186 • Total Fat 5.0 g • Saturated Fat 1.0 g • Trans Fat 0.0 g
Polyunsaturated Fat 1.5 g • Monounsaturated Fat 2.5 g • Cholesterol 49 mg
Sodium 70 mg • Carbohydrates 29 g • Fiber 2 g • Sugars 20 g • Protein 7 g
DIETARY EXCHANGES: ½ fat-free milk, ½ fruit, 1 other carbohydrate, ½ fat

½ cup fat-free sweetened
  condensed milk

½ teaspoon grated Key
  lime zest or lime zest

1 tablespoon Key lime
  juice or fresh lime juice

½ teaspoon vanilla
  extract

1 cup diced pineapple

1 medium mango, peeled
  and diced

1 medium Key lime
  or lime, cut into 4
  wedges (optional)

Key Lime Cream and Fresh Fruits

If you're a fan of Key lime pie, then you'll love the flavor and tartness of this cream. Luscious pieces of pineapple and mango top off this dessert for even more tropical flavor.

1. In a small bowl, whisk together the condensed milk, lime zest, lime juice, and vanilla. Spoon into 4 ramekins, custard cups, or dessert bowls.

2. Spoon the pineapple and mango onto the cream. Serve with the lime wedges.

TIPS, TRICKS & TIMESAVERS: This dessert can be made up to 24 hours in advance. Cover and refrigerate the cream. Just before serving, top with the pineapple and mango.

COOK'S TIP: Be sure to use fat-free sweetened condensed milk rather than fat-free evaporated milk. The sweetened condensed milk is much thicker and sweeter.

PER SERVING: Calories **184** • Total Fat **0.5 g** • Saturated Fat **0.0 g** • Trans Fat **0.0 g** Polyunsaturated Fat **0.0 g** • Monounsaturated Fat **0.0 g** • Cholesterol **5 mg** Sodium **41 mg** • Carbohydrates **42 g** • Fiber **2 g** • Sugars **40 g** • Protein **4 g** DIETARY EXCHANGES: 1½ fruit, 1½ other carbohydrate

Red Apple and Cranberry Roast

This fruity, nutty dessert is the perfect ending to an autumnal meal. The cranberries soak up the sweetness of the apples and sugar as they roast, and the pecans laced with brown sugar and cinnamon add a rich, toasted crunch.

SERVES 4
¾ cup per serving

PREP TIME
5 minutes

COOKING TIME
20 minutes

1. Preheat the oven to 350°F. Line a baking sheet with aluminum foil. Lightly spray the foil with cooking spray.

2. Arrange the apples in a single layer on the foil. Sprinkle the cranberries, pecans, brown sugar, and cinnamon over the apples. Roast for 17 minutes, or until the apples are tender-crisp.

3. In a small bowl, stir together the margarine and vanilla and almond extracts. Using a rubber scraper, gently fold the mixture into the apples on the baking sheet until well blended.

Cooking spray

2 medium unpeeled red apples, such as Gala or Jonathan (about 8 ounces each), each cut into 4 wedges

½ cup cranberries, coarsely chopped

¼ cup chopped pecans

3 tablespoons firmly packed dark brown sugar

1 teaspoon ground cinnamon

1 tablespoon light tub margarine

1 teaspoon vanilla extract

¼ teaspoon almond extract

COOK'S TIP: The residue that builds up on the foil during roasting contains a lot of concentrated flavor. It's important to add the margarine and extracts to help liquefy the residue and release that flavor so it can be incorporated into the apple mixture.

TIPS, TRICKS & TIMESAVERS: To chop nuts quickly, use a mini food processor or seal them in a plastic bag and crush them with a rolling pin or the flat side of a meat mallet.

PER SERVING: Calories **168** • Total Fat **6.5 g** • Saturated Fat **0.5 g** • Trans Fat **0.0 g**
Polyunsaturated Fat **2.0 g** • Monounsaturated Fat **3.5 g** • Cholesterol **0 mg**
Sodium **27 mg** • Carbohydrates **29 g** • Fiber **4 g** • Sugars **23 g** • Protein **1 g**
DIETARY EXCHANGES: 1 fruit, 1 other carbohydrate, 1½ fat

SERVES 4
6 pear wedges
per serving

___

PREP TIME
10 minutes

___

COOKING TIME
10 to 15 minutes

Cooking spray

⅓ cup pure maple syrup

¼ teaspoon ground
cinnamon (Vietnamese
preferred)

3 firm but ripe pears, such
as Bartlett, Anjou, or
Bosc, peeled and cut
into 8 wedges each

Butter-flavor cooking
spray

2 tablespoons coarsely
chopped pecans,
dry-roasted

Maple-Cinnamon Grilled Pears

After you've finished cooking dinner on the grill, keep it fired up to make this delectable dessert. Grilling caramelizes the pears and intensifies their sweetness.

1. Lightly spray the grill rack with cooking spray. Preheat the grill on medium.

2. In a small saucepan, stir together the maple syrup and cinnamon. Bring to a boil over medium heat. Boil for 30 seconds to 1 minute, or until thickened and slightly reduced (to about ¼ cup), stirring constantly. Set aside.

3. Place the pears on a large rimmed baking sheet. Lightly spray both sides of the pears with the butter-flavor cooking spray, turning with tongs. Transfer the pears to the grill. Grill for 6 to 10 minutes, or until tender and lightly browned, turning occasionally and brushing with half the syrup mixture during the last 3 minutes of grilling.

4. Fan the pears on dessert plates. Drizzle with the remaining syrup mixture. Sprinkle with the pecans.

SHOP & STORE: Don't use color to determine the ripeness of pears. Instead, gently press the top of the fruit next to the stem. If the pear gives slightly, it's ripe and ready to eat.

SHOP & STORE: Vietnamese cinnamon, also known as Saigon cinnamon, contains more essential oil and is stronger and sweeter than other cinnamon varieties. Look for it in the spice section of your grocery store.

PER SERVING: Calories 172 • Total Fat 2.5 g • Saturated Fat 0.0 g • Trans Fat 0.0 g
Polyunsaturated Fat 1.0 g • Monounsaturated Fat 1.5 g • Cholesterol 0 mg
Sodium 5 mg • Carbohydrates 40 g • Fiber 5 g • Sugars 30 g • Protein 1 g
DIETARY EXCHANGES: 1½ fruit, 1 other carbohydrate, ½ fat

Ruby-Red Compote

SERVES 4
½ cup per serving

PREP TIME
5 minutes

COOKING TIME
10 to 15 minutes

STANDING TIME
5 minutes

This dessert, lightly flavored with vanilla and a hint of fresh mint, celebrates early-summer red berries and rhubarb. Serve the compote with low-fat frozen yogurt or meringue cookies, or just enjoy it on its own.

1. In a small saucepan, stir together the rhubarb, water, and sugar. Bring to a boil over medium-high heat. Reduce the heat and simmer for 5 to 8 minutes, or until the rhubarb is soft, stirring frequently. Stir in the vanilla extract.

2. Meanwhile, in a medium bowl, gently stir together the strawberries, raspberries, and mint. Pour the hot rhubarb mixture over the strawberry mixture, stirring until combined. Let stand for 5 minutes, or until the compote cools to room temperature.

1 cup sliced rhubarb (½-inch pieces)

⅔ cup water

¼ cup sugar

½ teaspoon vanilla extract

1 cup sliced hulled strawberries

1 cup raspberries

2 tablespoons coarsely chopped fresh mint

HEALTHY SWAP: Numerous varieties of fresh mint are available to plant in your garden, including peppermint, apple mint, chocolate mint, and lime mint. Any of these would be perfect in this compote. Avoid using spearmint, however, because its strong flavor will overpower this subtle dessert.

SHOP & STORE: Rhubarb stalks require little preparation before cooking. Just discard any leaves, which are toxic, and trim the ends; peeling isn't necessary. You can refrigerate the stalks (just don't wash them first) for five to seven days in a resealable plastic bag or airtight container.

PER SERVING: Calories **87** • Total Fat **0.5 g** • Saturated Fat **0.0 g** • Trans Fat **0.0 g**
Polyunsaturated Fat **0.0 g** • Monounsaturated Fat **0.0 g** • Cholesterol **0 mg**
Sodium **5 mg** • Carbohydrates **21 g** • Fiber **4 g** • Sugars **16 g** • Protein **1 g**
DIETARY EXCHANGES: ½ fruit, 1 other carbohydrate

8 ounces dark sweet
cherries, halved

1 medium red apple,
such as Jazz or Gala,
chopped

¼ cup 100%
pomegranate juice

1 teaspoon cornstarch

½ teaspoon vanilla
extract

¼ teaspoon almond
extract

8 low-fat gingersnaps,
coarsely crumbled

¼ cup pecans, dry-
roasted and finely
chopped

Dark Cherry and Apple Crumble

Why buy frozen or store-bought crumbles when you can make your own hot, fresh fruit version in just minutes? And because you can microwave it, you don't have to heat up the entire house by using the oven.

1. In a medium bowl, stir together the cherries, apple, pomegranate juice, cornstarch, and vanilla and almond extracts until the cornstarch is dissolved. Spoon the cherry mixture into microwaveable ramekins, custard cups, or dessert bowls.

2. Microwave, covered, on 100 percent power (high) for 5 to 7 minutes, or until the mixture is slightly thickened.

3. Sprinkle the cherry mixture with the gingersnaps and pecans.

PER SERVING: Calories **174** • Total Fat **6.5 g** • Saturated Fat **1.0 g** • Trans Fat **0.0 g**
Polyunsaturated Fat **1.5 g** • Monounsaturated Fat **3.5 g** • Cholesterol **0 mg**
Sodium **55 mg** • Carbohydrates **28 g** • Fiber **3 g** • Sugars **19 g** • Protein **2 g**
DIETARY EXCHANGES: 1 fruit, 1 starch, 1 fat

Soft-Serve Blueberry-Cinnamon Ice Cream

SERVES 4
½ cup per serving

PREP TIME
5 minutes

STANDING TIME
10 minutes

Enjoy a delightful contrast of creaminess, tartness, and crunchiness all in one bowl, thanks to the trio of ice cream, blueberries, and almonds. A touch of cinnamon adds a hint of sweet spice. For a patriotic red, white, and blue look, try substituting raspberries or sliced hulled strawberries for some of the blueberries.

Put the ice cream in a medium bowl. Let stand for 10 minutes to soften slightly. Fold in the remaining ingredients. Spoon into dessert bowls.

2 cups fat-free vanilla ice cream

1 cup blueberries

2 tablespoons slivered almonds, dry-roasted

½ teaspoon ground cinnamon

TIPS, TRICKS & TIMESAVERS: You can make this dessert up to two days in advance. Just cover it with plastic wrap and freeze it. Remove it from the freezer 15 minutes before serving and let it stand so the ice cream will soften slightly.

PER SERVING: Calories 135 • Total Fat **2.0 g** • Saturated Fat **0.0 g** • Trans Fat **0.0 g**
Polyunsaturated Fat **0.5 g** • Monounsaturated Fat **1.0 g** • Cholesterol **0 mg**
Sodium **65 mg** • Carbohydrates **27 g** • Fiber **2 g** • Sugars **8 g** • Protein **4 g**
DIETARY EXCHANGES: 2 other carbohydrate, ½ fat

4 ripe medium peaches,
halved

2 tablespoons light brown
sugar and ¼ cup firmly
packed light brown
sugar, divided use

2 tablespoons light tub
margarine, melted

2 tablespoons fresh
lemon juice

1 teaspoon vanilla extract

2 tablespoons water

2 large egg whites

⅛ teaspoon cream of
tartar

Broiled Vanilla Peaches Topped with Meringue

Aromatic vanilla enhances the sweetness of these peach halves
while broiling caramelizes the sugars, giving them a rich, toasty
flavor. *(See photo insert.)*

1. Preheat the broiler. Put the peaches with the cut side up in
   a 9-inch square baking pan or 11 × 7 × 2-inch broilerproof
   baking dish.

2. In a small bowl, stir together 2 tablespoons brown sugar,
   the margarine, lemon juice, and vanilla. Pour over the peach
   halves (some of the mixture may spill into the pan). Broil
   about 4 to 6 inches from the heat for 20 minutes.

3. Meanwhile, in a small saucepan, stir together the water
   and the remaining ¼ cup brown sugar. Bring to a boil over
   medium-high heat. Boil rapidly for 2 minutes, or until slightly
   thickened, stirring occasionally. Set aside to cool.

4. About 5 minutes before the peaches are done, in a medium
   stainless steel mixing bowl, using an electric mixer on
   medium-low speed, beat the egg whites for 30 seconds, or
   until foamy. Beat in the cream of tartar. Increase the speed
   to high. Beat for 1 minute, or until the egg whites begin to
   form soft peaks. While continuing to beat, slowly pour in the
   cooled brown sugar syrup in a thin, steady stream. Beat for
   1½ minutes total, or until the meringue looks glossy.

5. When the peaches are done, remove them from the oven.
   Turn off the broiler. Preheat the oven to 350°F.

6. Top each peach half with a generous ¼ cup of meringue.
   Bake for 5 to 7 minutes, or until the meringue is lightly
   browned and crisp on the outside. Serve immediately.

TIPS, TRICKS & TIMESAVERS: For the best volume in the shortest beating time, let the egg whites stand for 30 minutes to bring them to room temperature before beating. Remember, even a single drop of egg yolk will prevent egg whites from forming peaks when beaten, so separate eggs very carefully.

SHOP & STORE: Ripe peaches will feel soft but not mushy and will smell sweet. To ripen peaches at home, put them in a paper bag and close, but don't seal, the bag. Leave the peaches at room temperature for two or three days until they're ripe.

PER SERVING: Calories 85 • Total Fat **1.5 g** • Saturated Fat **0.0 g** • Trans Fat **0.0 g**
Polyunsaturated Fat **0.5 g** • Monounsaturated Fat **0.5 g** • Cholesterol **0 mg**
Sodium **39 mg** • Carbohydrates **18 g** • Fiber **1 g** • Sugars **16 g** • Protein **2 g**
DIETARY EXCHANGES: ½ fruit, ½ other carbohydrate

APPENDIX A: AT-A-GLANCE FOOD STORAGE GUIDE

To maintain the quality and safety of fresh foods, proper handling and storage are important. Make sure your hands, storage containers, and the refrigerator and freezer themselves are clean to prevent bacteria from entering and spoiling your food. Check the temperature in your fridge and freezer periodically. Your refrigerator should register between 37°F and 40°F and your freezer at 0°F or below. The back of your fridge is the coldest part; the front and door areas are the warmest.

Freezing keeps food safe to eat indefinitely but quality can suffer over time, depending on the length of storage and the type of food. The times given here are for fresh foods from date of purchase; once a food is frozen, the sell-by dates are no longer relevant. Unless otherwise noted, the recommended freezer times are for prepped raw vegetables or fruit stored in airtight containers.

VEGETABLES	LOCATION	DURATION, REFRIGERATED	DURATION, FROZEN
ARTICHOKES	Crisper	5–7 days	NR
ASPARAGUS	Crisper	3–5 days	8–12 months
BEANS, GREEN	Crisper	3–5 days	8–12 months
BEETS	Crisper	2 weeks	8–12 months
BELL PEPPERS	Crisper	5–7 days	3–4 months
BROCCOLI	Crisper	3–5 days	8–12 months
BRUSSELS SPROUTS	Crisper	3–5 days	8–12 months
CABBAGE	Crisper	2 weeks	NR
CARROTS	Crisper	2 weeks	8–12 months
CAULIFLOWER	Crisper	5–7 days	8–12 months
CELERY	Crisper	5–7 days	8–12 months

VEGETABLES	LOCATION	DURATION, REFRIGERATED	DURATION, FROZEN
CORN, ON THE COB	Front of fridge	1–2 days	8–12 months
CUCUMBERS	Crisper	3–5 days	NR
EGGPLANTS	Crisper	3–5 days	NR
GARLIC	Dark, cool, dry, well-ventilated area	1–2 months; discard once sprouted	3–4 months
GREEN ONIONS	Crisper	3–5 days	NR
GREENS: COLLARDS, KALE, SPINACH, SWISS CHARD	Crisper	3–5 days	8–12 months
LEEKS	Crisper	3–5 days	3–4 months, chopped
LETTUCES	Crisper	5–7 days	NR
MUSHROOMS	Front of fridge	1–2 days	8–12 months
OKRA	Front of fridge	3–5 days	8–12 months
ONIONS, SHALLOTS	Dark, cool, dry, well-ventilated area	2–4 weeks	3–4 months
PARSNIPS	Crisper	3 weeks	8–12 months
PEAS, GREEN	Front of fridge	3–5 days	8–12 months
PEPPERS, HOT	Crisper	5–7 days	8–12 months
POTATOES, SWEET POTATOES	Dark, cool, dry, well-ventilated area	1–2 weeks	Best if cooked; 8–12 months
RADISHES	Crisper	2 weeks	NR
SNOW PEAS	Crisper	2 weeks	8–12 months
SQUASH, SUMMER (YELLOW, ZUCCHINI)	Crisper	3–5 days	8–12 months
SQUASH, WINTER (ACORN, BUTTERNUT)	Dark, cool, dry, well-ventilated area	3 months	8–12 months

NR indicates not recommended.

FRUIT	LOCATION	DURATION, REFRIGERATED	DURATION, FROZEN
APPLES	Back of fridge	2–3 months	NR
APRICOTS	Countertop*	1–2 days after ripened	6 months
AVOCADOS	Countertop*	1–2 days after ripened	NR
BANANAS	Countertop*	1 week	6 months
BERRIES	Front of fridge	1–2 days	6 months
CHERRIES	Back of fridge	3–5 days	6 months
CRANBERRIES	Crisper	4 weeks	8–12 months
GRAPEFRUIT	Front of fridge	2 weeks	4–6 months
GRAPES	Back of fridge	2 weeks	6 months
KIWIFRUIT	Countertop*	3–5 days after ripened	NR
LEMONS	Front of fridge	3–4 weeks	Juice and zest: 8–12 months
LIMES	Front of fridge	3–4 weeks	Juice and zest: 8–12 months
MANGOES	Front of fridge	5–7 days	6 months
MELONS	Countertop*; front of fridge once cut	1–2 days once cut	8–12 months
NECTARINES	Countertop*	3–5 days after ripened	6 months
ORANGES	Front of fridge	3–4 weeks	4–6 months
PEACHES, PEARS, PLUMS	Countertop*	3–5 days after ripened	6 months
PINEAPPLES	Countertop*; front of fridge once cut	3–5 days after ripened	8–12 months
TOMATOES	Countertop, away from sunlight and ventilated; in crisper once cut*	1–2 days	3–4 months (wedges; use for cooking only)

NR indicates not recommended.

*Once ripened, store in the refrigerator to slow spoilage. Some flavor loss, drying, and/or discoloration can occur.

FISH, POULTRY, MEAT, AND DAIRY**	DURATION, REFRIGERATED	DURATION, FROZEN
LEAN FISH (SUCH AS COD, FLOUNDER, SOLE)	1–2 days	6 months***
FATTY FISH (SUCH AS SALMON, BLUEFISH, MACKEREL, SALMON)	1–2 days	2–3 months***
SHELLFISH (SUCH AS SHRIMP, SCALLOPS)	1–2 days	3–6 months
CHICKEN OR TURKEY, WHOLE	1–2 days	1 year
CHICKEN OR TURKEY, PIECES	1–2 days	9 months
GROUND POULTRY OR MEAT	1–2 days	3–4 months
STEAKS	3–5 days	6–12 months
CHOPS	3–5 days	4–6 months
ROASTS	3–5 days	4–12 months
BUTTERMILK	1–2 weeks	1 month; thaw in refrigerator (best used for cooking)
CHEESE, GRATED (SUCH AS PARMESAN)	6 months, unopened; 3–4 weeks, opened	1–2 months
CHEESE, HARD (SUCH AS CHEDDAR, SWISS)	6 months, unopened; 3–4 weeks, opened	6 months; thaw in refrigerator
CHEESE, SOFT (SUCH AS BRIE)	1 week	6 months
CREAM CHEESE	2 weeks	NR
MARGARINE, SPREAD SUBSTITUTES	4–5 months	12 months; leave in original wrapping and overwrap
MILK	1 week	1 month; thaw in refrigerator (best used for cooking)
SOUR CREAM	1–3 weeks	NR
YOGURT	1–2 weeks	NR
EGGS, IN SHELL	4–5 weeks	NR
EGGS, HARD-COOKED	1 week	NR

NR indicates not recommended.

**Keep all fish, poultry, meat, and dairy products in the coldest parts of the refrigerator.

***Wrap well or use ice method: Place fish on a foil-covered cookie sheet. Freeze. Dip in water several times; freeze to form thin ice glaze; wrap well, then wrap well again.

APPENDIX B: AT-A-GLANCE VEGETABLE COOKING TIMES

VEGETABLE	COOKING TIME IN MINUTES					
	STEAM	BOIL OR SIMMER	SAUTÉ OR STIR-FRY	MICROWAVE	BAKE OR ROAST	GRILL
ASPARAGUS	8–10	5–10	5–7	4–6	15–25 at 400°F	8–10
BEANS, GREEN	5–15	10–20	3–4	6–12	12–15 at 425°F	**10–15**
BEANS, LIMA	10–20	20–30	15–20	8–12	NR	NR
BEETS, WHOLE	40–60	30–60	NR	20–30	45–60 at 350°F	25 in foil
BELL PEPPER, STRIPS	2–4	4–5	2–3	2–4	NR	NR
BROCCOLI, FLORETS	5–6	4–5	3–4	4–5	10–15 at 425°F	8–10
BRUSSELS SPROUTS	6–12	5–10	3–4	7–8	35–40 at 400°F	Blanch; then 10 in foil
CABBAGE, SHREDDED	5–8	5–10	3–4	8–10	30–45 at 425°F	NR
CARROTS, SLICED	4–5	5–10	3–4	4–7	30–40 at 350°F	NR
CAULIFLOWER, FLORETS	6–10	5–8	3–4	5–10	20–30 at 450°F	30 in foil
CORN ON THE COB	6–10	4–7	NR	3–4	30–35 at 350°F	15–20
EGGPLANT, SLICED	8–10	5–10	5–6	6–8	10–15 at 425°F	5–6

VEGETABLE	COOKING TIME IN MINUTES					
	STEAM	BOIL OR SIMMER	SAUTÉ OR STIR-FRY	MICROWAVE	BAKE OR ROAST	GRILL
GREENS: KALE, COLLARD	4–6	5–8	2–3	8–10	NR	NR
LEEKS, HALVED	5–10	10–15	5–10	6–8	35–45 at 400°F	15–20 in foil
MUSHROOMS, SLICED	NR	NR	4–5	3–4	20–25 at 450°F	Whole: 4–5
OKRA, SLICED	8–10	NR	5–10	2–3	25–35 at 400°F	10–15
PARSNIPS, CUBED	10–15	NR	NR	4–6	20–30 at 350°F	10–15 in foil
PEAS, GREEN	3–5	8–12	2–3	5–7	NR	NR
POTATOES, WHOLE	NR	20–30	NR	6–8 for 1; +2 each added	40–60 at 400°F	45–60 in foil
SNOW PEAS	3–5	2–3	5–7	3–4	NR	NR
SPINACH, SWISS CHARD	5–6	2–5	3–5	3–4	NR	NR
SQUASH, SUMMER, SLICED	5–10	5–10	3–5	3–6	10–15 at 450°F	10–15
SQUASH, WINTER, CUBED	15–20	NR	NR	8–10	45–60 at 400°F	15–20 in foil
SWEET POTATOES, WHOLE	NR	20–30	NR	10–15	40–60 at 425°F	45–60 in foil

NR indicates not recommended.

APPENDIX C: INGREDIENT EQUIVALENTS

VEGETABLES	
ASPARAGUS	1 lb = 16 to 20 ¾-inch spears = 2 cups chopped
AVOCADOS	1 lb = 2 medium = 2½ cups sliced, diced, or chopped
BEANS, GREEN	1 lb = 3 to 3½ cups whole and trimmed = 3 cups sliced
BEETS (WITHOUT TOPS)	1 lb = 5 to 6 medium = 2 cups chopped or sliced 1 medium = ⅓ cup chopped or sliced
BELL PEPPERS, ALL COLORS	1 lb = 5 medium or 3 large 1 large = 1 cup chopped
BROCCOLI	1 lb = 2 cups chopped or sliced = 3½ cups florets
BRUSSELS SPROUTS	1 lb = 4 cups whole
CABBAGE	1 lb = 3½ to 4 cups shredded
CARROTS	1 lb = 6 to 8 medium = 3 cups chopped or sliced = 2½ cups shredded 1 medium = ½ cup chopped or sliced = 6 baby carrots
CAULIFLOWER	1 lb = 1½ cups chopped or sliced = 1½ cups florets
CELERY	1 medium rib = ½ cup chopped or sliced
CORN	1 medium ear = ½ to ¾ cup kernels
CUCUMBERS	1 lb = 2½ to 3 cups chopped or sliced 1 medium = 1 cup chopped or sliced
EGGPLANTS	1 lb = 2½ to 3 cups diced = 5 to 6 cups cubed
FENNEL	1 lb = 2 medium bulbs = 3 cups sliced
GARLIC	1 head = 2 oz = about 10 cloves 1 clove = 1 tsp minced
GINGERROOT	½ oz = 1 inch = 1 Tb grated or minced
GREEN PEAS	1 lb in pod = 1 cup shelled
JÍCAMA	1 lb = 4 cups shredded

VEGETABLES	
KALE	1 lb = 6 cups leaves
LEEKS	1 lb = 2 large or 3 medium = 2 cups chopped or sliced (white part)
LETTUCES	1 lb Boston, Bibb, butter = 1 medium head = 4 cups torn 1 lb iceberg, romaine = 1 medium head = 6 to 8 cups torn = 4 cups shredded
MUSHROOMS, BUTTON	1 lb = 20 to 24 whole = 4 to 5 cups chopped or sliced
OKRA	1 lb = 35 pods = 1½ cups sliced
ONIONS, GREEN	1 bunch = 7 to 9 bulbs (green and white parts) = 1 cup sliced = ¾ cup diced
ONIONS (YELLOW, WHITE, RED)	1 lb white/yellow = 4 medium or 3 large 1 medium = ½ to ⅔ cup chopped 1 large = 1½ cups chopped
PARSNIPS	1 lb = 4 medium = 2½ cups chopped 1 medium = ⅔ cup chopped
POTATOES	1 lb = 3 to 4 medium white 1 lb = 7 to 9 medium red = 12 to 15 small red 1 medium white = ¾ cup chopped or sliced = 1 cup shredded
PUMPKINS	1 lb = 3 cups shredded = 4 cups cubed = 1 cup cooked and mashed
RADISHES	½ lb = 1⅔ cups sliced
SHALLOTS	1 medium = ½ to 1 oz = 1 Tb minced
SNOW OR SNAP PEAS	14 to 18 medium pods = 1 cup whole or chopped
SPINACH	1 lb = 6 cups raw, loose = 4 cups raw, packed
SQUASH, SUMMER (YELLOW, ZUCCHINI)	1 lb = 3 medium = 2½ to 3 cups sliced 1 medium = ⅔ cup grated = 1 cup sliced
SQUASH, WINTER (ACORN, BUTTERNUT)	1 lb = 2 cups sliced or cubed
SWEET POTATOES	1 lb = 3 medium or 2 large = 2 to 3 cups cubed or sliced 1 medium = ⅔ cup cubed = ¾ cup sliced
SWISS CHARD	1 lb = 4 cups stalks and 5 to 6 cups leaves
TOMATILLOS	1 lb = 12 to 16 medium
TURNIPS	1 lb = 3 to 4 medium = 2½ to 3 cups sliced

FRUIT	
APPLES	1 lb = 3 to 4 medium = 2½ to 3 cups chopped or sliced 1 medium = ¾ cup chopped = 1 cup sliced
APRICOTS	1 lb = 8 to 12 medium = 2 to 2½ cups sliced or halved 2 medium = ½ cup sliced
BANANAS	1 lb = 3 to 4 medium = 2 to 3 cups sliced = 1¾ cups mashed
BERRIES: BLUE, BLACK	1 pint = 2 cups
CHERRIES	1 lb unpitted = 2½ to 3 cups pitted
GRAPES	1 lb = 2½ to 3 cups
KIWIFRUITS	1 medium = 5 to 6 slices = ½ cup sliced
LEMONS	1 lb = 4 to 6 medium or 2 to 3 large = 1 cup juice 1 medium = 2 to 3 Tb juice = 2 to 3 tsp zest
LIMES	1 lb = 6 to 8 medium = ½ to 1 cup juice 1 medium = 1 to 2 Tb juice = 1 to 2 tsp zest
MANGOES	1 medium = 12 oz = ¾ cup chopped
ORANGES	1 lb = 3 to 4 medium 1 medium = ⅓ to ½ cup juice = 2 Tb zest = ½ cup sections
PEACHES, NECTARINES	1 lb = 3 to 4 medium = 2 to 2½ cups chopped or sliced 1 medium = ⅔ to ¾ cup chopped or sliced
PEARS	1 lb = 3 to 4 medium = 2 cups sliced
PINEAPPLES	1 medium = 1½ to 2 lbs = 3 cups chunks
PLUMS	1 lb = 6 medium or 5 large = 2 cups pitted and quartered
RAISINS	1 lb = 2¾ to 3 cups
RASPBERRIES	½ pint = scant 1 cup
RHUBARB	1 lb = 4 to 8 stalks = 2 cups chopped and cooked
STRAWBERRIES	1 pint = 24 to 26 medium = 2 cups chopped or sliced
TOMATOES	1 lb = 3 medium = 1½ to 2 cups chopped 1 medium = ½ cup chopped 1 medium Roma (plum) = 3 oz = ⅓ cup chopped 1 lb cherry = 1 pint = 25 to 35

HERBS	
BASIL	1 bunch = 2½ oz = 60 sprigs = 1 cup packed = 2 cups loose ½ oz = 1 cup chopped
CILANTRO	1 bunch = 3 oz = 95 sprigs = ¾ cup packed = 1½ cups loose
MINT	1 bunch = 3½ oz = 80 sprigs = ½ cup chopped = ⅞ cup loose
OREGANO	1 bunch = 1 oz = 40 sprigs = ¾ cup chopped
PARSLEY	1 bunch = 2 oz = 48 sprigs = ¾ cup chopped
MISCELLANEOUS	
ALMONDS, PECANS, WALNUTS	1 lb = 4 cups whole or halved = 3½ cups chopped 1 oz = ¼ cup chopped or slivered
PEANUTS	1 lb shelled = 3½ to 4 cups unshelled
CHEESES, HARD (SUCH AS PARMESAN) AND SEMIHARD (SUCH AS CHEDDAR, SWISS)	3½ ounces = 1 cup shredded 4 ounces = 1 cup grated
CHEESES, SOFT (SUCH AS BLUE, FETA, GOAT)	1 ounce = ¼ cup crumbled
RICES	white: 1 cup uncooked = 3 cups cooked white instant: 1 cup uncooked = 2 cups cooked brown: 1 cup uncooked = 4 cups cooked brown instant: 1 cup uncooked = 2½ cups cooked

INDEX

Note: **Bold** page references indicate recipe has a photo in color insert pages.